10/73

SO-DVF-681

(24.75)

MANAGING STRESS
A Guide for Health Professionals

Rita E. Numerof, Ph.D.

Assistant Professor, The George Warren
Brown School of Social Work

Adjunct Professor, Health Administration
and Planning, School of Medicine

Washington University
St. Louis, Missouri

AN ASPEN PUBLICATION®
Aspen Systems Corporation
Rockville, Maryland
Royal Tunbridge Wells
1983

Library of Congress Cataloging in Publication Data

Numerof, Rita E.
Managing stress.

Includes index.
Bibliography: p. 317.
1. Health facilities—Administration—Psychological
aspects. 2. Health services administrators—Job
stress. 3. Medical personnel—Job stress. 4. Professional socialization. 5. Organizational behavior.
I. Title. [DNLM: 1. Stress, Psychological. 2. Personnel, Hospital—Psychology.   WX 159 N971m]
RA965.3.N85   1983   362.1′068′3   83-11944
ISBN: 0-89443-939-1

Publisher: John Marozsan
Editor and Chief: Michael Brown
Executive Managing Editor: Margot Raphael
Editorial Services: Martha Sasser
Printing and Manufacturing: Debbie Collins

Copyright © 1983 by Aspen Systems Corporation

Library of Congress Catalog Card Number: 83-11944
OCT 1 3 1983   ISBN: 0-89443-939-1

Printed in the United States of America

1 2 3 4 5

To Michael

whose patience and understanding helped make this possible.

Table of Contents

Preface ix

Acknowledgments xi

PART I—STRESS AND ITS EFFECTS 1

Chapter 1—The Physiology of Stress 5
    Physiological Mechanisms and Stress 6
    Fight-Flight and the Adaptation Syndrome 14

Chapter 2—The Socioemotional Components of Stress 17
    Individuals and Psychological Causes 18
    Stress and Productivity 27
    Elastic Limits 29
    Socioemotional Vulnerability and Stress 32
    Life Events and Stress 37

Chapter 3—Sources of Stress 41
    Stress: Management or Personal Problem 41
    Stress in the Physical Environment 42
    Stress in the Interpersonal Environment 45
    Evaluation and Defensive Behavior 52
    Passive-Aggressive and Aggressive 56
    Stress at the Organizational Level 57
    Key Sources of Problems 64
    Stress at the Personal Level 67

**PART II—THE CASE OF THE HEALTH CARE
          PROFESSIONAL** **73**

Chapter 4—Stress in the Health Care Environment **75**
    An Environment Ripe for Stress 75
    Hass: Health Administrators Stress Study 78
    The Sample 81
    Stress Situations 82
    Stress as a Function of Sex and Position 86
    Stress Events, Outcomes, and Symptoms 102
    Symptomatology and Situational Stress 107
    Stress Situations and Coping Strategies 111
    Stress, Symptoms, Demographics 115
    Stress and Vulnerability—IPS Results 125
    Summary of Important Findings 129
    Building a Model 131

Chapter 5—The Physician Experience **135**
    Training in Stress? Residency Experience 135
    Beyond Residency: Stress and Impairment 140
    Vulnerability: The Person or Profession? 143
    The Role of the Health Care System 143
    Changing Values as a Source of Stress 146
    Clinical vs. Administrative Perspectives 146
    Issues for the Physician as Manager 148
    Holistic vs. Disease Models of Medicine 151

Chapter 6—The Nurse Experience **157**
    Professional Socialization and Nurses' Role 158
    Beyond Socialization: Sources of Stress 164
    Hypotheses and Discussion 167
    Stress: National Commission on Nursing View 177
    Nurse-Physician-Administrator Relationship 178
    Union Bargaining: Issues and Prospects 180
    The Nurse as Manager: Promotion Problems 186

Chapter 7—The Administrator's Experience **191**
    The Evolution of the Administrator 192
    Mediating Across Value Systems 193
    The Administrator as Conflict Negotiator 197
    Administrators and Boards 200
    'Loneliness at the Top' 204

PART III—MEETING THE CHALLENGE 207

Chapter 8—Recognizing Signs of Stress 209
    Burnout 210
    Problems of Addiction: Alcohol 217
    Drug Addiction: Causes and Symptoms 221
    Signs of Emotional Disturbance 226
    Confronting the Problems of Stress 232

Chapter 9—The Organizational Response 235
    Preventive Mechanisms in Alleviating Stress 237
    Reducing Organizational Stress 248
    Rethinking Socialization 259
    Monitoring and Control Mechanisms 263

Chapter 10—The Personal Response 273
    Individual Stress Reduction Techniques 273
    Cognitive and Behavioral Approaches 278
    Employee Assistance Programs 285
    In Retrospect 288

Appendix A—Questionnaire Used in Health Administrators
    Stress Study 289

Appendix B—Personal Stress System Assessment 299

Appendix C—Coping Strategies 303

Appendix D—Individual Profile of Stressors 313

References 317

Index 335

Preface

In recent years the topic of stress has almost become a cliché. The popular literature abounds with articles and books alerting the public to the dangers of stress and advocating a variety of remedies to counteract its evil effect. Often, these "sure cures" are based on anecdotal evidence—testimony of those who struggled with stress and managed to find relief and now are sharing it with others.

The professional literature, also extensive, is by no means immune to such testimonial writing. In addition to a great variety of works over the last 20 years describing the human stress response and its effects, there has been a surge of interest in job-related stress. It is this literature in particular that presents an often confusing array of conceptualizations of that elusive phenomenon called stress and a wealth of anecdotal remedies on ways of contending with it.

Given this murky state of affairs, what, then, is the orientation of this book and how does it relate to what has preceded it? The purpose here is to discuss stress from the perspective of the organization, specifically the health care organization and the three major professional groups that dominate it: administrators, nurses, and physicians.

Based on research on responses to stress, it clarifies the physiological, social, and emotional effects of stress on individuals, then explores the implications for health care organizations, particularly hospitals.

To understand the impact of stress and institutions' responsibility in monitoring and controlling it, the impact of what individuals and professional groups bring to the situation in terms of their own socialization experiences must be analyzed. What is a source of stress to one individual may not be to another. Thus, a major contribution of this work is to examine the influence of professional socialization and role on perceived organizational stress. Coping strategies used by different professionals and the relationship of these tactics to stress symptomatology and vulnerability also are explored.

All this should help readers achieve a better understanding of the complexity of the problem of organizational stress and be stimulated to think creatively in terms of the organization's responsibility in managing it effectively.

It is important, of course, to recognize that organizations cannot be blamed totally for the stress that individuals working within them experience. Organizations do, indeed, precipitate stress, some of which is exhilarating and challenging for their employees. However, they also are responsible for employees' incurring unnecessary, harmful stress.

It must be recognized that individuals themselves may be a source of stress to themselves and their colleagues. While organizations have climates and cultures that impinge on their employees, those people bring with them their self-images, values, expectations, nonwork-related stresses, and a whole host of vulnerabilities that interact with the organizational environment.

To understand stress, it is necessary to understand the peculiarities of the organization, the individual, and the relationship that exists between them.

Rita E. Numerof, Ph.D.
St. Louis, Missouri
LaJolla, California
September 1983

Acknowledgments

The author wishes to acknowledge the assistance of the many persons who participated in the health administrators stress study reported in Chapter 4, particularly Dr. Sandra A. Shachar Hendin and Dr. Kathryn D. Cramer, my coinvestigators in that project. Support for that research was provided by The George Warren Brown School of Social Work, Washington University, St. Louis; The Stress Center, St. Louis University School of Medicine; and The Missouri Institute of Psychiatry, University of Missouri, St. Louis, Mo.

In addition, I would like to thank those who participated in the many stress workshops I have conducted in the last several years. For confidential reasons, these individuals must remain unidentified here.

Portions of five of the chapters are adapted from earlier works in which the author participated, as follows:

Chapter 3: Parts of the section "Problems in Communication" are adapted from the author's book, *The Practice of Management for Health Care Professionals,* published by AMACOM, the American Management Associations, 1982.

The section on "Stress at the Organizational Level" is adapted from a presentation by the author to the Society of Hospital Personnel Directors and the Council of Nursing Directors, St. Louis, June 16, 1982.

Chapter 4: The section on "The HASS: Health Administrators Stress Study," is mentioned above.

Chapter 5: Parts of this chapter are adapted from an article by the author and Michael N. Abrams, "Before Impairment: Physician Stress and the Organization's Responsibility," *Health Care Management Review,* Fall 1981, 6(4), 77–82.

xi

Chapter 6: Parts of the section on "Union Bargaining: Issues and Prospects" are from a paper by the author and Michael Abrams, *Collective Bargaining Among Nurses in Health Care: Current Issues and Future Prospects,* Washington University, St. Louis, 1982.

Chapter 9: The approach discussed in the section on "Integrated Management Development" was designed by Numerof and Associates, Inc., 1981.

I would like to acknowledge the work of Teresa Danik, in collecting the data for the nurses study reported in Chapter 6.

Special thanks go to my copy editor, Sam Sharkey, whose painstaking efforts have enhanced the clarity and accuracy of this book, and to the others at Aspen who helped to make this book a reality.

A special word of thanks is extended to my secretary at Washington University, Keith Morton, for managing the typing and production of what was in many ways a complex and very stressful project, and to all the others in the GWB Secretarial Center who contributed their talents in some special way.

Finally, a special note of appreciation to my husband, Michael, for his excellent editorial comments and his continued encouragement and support throughout the time I researched and wrote this manuscript.

Part I

Stress and Its Effects

Stress is perhaps one of the most frequently discussed and studied phenomena today. Despite its popularity, the term is surrounded with confusion. It is used to describe a wide variety of symptoms and experiences. While most people think they know what it is, the definitions of stress remain vague and imprecise. In large part, what is considered "stress" depends on the perspective of the researcher.

From the perspective of Hans Selye, a pioneer in psychosomatic medicine and a recognized leader in the field, stress in its simplest form can be understood as the "rate of wear and tear within the body" (Selye, 1956). From a more technical, medical perspective Selye defines stress as a specific syndrome consisting of all nonspecifically induced changes within the human organism. This latter definition has produced the commonly accepted view of stress as any nonspecific demand on the body requiring the individual to respond or change.

Regardless of how it is defined, there is general consensus that stress is an integral part of all life. All living organisms come equipped with innate warning signals—stress reactions—that help them cope effectively with the demands of their environments. Without challenge, without stress, it is questionable whether constructive activity or growth could occur. However, the degree to which people experience stress in today's society has become excessive and harmful. In competitive work environments with limited financial and human resources, individuals are under pressure to accomplish more and more in less and less time. Often, they perceive themselves as caught in an inescapable maze, with the only alternative being to adapt.

For purposes of clarity, stress is defined here as the state in which any nonspecific demand requires an individual to respond or to take action. Stressor refers to any event or condition, perceived as positive or negative, that triggers a stress reaction—the response to the demand. These responses,

1

in turn, have far-reaching consequences in physiological, psychological, and emotional terms. These are referred to as stress effects.

The effects of stress are nondiscriminatory with respect to sex, age, race, or religion. Nor is stress the exclusive domain of the stereotypic harried executive. For example, adolescents and young adults may be accumulating negative stress effects that they may not manifest until they reach midlife. Stress-related disorders do not spring up spontaneously but are the result of the gradual accumulation of reactions over a lifetime. Some persons are vaguely aware of the negative effects of stress on their lives. Others are conscious of it and take active steps to ameliorate its deleterious effects and modify their life styles. Still others become aware of these harmful results only when hit over the head with serious, stress-related illness.

Stressors, often referred to as stress triggers, are ubiquitous. While Chapter 3 focuses more specifically on the sources of stress, some mention of these triggers here will help lay the groundwork for what follows. General environmental stressors present demands with often subtle and powerful effects: noise and air pollution, overcrowding in cities, the pressure of deadlines at work, the continual sense of competition in most aspects of life. Other sources may involve social and personal relationships: the difficult and demanding boss, the spouse, child, friend, or relative who presents demands to be met. Other events easily identifiable as stressors include the death of a loved one, financial pressures, serious illness, loss of a job. These are the negative stressors, what Selye refers to as "distress."

However, stress is by no means the exclusive domain of events laden with negative affect. There also is the stress of positive events—marriage, the birth of a child, a promotion, an inheritance, even holidays and vacations. Selye (1956) refers to these positive stressors as "eustress." The life-events research of Holmes and Rahe (1967) demonstrates rather convincingly that events that people typically regard as positive can induce as much stress as those regarded as negative. Essentially, the body does not know the difference between distress and eustress. It responds the same way to pleasurable events as it does to unpleasant ones. Anything, then, that changes an existing homeostatic balance can be seen as a source of stress.

What is common to all stressful events is the requirement that individuals change or adapt, thus taxing their physical and emotional adaptive mechanisms. It is the change and rapid adaptation required by both positive and negative stressors that plays havoc with humans' systems. Any alteration in life requires a change. When the changes occur too frequently over a short space of time, negative results are likely. To compound the problem further, many reactions to a stressor themselves become stressors. Changes in eating or sleeping habits, muscle tension and spasms, and anxiety can feed back on the human system, causing more complex and harmful stress reactions.

Obviously, not all stress reactions can be harmful, especially since stress is indeed a vital part of a vital life. Pelletier (1977) offers a lucid explanation differentiating the harmful from the harmless:

- A normal stress reaction that facilitates adaptation occurs when the stressor (i.e., the source of stress) is clear and identifiable. Under these conditions the stress response is invoked to meet the challenge and the individual returns to a normal level of functioning following a brief rest period.
- An abnormal reaction occurs when the stressor is unclear (i.e., undefined or ambiguous), exists over a prolonged period, or is part of a constellation of stressors existing at once. The individual does not return to normal physiological or emotional functioning as rapidly. Instead, the stress reaction continues and becomes potentially damaging.

As Pelletier notes, it is this notion that is critical to the understanding of psychosomatic illness. Rather than the trembling and exhilaration followed by the sigh of relief and relaxation that individuals experience facing a specific life-threatening situation, a stressful day leaves them feeling exhausted. There has been no immediate life-threatening situation, no particular source of stress from which to recover. The stressors have been ambiguous and are chronic. The individuals have had little, if any, respite from them, and thus have not recovered from the stress-alarm reaction brought about to deal with them.

While the day of chronic stressors may seem very different from the short-lived life-threatening crises, the difference exists only from a psychological standpoint. Neurophysiologically, the pattern of the stress response is the same for both situations. It is the effect of the more chronic, unremitting stressors that is particularly relevant to psychosomatic illness and to this exploration of organizational stressors and their effects.

To pinpoint the relationship between stressors and their consequences, Part I examines the physiological and socioemotional components of stress separately. It should be understood that in actuality these components are intricately interwoven. Together with life style, nutrition, and a host of other factors to be explored, they form a response to the stressor that has consequences of its own. Chapter 1 explores the physiology of stress. Chapter 2 examines the socioemotional components of stress—the "burnout syndrome,'' the role of stress in creativity, motivation, and productivity, and the effects of excessive or uncontrolled stress. Chapter 3 studies major sources of stress—physical, personal, social, and organizational—and discusses their manifest and latent effects.

The Physiology of Stress

While the influence of stress in the development of disease has been recognized for centuries, it is only within the last several decades that society really has begun to understand its significance and appreciate how it works.

Perhaps the earliest scientific investigations of stress can be traced back to the observations of Dr. Walter B. Cannon, a Harvard physiologist who noted in his classic research of 1939 that emotions produced bodily changes. The relationship between emotions (psychology) and the body (physiology) is not universally accepted, however. Debates have raged for centuries concerning the relationship between physical and psychological well-being. On one end of the continuum is the philosophical and clinical medicine school that believes that health and disease are merely the result of physiological processes. Psychological factors should be dismissed summarily in studying illness, according to this viewpoint. At the other end of the continuum is the Calvinist-influenced view that suggests that all illness is the end product of a psychological or spiritual defect of the individual.

The problem with both orientations is their inherent separation of mind and body. Obviously, the truth lies somewhere in between. Health or illness is the result of an exceedingly complex interaction between individuals and their psychosocial environment. It is this concept that forms the core of the holistic approach to health care and is the orientation adopted in this book. The holistic approach sees the mind and body as parts of an integrated whole. Health exists to the extent mind and body operate in harmony; illness or disease results when the balance is disrupted, as in exposure to excessive stress. In the context of holistic medicine, psychosomatic illness conveys the idea that an interaction between mind and body exists in all diseases, in all processes affecting health.

According to Pelletier (1977), all illness is the result of a complex interaction of physical as well as psychological stress, social factors, the per-

5

sonality of the individual experiencing these stresses, and the resources available to that person to cope with the stress. In this framework physical symptoms of illness are best understood as early warnings of excessive stress or strain being experienced by the "mind-body system." While it is not known precisely how psychological phenomena are translated into physical responses, it is useful to explore what is known about the physiological response to stress and how it affects the body's ability to cope with disease under conditions of prolonged pressure.

A basic premise in stress research is that individuals operate at a homeostatic level of stress considered nonpathogenic. This homeostasis differs from individual to individual but in all cases the equilibrium achieved contributes to overall functioning and productivity in positive ways. Deviations from this baseline become problematic and generally are associated with heightened activity designed to cope with impending danger. As will be discussed, the physiological response that prepares individuals to deal with the situation often is inappropriate to the danger as it is perceived.

PHYSIOLOGICAL MECHANISMS AND STRESS

The brain and neuroendocrine system pick up stress messages, relaying the information throughout the body to mobilize it to deal effectively with the challenge of the stressor. The stress response is part of humans' instinctual heritage, left over from the years when their physical makeup more closely resembled that of the lower animals.

The Brain: Components and Functions

The brain consists of two major components: the upper part or cerebral cortex and the lower part or subcortex. The subcortex regulates vital bodily functions and houses the control center for the autonomic or involuntary nervous system. It is the autonomic nervous system that is responsible for the majority of physiological changes that occur during the stress response. Within the subcortex are three major structures of significance in the stress response: (1) the cerebellum, which coordinates the timing and integration of bodily movements; (2) the medulla oblongata, which regulates basic physiological processes, including heartbeat and perspiration rate; and (3) the pons, which helps regulate sleep.

The next region of the subcortex (diencephalon) regulates emotions (e.g., sadness, joy, fear, rage, passion, fury). This region houses the hypothalamus, a small gland that is of primary importance in the stress response. The hypothalamus controls body temperature and hunger. Regulating the pituitary gland, the major endocrine gland, it translates neu-rological stimuli into endocrine processes during stress reactions, is a primary activator of the autonomic nervous system, and serves as a strong pleasure center. It tends to be a somewhat volatile gland and is brought under control by the cerebral cortex. Without such control, individuals would find themselves experiencing a wide range of quickly changing emotions. The relationship between the hypothalamus and the endocrine system is important in the etiology of psychosomatic disorders.

Higher in the brain is the limbic system, often referred to as the visceral brain in that it regulates basic biological functions. Like the diencephalon, it is concerned with various aspects of emotion. In this case, it regulates some kinds of actual emotional expression. It also connects with the temporal lobes, receptive areas for hearing that also mediate sexual behav-ior and control the degree to which emotions are expressed or withheld. Another part of the limbic system governs smell. Lesions in the limbic system have been known to produce hallucinations, reality disturbance, psychomotor epilepsy, and disturbed recognition and memory (Gardner, 1968).

At the top of the brain and surrounding most of the other structures is the cerebral cortex—the part of the brain commonly referred to as "gray matter." It governs higher order abstract functioning and exerts control over more primitive responses of the brain. It is the center for such functions as language, judgment, reasoning, and memory. The right por-tion of the cerebral cortex houses artistic, perceptual functions, while the left is the center for logic and intellectual functions such as reading.

The cerebral cortex is connected to the subcortex by the sensory motor cortex. Pelletier (1977) describes this connection as a one-inch-wide band extending inside the top of the head from one ear to the other. Impulses that govern the voluntary muscular system originate in the sensory motor cortex, are sent down pathways to the bottom of the cortex, pass through the medulla, and move down the spinal column, sending specific messages to the appropriate muscles (Pelletier, 1977). Research with electrical activ-ity in this area of the brain suggests that epileptic seizures become likely when activity decreases sufficiently or is poorly synchronized. Sterman (1974) finds that epileptics who are taught to monitor electrical activity through biofeedback techniques can recognize such electrical impulse changes and can act in such a way as to reverse the process preceding the seizure, thus preventing it from occurring.

Perhaps one of the most important structures is the reticular activating system, a system of nerves located in the center of the brain extending to the region of the thalamus. Messages are sent to this central system of nerves through other nerve tracts taking impulses from the cortex and subcortex. Essentially, neurological channels between the cortex and sub-cortex make it possible for the cerebral cortex to control the hypothalamus and subcortical areas (i.e., autonomic or involuntary nervous functions) of the brain and regulate them through elaborate neurological feedback loops. It is the reticular activating system that provides concrete evidence of the mind-body interconnection.

Physiological Key to Stress

Dr. J. D. French, a neurosurgeon at UCLA, in 1957 described the basic purpose of the reticular activating system as: (1) an arousal function through which the cortex is activated to receive visceral stimulation and (2) a transmitting function sending impulses from the cortex to the muscles and involuntary nervous system. Thus, its role is critical in understanding stress. Through the feedback system, purely intellectually or cognitively perceived stressors may precipitate physiological reactions while purely physical stressors will affect cognitive centers and processes. In addition, the reticular activating system selects and screens stimuli transmitted from the autonomic nervous system before these stimuli are recorded by the cortex or conscious part of the brain.

This occurrence accounts for the fact that environmental noise, unpleasant odors, or other stimuli perceived subliminally can produce irritability, tension, or anxiety in individuals without their knowing why the condition exists. Background noises and visceral stimuli as seen in lighting and temperature changes may not be recorded consciously but they do affect people's behavior (Pelletier, 1977; Shevrin, 1973). In one sense the reticular activating system is the gatekeeper of consciousness, monitoring stimuli in the environment, accepting what is to be perceived, rejecting what is not, and focusing attention, introspection, reasoning, and bodily movements (French, 1957).

Given the interrelation of the subcortical and cortical regions of the brain, it is known that a cognitively perceived stressor (cortical activity) will result in a stress message's being sent through nerve endings to the subcortex, which initiates a series of physiological reactions. The two networks so activated by the subcortex are the autonomic or involuntary nervous system and the endocrine system. Both of these are controlled by the hypothalamus—the gland in the brain believed to be the center governing human emotions (Pelletier, 1977). The hypothalamus not only activates the involuntary and endocrine systems and controls the emotions, it also responds to cortical messages (i.e., cognitively perceived stress) and thus is the critical link in the process by which a psychological stressor produces a physiological reaction (Pelletier, 1977).

The functions of the autonomic nervous system are important to an understanding of stress. This system controls "involuntary" functioning—gastrointestinal, reproductive, cardiovascular, and pulmonary processes. (By contrast, the voluntary nervous system controls voluntary muscles and all movement that requires human will, including posture.) The name autonomic derives from the belief that these functions operate independently of human will.

It now is known, in part through biofeedback research, that this notion of pure independence is erroneous. People can and do learn to exercise control over autonomic functions. Under most circumstances, internal sensory receptors and visceral impulses activate the autonomic nervous system, which transmits responses back to the appropriate organs by reflex once it receives the impulses (Pelletier, 1977). When confronted with any type of stressor, mental or physical, the autonomic nervous system automatically initiates a variety of physiological and chemical changes in the body.

The 'Fight-Flight' Response

One part of the autonomic nervous system, the sympathetic nervous system, tenses and constricts involuntary muscles and induces endocrine changes. It responds through a general discharge, stimulating many parts of the body at once. This "mass discharge" (Guyton, 1971), or excitation of the body also is popularly known as the "fight-flight" response, first described by Cannon (1953). This general response is a comprehensive physiological response of the human body to stress, a response that is identical to that in animals.

For example, when an animal perceives a dangerous or threatening situation (i.e., a stressor), its reflexive reaction is a highly complex, integrated physiological one that prepares it to do one of two things: fight the perceived enemy or flee. The response is characterized by coordinated increases in oxygen consumption (metabolism), rate of breathing, heartbeat rate, blood pressure, the amount of blood pumped by the heart and to the muscles, contraction of leg muscles, sweating palms, tense neck and upper back, and dilated pupils.

The parasympathetic nervous system, on the other hand, stimulates dilation of the smooth muscle, generally referred to as involuntary (Thompson, 1967), and brings about the state known as relaxation. The parasympathetic responses follow those of the sympathetic nervous system under "normal" circumstances, thus providing the body with much-needed rest—a nutriment following the superwork period during the fight-flight response. Figure 1-1 shows the relationship between homeostasis, fight-flight, and

Figure 1-1 Homeostasis, Fight-Flight, Relaxation

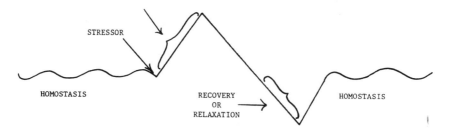

relaxation at its most basic level. Homeostasis is interrupted by a perceived stressor; the fight-flight response is engaged, allowing the organism to run or fight. After discharging the available energy and following the solution to the stress situation (i.e., fighting or running), the parasympathetic nervous system induces the relaxation response, a term coined by Herbert Benson (1974), in which the organism rests at a point below normal homeostatic functioning.

A human situation demonstrates this process:

Imagine that you meet what you think might be a mugger in the park. Your heart starts beating faster, you can feel your blood pressure go up, your muscles tighten, you breathe faster, and you are vaguely aware that a number of processes are occurring within your body that are giving you energy. You are ready to fight off an attack or run away. You immediately spring into action, running away. As you realize you are safe, you begin to relax, feel warm, your heart stops pounding, you feel unable to move for a few minutes. Then you begin to function normally.

What might also be experienced during the early phase of this process are psychological counterparts to the physiological changes occurring in the body. "Cold feet" really reflect the fact that blood diminishes at the extremities in favor of the head and trunk. A similar effect results from reduced blood flow around the stomach and has been described as a "knot in the stomach."

Role of the Endocrine System

At the same time the sympathetic nervous system is creating changes in the cardiovascular and other systems described, it is working closely with the endocrine system. Here the relationship between the hypothalamus and the pituitary gland, which controls the endocrine system and in turn is regulated by the hypothalamus, is critical. One portion of the hypothalamus serves to inhibit both the release of stress hormones from the pituitary and the activation of sympathetic responses of the autonomic nervous system. The other part of the hypothalamus has the opposite function. It stimulates the release of the stress hormones produced by the pituitary and activates the sympathetic nerve responses.

When pituitary stress hormones are released, they are discharged into the bloodstream, sending messages to other endocrine glands. Vasopressin, one of these hormones, is released from the posterior lobe of the pituitary, contracting arterial walls and raising blood pressure. Hormones released from the anterior lobe are the adrenocorticotropic hormone (ACTH), thyrotropic hormone (TTH), and the gonadotropic hormones (GTH), which influence the genital glands and sexual functioning. ACTH and TTH help the body prepare to cope with a stressor through a temporary increase in heart rate, circulation, metabolism, and the related processes noted previously. The action of ACTH upon the adrenal glands is considered the most important of these reactions in relation to the stress response. While ACTH is acting upon the adrenals, the pituitary simultaneously is releasing TTH, causing the thyroid gland to secrete thyroxine, a hormone that influences the rate of metabolism and governs physical, sexual, and mental growth and development.

During the stress response, metabolism is speeded greatly, leaving the person with a host of fairly unpleasant symptoms. The individual sweats easily, becomes tired quickly, and has rapid heartbeat and deep, rapid breathing (Pelletier, 1977). This state of hyperactivity, unpleasant even in the short run, can cause chronic fatigue and insomnia over extended periods of time. Increased levels of thyroxine tend to make the system more responsive to adrenalin, with both of these hormones producing essentially the same subjective effects. With regard to the third type, the gonadotropic hormones, it is important to note that while ACTH and TTH are being released during a stress response, the production of gonadotropic hormones decreases. This offers additional credence to research (Sandler, 1960; Harrison, O'Moore, and McSweeney, 1980) suggesting that stress is an important component in many problems of infertility, including those of "undetermined origin." (Although relatively little has been written on the subject, the link between psychological stress and infertility has long been recognized. Sandler (1960) noted that approximately 25% of infertility in couples was stress-related. The fact that a large percentage of couples attending infertility clinics conceive without an attributable treatment (46% in Harrison et al., 1980) or from placebo suggests that another variable (e.g., stress) is operative. Harrison et al. (1980) note that psychological stress must be recognized as an important variable in the pharmacological treatment and study of infertility.)

Another set of endocrine glands directly stimulated by the sympathetic nervous system during the stress response is the adrenal, located immediately over the kidneys. Messages from the sympathetic nervous system stimulate the adrenals to produce adrenalin, also known as epinephrine, and noradrenalin, also known as norepinephrine. These substances are secreted in the intersection of the adrenal glands, the medulla. The medulla receives stress messages directly from and through the sympathetic nervous system and is surrounded by the outer section of the adrenal glands, the adrenal cortex. In a stress response adrenalin quickly enters the bloodstream and is distributed to all parts of the body. The release of adrenalin in combination with the hypothalamus stimulates the pituitary, and together they affect the other endocrine glands of the body.

Most everyone at one time or another has experienced a tremendous surge of energy and power, a flush of excitement called an "adrenalin rush." This reaction occurs when the medulla releases great amounts of adrenalin into the system, often enabling people to perform apparently miraculous feats of strength that, under usual circumstances, would be impossible. The adrenalin thus released acts through the liver, mobilizing glucose in the bloodstream, providing a quick energy source for the cells to use in response to the stressor (Pelletier, 1977). In addition, adrenalin increases the metabolism of carbohydrates, dilates arteries in the skeletal muscles and heart, stimulates heart rate and adds to the amount of blood circulating in the body, elevates body temperature, and increases oxygen consumption and the production of carbon dioxide (Pelletier, 1977). Simultaneously it relaxes smooth gastrointestinal muscles, constricts the sphincter, and dilates respiratory muscles.

Noradrenalin, on the other hand, constricts arteries and raises blood pressure. It also has considerably less effect on blood glucose and heart rate than adrenalin (Schildkraut & Kety, 1967). Under certain stress conditions, adrenalin is released, while in others noradrenalin is released. The reasons for this difference are not understood clearly. However, adrenalin generally is associated with fear responses, noradrenalin with anger (Pelletier, 1977).

The Adrenocortical Involvement

Hormones secreted by the adrenal cortex and stimulated by ACTH have functions somewhat different from adrenalin and noradrenalin. The adrenocortical hormones are important in maintaining body functions at a time of nonstress—that is, maintaining homeostatic functioning. Some of these hormones, the glucocorticoids, can raise blood sugar levels and also inhibit inflammation (Pelletier, 1977). Another group of adrenocortical hormones is called mineralocorticoids. They increase the amount of sodium and chloride retained in the body, decrease potassium levels, and promote inflammation.

The adrenocorticoids tend to be associated with long-term chronic stress reactions and can do serious, irreversible damage to the kidneys. This set of hormones also is important in monitoring and controlling the body's immune system that, in turn, is strongly related to the degree of health or illness an individual experiences (Pelletier, 1977).

The Immune System at Risk

An impressive array of studies investigating the role of the immune system in the development of and resistance to disease has been conducted over the last several decades (Solomon, 1969; Solomon, Amkraut, and Kasper, 1974; Stein, Schiavi, and Camerino, 1976). It is generally accepted among these researchers that one of the most pernicious effects of prolonged, excessive stress is the impact on the immune system (Pelletier, 1977).

The evidence linking psychological stress events with immune disorders is not precise in explaining how this occurs but it seems fairly clear that a connection exists. George Solomon of the Stanford University School of Medicine, for example, has examined the relationship of stress and immunity, particularly in relation to cancer (1969). He and his colleagues (Solomon, Amkraut, and Kasper, 1974) recognize the multifaceted interactive system of stress, environment, genetic constitution, and the immune system. Despite the complexity, these researchers believe there are links between immunity and the central nervous system, particularly in the case of infectious disease, allergy, and cancer.

More specifically, Solomon believes that personality factors, stress, and psychological defense failure at the onset of illness are related to the pathogenesis of cancer (Amkraut & Solomon, 1975; Solomon, 1969). The changes in immune reactions brought about by stress are relatively quite small. In spite of their small magnitude, however, they can shift the entire immune system balance and predispose an individual to develop a severe disorder (Pelletier, 1977).

For example, stressful life changes that produce "extreme emotional reactivity" may be sufficient to produce dysfunction in the brain that, in turn, disrupts the immune balance (Pelletier, 1977). It is to be hoped that future research will further illuminate the linkages and feedback loops between emotions, the endocrine system, and the immune system.

FIGHT-FLIGHT AND THE ADAPTATION SYNDROME

What should be clear at this point is the complexity of the stress response and the interconnectedness of emotional and cognitive processes and physiological reactions. Psychological stress can initiate responses of the hypothalamus that trigger pituitary activity that in turn stimulates further endocrine activity in other glands. Feedback mechanisms from the endocrine system to the brain further stimulate the hypothalamus and provide indicators to individuals as to the accuracy of their perception of the given stressor. Sympathetic nervous system discharges, together with the hypothalamus and endocrine glands, function in a highly synchronized effort to cope with stress. These systems are constantly in a dynamic state. However, most fluctuations are aimed at keeping the organism in a state of homeostasis with little variation.

Given humans' sophisticated apparatus to help them survive in the face of stress and danger, why should this intricate survival system be the cause of bodily harm and destruction? The answer lies partly in the advance of human civilization and psychological development. People are equipped physiologically to respond to stress in the same way that animals do. However, unlike the experience of animals, which is limited to physiological dangers, humans perceive cognitive and emotional stressors through their higher brain centers that also trigger physiological reactions. Although this information may be emotional or psychological in nature, it still generates a physical response—the fight-flight syndrome.

Unfortunately, in most of these situations, neither fighting nor running away is an appropriate response, although it may indeed be an initial impulse. People have been socialized to view running from stress or engaging in flight as unacceptable. For example, an individual can imagine sitting in the office with the boss who has just announced that a hoped-for salary increase will not be forthcoming. It would not be acceptable to respond to the stress by punching the superior or by running out of the office. Instead, the employee may express displeasure but remain outwardly calm while internally the person's body is prepared to do battle. This is unlike the animal in the "ready" state that quickly discharges its energy. Its stress response subsides, its body goes into deep relaxation, then returns to an even keel—to a state of equilibrium.

Because humans cannot physically discharge their energy, they continue to experience negative stress in the boss's office. Their physiological readiness or stress response continues. They are "up tight" and have no way of expending their excess energy. They know that a certain amount of stress is good for them. It stimulates them to action. But when it becomes prolonged or excessive, they have problems adapting to it. If they experience a prolonged stress response without a discharge, the biochemical changes in their bodies that result from the stress response can endanger their health seriously.

Much of the theory about what exactly occurs under conditions of prolonged stress reaction is speculative, but one model (Selye, 1956) serves as the generally accepted cornerstone on which later work has been built. In *The Stress of Life,* Selye defines stress as a state characterized by a "specific syndrome" consisting of all the nonspecifically induced changes that occur within the biological organism. Thus, stress is a specific configuration of physiological processes that are triggered by any one of many factors. The specific series of processes and their effect he calls the General Adaptation Syndrome. Figure 1-2 presents its three phases.

The alarm (fight-flight) phase (Phase I) is the initial and most dramatic response to the stressor, mobilizing the body's entire psychophysiological apparatus. In this model, a primary function of the General Adaptation Syndrome is to select the organ or system most appropriate for dealing with the stressor.

The syndrome then moves into Phase II, resistance. During this phase the adrenocortical hormone activity decreases and dealing with the stressor becomes the task of the specific organ or system selected for the job. Resistance to the stressor is high at this point but because vital resources have been diverted from other areas of the body, resistance to a disease is likely to be low.

In Phase III, exhaustion, the system or organ coping with the stressor becomes worn out and breaks down. Once again, the more general response

Figure 1-2 Selye's General Adaptation Syndrome

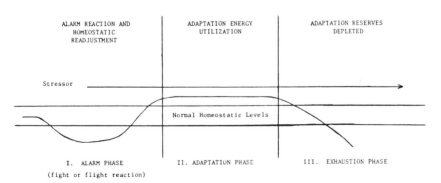

Source: Adapted from *The Stress of Life* by Hans Selye. New York: McGraw-Hill Book Company, © 1956, p. 87.

of Phase I becomes activated, removing the burden from the now worn system and starting the three-phase cycle again.

Selye believes that the General Adaptation Syndrome works to maximize the body's resistance to stress. Even the exhaustion phase does not necessarily result in psychosomatic illness. After a system or organ is exhausted from being called to respond to a stressor, the responsibility for coping with this or other stressors is shifted onto other organs and systems. Some moderate or not-too-frequent amounts of stress may, in the process of transferring responsibility for the attack, lead to a more effective response to the stressor and help to stimulate the production of new cells to the exhausted area.

Under conditions of prolonged, unabated stress, however, the exhaustion phase is associated with disease since the body is worn out and resistance is poor. What Selye refers to as "diseases of adaptation" are the likely result. These ordinary diseases are the result of continuous General Adaptation Syndrome response. Selye notes that the diseases are not purely the result of stress but result from the fact that in the body's attempt to adapt to continuing stress, physiological conditions are brought about that precipitate disorders or predispose the individual to disease. What disorder or disease occurs is in large part a multidetermined phenomenon, the result of constitutional and hereditary factors, environment, behavior, health practices, previous illness, and the like.

The key factor is that prolonged, nonspecific, unremitting occurrences of stress put the individual in a state of disequilibrium, thus increasing susceptibility to a wide array of illnesses. Because of the manner in which cognitive and emotional information is perceived by the cerebral cortex, transmitted to the lower emotional centers of the brain, and to the hypothalamus (which stimulates physiological mechanisms with far-reaching effects throughout the body), unabating psychosocial pressures also can be expected to lead to a breakdown of the body's coping ability, thus resulting in or predisposing the individual to psychosomatic illness.

Chapter 2

The Socioemotional Components of Stress

Even though the physiological evidence presented in Chapter 1 indicates a strong relationship between stress and psychosomatic illness, an understanding of neurophysiological and biochemical processes still does not make it possible to predict how specific individuals will respond to stressors or who will become ill and who will not. One commonly accepted fact among stress researchers is that there is great variation in people's responses to events that are potential stressors. Different "stress situations" have different effects on different persons. The same individual may even react differently to the same event at another time.

The reason for these differences rests in the fact that personality and emotional factors, physical condition, heredity, previous experience, and current life situation all influence how a person responds to an event and copes with stressors. It is only when all of these factors are understood and taken into account that the biology, prognosis, and prevention of psychosomatic disorders can be comprehended. Seen in that context, a specific disease may be symptomatic of a much larger constellation of problems and life circumstances.

In exploring various aspects of the socioemotional side of stress it is useful to keep in mind a number of hypotheses that underlie much of the research in this area. Appley and Trumbell (1967) summarize these well:

- Stress is best understood as a state of the whole organism under extenuating circumstances rather than as a specific event occurring in the environment.
- Many different environmental events or conditions are capable of producing a "stress state."
- Reactivity to such events varies widely from person to person. An individual may experience a stress state in response to one event and not to another.

- Different individuals experience the same event differently: one may be immune to the event, another may become confused and overwhelmed, still another may appear alert and challenged, resulting in improved performance.
- The psychophysiological response pattern of an individual in the stress state tends to be consistent over time; however, such patterns vary from person to person. It is important to reexamine the notion of a universal stress reaction.
- An understanding of the stress reaction—its intensity and related behaviors—may not be possible from an analysis of the stressor event or precipitating conditions by themselves but may require looking at the individual's underlying motivations and the meaning and context of the stress event.
- Situational factors are likely to determine the salience of any given stressor and thus the intensity and extent of the stress state.

Given such individual variation with regard to stressors and stress states, it is almost impossible to predict with any degree of certainty which specific ones will result in a physiological or psychological disorder. However, an understanding of factors that contribute to these outcomes will facilitate practitioners' ability to understand their own and their colleagues' sources of vulnerability so they can begin to explore avenues to effectively reduce such vulnerability.

INDIVIDUALS AND PSYCHOLOGICAL CAUSES

It would be most helpful to begin this exploration of the socioemotional aspects of stress with an examination of the individual system and various psychological causes of stress. Figure 2-1 demonstrates the relationships among key components in this system. It indicates that events in the environment that are perceived consciously or subconsciously enter into the system and influence the degree to which a stressor is experienced as stressful. (Specific sources of stress are discussed in Chapter 3.) To clarify the difference between perceived and nonperceived events: the former consist of all behaviors in the environment that are observed by the individual; the latter, while not observed, do influence behavior through unconscious processes.

Both perceived and nonperceived events are sources of information for the sensory receptors. Humans' sensory apparatus includes the senses of touch, taste, hearing, smell, and sight. This apparatus transmits a variety of neural signals to various centers of the brain, where they are processed.

Figure 2-1 The Individual System and the Psychological Process of Stress

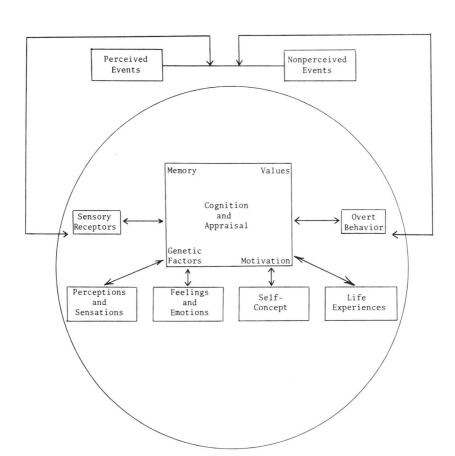

Source: Reprinted from *Managing Organizational Stress: A Systems Perspective,* with permission of Numerof and Associates, Inc., © 1981.

This processing in the brain is what differentiates variety and intensity of signal. It also is what frequently gives meaning to the context of the signal and determines whether or not the signal will be a stressor.

Based on previous experience, certain sounds or odors may trigger unpleasant associations and become sources of stress. Differences in sensory sensitivity across individuals help to explain why a particular stimulus is a stressor to one person and not to another. Night driving is a serious stressor for a person with cataracts because of the bright lights of oncoming cars but is unlikely to be for a person without cataracts. Bright sunlight generally is more stressful for blue-eyed people than for brown-eyed.

The Major Influence of Values

The box in the center of Figure 2-1 represents the cognition and appraisal apparatus of the brain in addition to a constellation of constitutional and learned elements that influence subsequent perceptions, feelings, and behavior.

Values are perhaps one of the most important and most frequently overlooked learned influences on behavior. Because they have great relevance to this discussion of organizational stress in Part II they are discussed here.

Values are essentially intangible beliefs about what each person thinks and feels is important in life. Every decision individuals make, opinion they give, or action they take is based on these values. Some of them are held consciously. People are very much aware of what these are, why they are, and how they influence them. Others are held unconsciously. They influence decisions without individuals' direct knowledge of how. Often people are unaware of these values' existence even as they influence them. Given that values play an extremely important part in everyone's lives, it is important to know how they got there, what they are, and how they exert influence.

Values are first transmitted when individuals are young children through their families, in the classroom, through religious teachings. They often are handed on in the form of moralizing by adults who reinforce behaviors that they believe are "right" and discourage those they believe are "wrong." A similar process occurs in professional training when individuals are socialized to accept and promote the values of the particular career structure with which they identify and to reject those that conflict. The subsequent values held—what people believe is important—guide behavior and tend to be associated with strong feelings about right and wrong. What people value, they tend to see as "right" and "good"—the way things ought to be. When they feel their values or value system are being challenged, violated, or attacked, they tend to react defensively, as though they have been attacked physically. It is this socioemotional definition of the situation that is translated into a source of stress and initiates the reaction.

What is forgotten here is that values are essentially a personal matter, differing from one person to another, from one profession to another. What is "right" for one is not necessarily "right" for another. The fact that people see situations differently and hold different values can lead to much conflict and stress—not so much because the values are different as because some individuals have difficulty accepting the fact that others do not share the same concepts.

Motivation: Process and Problems

Motivation is another key element in the cognition and appraisal system—a topic that has been of great interest to theoreticians and philosophers for centuries. Motivation is essentially the desire of an individual to do things to accomplish certain goals. It is an inner process that affects performance but it also can be affected by external events. These external events include pressures or demands to perform certain activities to avoid bringing about possible negative consequences. Thus, a person may obediently follow the orders of a superior instead of risking displeasure and a possible negative appraisal. To the extent that this behavior puts individuals in conflict with personal or professional values they will experience stress. An external attraction also may serve to motivate behavior in a given direction.

While the external demand situation can be likened to the "stick approach" to motivation, the external attraction can be compared to the "carrot approach" (Numerof, 1982). Thus, a person may work harder for external recognition, a pay increase, or a promotion. Internal states, including the desire to perform excellent work for an inner satisfaction, can be extremely powerful motivators. As discussed in Chapters 3 and 4, internal states and expectations also may be the source of a significant amount of stress.

Another potential source of stress involving motivation results from the important relationship between internal needs and external motivators, whether they be rewards, incentives, or sanctions. Individuals' needs will decide, to a large degree, their motivation to perform different tasks. Needs create a drive or force to satisfy themselves; needs that have not been satisfied create inner tensions. The tensions created by the unsatisfied needs are translated into energy that, in turn, is directed into behavior that will satisfy the needs. Needs that continue to remain unsatisfied over long periods of time are a source of stress and may translate their energy in destructive ways.

Clinical experience and research (Ausubel, D.P., 1954; Reiner and Kaufman, 1959; Sperling, 1974; Mednik, 1979; Garmezy, 1981; Werner and Smith, 1982) suggests that children whose needs are not met will consistently translate their tensions into destructive behaviors and feelings that then become secondary stressors. These youngsters are likely to become apathetic, unfeeling, easily frustrated, insecure, fearful, and untrusting.

As adults, they are sources of stress in the work environment as colleagues, as superiors, or as subordinates. For adults, needs consistently not met at work tend to be associated with lowered morale and reduced productivity.

Memory and Genetic Factors

Any mental health professional will be quick to note that short term memory functions are impaired with increasing amounts of stress. The point at which memory and judgment are negatively affected differs from person to person, reflecting an individual threshold phenomenon. Under conditions of massive or traumatic stress, long term memory is likely to be impaired. Psychodynamic explanations of this occurrence point to the use of psychological defense mechanisms to ward off the experience of anxiety associated with the threat of a particular event (Dewald, 1971). With increasing stress experienced in relation to the event, defense mechanisms work to shut off subsequent anxiety such that the event and the feelings associated with it are modified and lost to conscious awareness. To the extent that anxiety generalizes from the specific situation to related events, the individual's perception is increasingly distorted. Both judgment and memory become further impaired. By the same token, as memory colors perception, it also influences present feelings and emotions, overall self-concept and life experiences.

Heredity also plays an important role in one's appraisal of events and the degree of stress associated with them. As noted in Chapter 1, certain organs may be genetically "weak" and thus vulnerable to the negative effects of stress. By the same token, genetic or constitutional "strength" may enable individuals to handle greater amounts of stress than would otherwise be possible. Higher levels of intelligence in children, for example, have been shown to facilitate their ability to cope with stress successfully.

Congenital defects and any hereditary illness cause the organism to experience stress. Most simply, every physiological difficulty causes stress because it imposes demands for adaptation and compensation on the organism. This is most dramatically seen in the case of blindness, hearing impairment, or other physical disability. While illness may be the result of stress in that one's responses to a particular virus or germ may be inadequate, illness itself becomes a stressor putting further strain on the individual's coping capacities.

Disability and illness can lower the individual's capacity to adjust to the environment, and affect perception of the environment. The child who contracted polio at an early age and was hospitalized for extensive periods of time must deal with the physiological trauma of the illness and its subsequent psychological effects. The world appears very different when one is prone or confined to a wheel chair as compared to when one is able to maneuver independently on foot. Issues of loss, abandonment, and blows to self-esteem are magnified for such individuals as children and clinical experience indicates that the effects are long-lasting. The effects for adults are no less significant. The effect of physiological characteristics can be seen in less extreme form in the case of body build, which is of utmost importance during adolescence and may have a long-term effect on perception, feelings, self-concept, and life experiences.

Perceptions and Sensations

Perceptions and sensations, feelings and emotional self-concept, and life experiences, the next part of this system, are separated out of the cognition and appraisal box for purposes of conceptual clarity. The development of these factors is influenced by the cognitive/appraisal system and, once formed, becomes a part of the cognitive/appraisal assessment. This interaction effect is indicated in Figure 2-1 by the two-directional arrows.

Perception and sensation are treated as the same phenomenon here. However, in some circles the term sensation is used to refer to specific neurophysiological impulses resulting from the stimulation of a sensory organ. Perception describes the higher level or cognitive interpretation of these sensations by the brain. Pain is an example of an important experience that can be understood as a sensation (e.g., gastrointestinal spasms translated as pain) or a perception that becomes a source of stress in itself.

Perception may be one of the most important and poorly understood aspects of human behavior that has tremendous relevance for experienced stress because how everyone views a particular situation plays an essential role in how it actually turns out. The idea of perceptual determination or influence is captured best in the concept of the "self-fulfilling prophecy." People have a tendency to act in ways that encourage things to turn out according to their own expectations.

Perception is another process that occurs within the individual through the sensory receptor-appraisal chain. Perception is the way people observe and understand the surrounding world by taking in information through the five senses. In the process of assimilating this information and assigning meaning to it—information about light, temperature, noise, smoke, bitterness, sweetness, obstacles—people learn about their environment and develop ways to respond and adapt to it. But the taking in of information is not as simple as it might first appear. What individuals take in regarding the immediate environment is very complex because the information about their present situation is added to and combined with what was previously learned, with needs and values, with life experience and self-concept, and with expectations about the future. The activity of combining happens very quickly and automatically, often without any awareness that it is occurring.

It is only after the information has been combined, however, that it is available for use. Part of the combining activity is similar to placing ideas into categories or generalizations. People try to match their present perceptions to ways of thinking that they have developed in the past. While such generalizing abilities are useful, people sometimes tend to change "reality" to fit into their categories, even when the match between them is not good. At one extreme, individuals tend to form stereotypes, a topic discussed later.

Here-and-now perceptions are influenced in still another way by previous experiences. The brain can only perceive a portion of all the information in any given situation. Because people are constantly being bombarded with information from their five senses and cannot handle all the information at once, they have developed a filtering process that allows them to ignore much of the stimuli and perceive only a small, manageable number.

For example, there is the first day on a new job, with a myriad of new stimuli demanding immediate attention—new faces, new tasks, new places, new routines, locating the bathrooms, the water fountain, the cafeteria, the closest exit to the parking lot. After newcomers become more comfortable and these stimuli are routine, they focus on other stimuli—learning what names belong to what faces, what kinds of tasks coworkers perform, what these people are like, etc.

Each person goes about perceiving in a different manner. Some concentrate on where things are, others on the people around them. These choices for concentration are not made randomly. People unconsciously select information on the basis of their own personalities and their past experiences. The process of seeing familiar things and not seeing other things is called "selective perception." It is this selectiveness that gives another bias to perceptions and becomes a source of stress in the interpersonal environment. Since no two people have had exactly the same experiences, the ways in which each selectively perceives will be different. Everyone has heard phrases such as "people see what they want to see" or "people hear what they want to hear." The phrases describe some processes of perception that can lead to problems in communicating with and understanding others, thus creating additional sources of stress.

Over their lifetime, people learn certain ways of thinking and behaving that are unique to each individual. This knowledge comes from observing the environment and by learning from others, learning that begins at birth. Some learning comes from repetition and imitation, some from the way in which people have been treated. If parents showed pleasure when caring for children, they learned to respond to pleasure and learned ways of experiencing it. If teachers became angry when students did not know the right answers, the youngsters learned how to respond to anger and how to express anger. As they grew older, the learning developed into more consistent patterns or habits.

The Role of Self-Concept

Individuals' special habits, or the particular ways in which they think and behave, make up their unique personalities. Personality affects perception of specific events since personality includes the way in which an individual views the world: as a challenging, exciting place to be; as a place to receive warmth and comfort; as a cold menacing place where people cannot be trusted; or as a competitive place where people must struggle. The part of the personality that most influences perception of the world is self-concept—what people see and think about themselves, how they organize their own goals, beliefs, values, and abilities. Self-concept is always there, influencing behavior, showing itself in various ways to others, and influencing how each person perceives and responds.

The way people think about themselves generally is internally logical and consistent even if it seems illogical to someone else or, at times, even to themselves. As with other parts of their personality, individuals first learn their self-concept from others. The significant people in their lives, such as parents, families, teachers, friends, help build self-concept by the way they talk and act with the individuals. Especially when they are young, people look for acceptance and approval. While they never completely outgrow those wants, their need for these elements is much stronger in childhood than in adulthood, when, in most cases, they have learned to give acceptance and approval to themselves.

As discussed in Chapter 3, one important source of stress is individuals' own negative self-concept and their expectation that the adult environment will meet needs that were unmet in childhood. From a psychoanalytic perspective this phenomenon is known as transference. (While the concept of transference technically refers to the client's distortions in the client-therapist interaction, transference elements are found in nontherapeutic encounters, as noted here.) In the process of transference an individual responds to others in the current environment as if they were significant people from the past. For example, a boss is experienced as though a parent, a co-worker as though a sibling. Transference influences interaction at a primarily unconscious level and causes varying degrees of inter-personal distortion to the extent that it is operative.

It is interesting to note that transference does not occur in a vacuum. The receivers of the transference needs and perceptions in reality have some quality (or qualities) similar to the historical figure. Because it creates a distortion in interpersonal relations, transference is a source of stress. On the positive side it is a phenomenon over which individuals can gain control as they increase insight into and control over their own needs and feelings, perceptions, behavioral responses, and tendencies toward distortion (Langs, 1974).

Feelings and Emotions

Feelings and emotions comprise another major influence in the socioe-motional component of stress. As discussed in Chapter 1, control over affective experience rests in the brain, specifically with the cerebral cortex, which exercises direction over the hypothalamus and the limbic system—seats of emotional activity. Visceral sensations were described as having an affective counterpart through neural transmissions in the brain. Exactly how the interpretation from physical sensation to emotional experience is made is not known. Suffice it to say that feelings and emotions result from the complex interactions of neural transmissions in the central nervous system involving a wide variety of feedback loops.

Although the pattern of emotional development is far from clear, some evidence suggests that the ability to experience and differentiate specific feelings is not innate in humans. Rather, it comes about as a result of the interactions between the normal process of biological maturation and environmental experience (Fraiberg, 1959; Mahler, Pine, & Bergman, 1975). In Chapter 3, a number of emotions frequently mentioned in the literature as being related to stress are explored. Among them are worry and anger. It should be noted that the development and experience of these separate emotions are in themselves a complex process involving neural currents, physiological organs, sensations, and feedback loops, with each part of the system stimulating and reinforcing another part.

Life Experiences

The last element in Figure 2-1 to be discussed is life experiences. This element consists of the entire set of events that makes up a person's unique history. Some of these events are considered to be traumatic at the point of occurrence. All of them have some impact and may or may not be sources of stress. All individuals share certain developmental stages through which they must pass as they live life. When these stages occur and how they will be experienced are subject to a great deal of variation.

Some determinants of the variations are cultural. Within cultures, some determinants may be familial, social, financial, or individual. No two people in the same family experience life in exactly the same way. Life experience, then, must take into account not only the actual events but also the psychological meaning and physiological effect they have had on the individual. A young woman who is accepted to medical school from a wealthy family that has encouraged her career choice experiences an event differently from the young woman who also is accepted but comes from a wealthy family that has held traditional, repressive views of a woman's role.

It should be readily apparent from this discussion that the psychological process involved in stress experiences is highly complex. Like the physiological process, it also is highly variable, differing from person to person.

STRESS AND PRODUCTIVITY

It is generally recognized that physical and emotional well-being—overall "fitness"—is conducive to productivity, cognitive effectiveness, and socioemotional stability. Similarly, it is recognized that high levels of stress are detrimental to physical and emotional well-being, thus are detrimental to productivity, and so forth. However, the opposite also is true. Too little stress has an adverse effect on performance.

The relationship between stress and productivity is generally understood as an inverted U-shape (Figure 2-2) whereby highest productivity is associated with moderate stress. What is seen as moderate differs from person to person. Such stress is best understood in terms of job challenge and motivation, whereby optimal levels of challenge and stimulation (i.e. stress) increase motivation and productivity. To the extent that research on job satisfaction shows some relationship between productivity and satisfaction (Brayfield & Crockett, 1955; Lawler & Porter, 1967; Vroom, 1964), such positive stress enhances job satisfaction as well. This, in turn, has positive implications for morale and organizational climate.

Thus, a positive snowball effect is set in motion in the organization when optimal levels of stress are maintained. Too little stress or challenge is associated with boredom, fatigue, and poor productivity, morale, and organizational climate. Conversely, too much stress, as in organizations with unrealistic deadlines, too rapid change, and lack of structure and clarity, results in the same negative performance cycle: frustration, low motivation, and poor productivity, morale, and organizational climate.

Figure 2-2 Levels of Stress and Job Performance

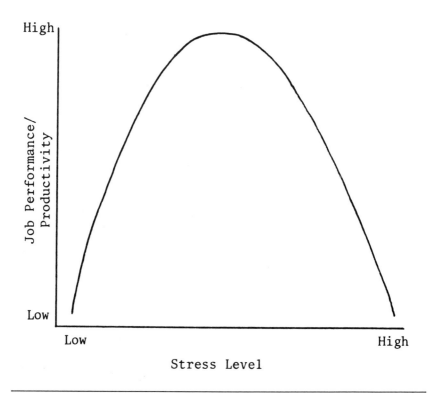

Managers who are not stimulated by the job (i.e., experience levels of stress too low for optimal functioning) are characterized as unambitious, display little or no enthusiasm for the work and the organization, and are passed over for advancement since the symptoms generally are attributed to the individuals rather than to a mismatch between them and their job demands.

This problem is an example of job underload, a serious form of organizational stress (also discussed more fully in Chapter 3). The same symptoms are likely to result under conditions of inappropriate or absent incentives to perform, where rewards are not tied to employee needs, where rewards are not executed as promised, and where the tie between rewards and performance is unclear or fluctuates constantly. Under those conditions the expenditure of effort toward a goal—characterized as motivation or ambition—seems pointless. Given this set of circumstances it is critical to diagnose the problem thoroughly, assessing how much of the problem is employee failure, how much organizational failure, and how much an interactional problem involving both.

At the other end of the spectrum is the problem of overload—where talented managers are placed in jobs in which work demands far exceed their capabilities or are blatantly unreasonable and unrealistic for any normal person to accomplish. Where goals are set too high, the normal reaction is greatly diminished effort (e.g., why bother trying?), resulting in poor performance.

Under some circumstances the individuals themselves can cause job overload through overly ambitious personal commitments. Performance deteriorates under unrealistic personal demands and expectations. The stress entailed in juggling the pressures drains these individuals' health, concentration, and vigor, and blurs their judgment and perspective. Signs of such overload are physical and mental fatigue, inability to make reasonable decisions, loss of objectivity, poor decisions, tendencies toward error, forgetfulness, irritability, and generally strained interpersonal relations.

While Figure 2-2 demonstrates the relationship between job performance and stress it does not speak to the issue of differences in individual tolerance to gross amounts of stress nor the problem of which stressor is likely to impede or stimulate performance for which individuals under what circumstances. Figure 2-3 identifies three hypothetical employees. The productivity curve of each follows the inverted U-shaped pattern. However, the amount of stress each requires for optimal performance varies greatly.

Ultimately, the assessment of what constitutes optimal stress magnitude in relation to consistently high productivity or performance is the manager's responsibility in relation to each employee. Such an assessment is possible only when the manager knows the needs of each employee, monitors continuing performance, and works to facilitate a climate that fosters maximum growth of all workers in a team effort. (Specific interventions aimed at establishing such a climate are the subject of Chapter 9.)

ELASTIC LIMITS

Another concept useful in underscoring individual differences to stress tolerance is called elastic limits. This concept can be regarded as part of the organism's physiological response to stress. Given the intricate relationship between physiological and socioemotional aspects of stress, it is discussed here, in part because individuals' psychological perception of their own stress tolerance has a bearing on elastic limits.

Figure 2-3 Variances in Stress and Job Performance

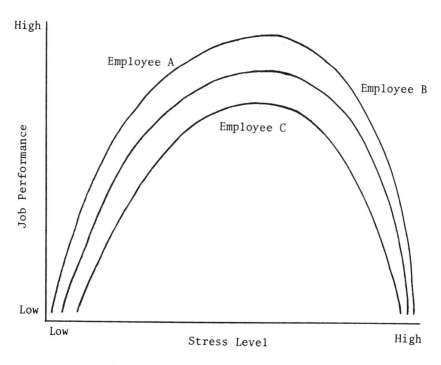

Conceptually, elastic limits derive from an analogy between the body's response to stress and the behavior of a rubber band. Individuals have different tolerances to how much stress they can absorb before they "snap." Some have genetic heritages that allow them to tolerate more stress than others. Some have learned over the years to develop resources to handle stressors effectively; these persons are able to tolerate more stress than those who have not developed such resources or coping strategies.

An important part of the elastic limit concept is the "yield point," which represents a slight change from normal behavior and serves as an early warning signal that the individual is rapidly approaching the limit or stress threshold. At this point a slight increase in stress will result in overriding the elastic limit. Irritability, rigidity, and intolerance may now have become usual attitudes. Beyond this point a rupture in behavior will occur, with serious maladjustment of a magnitude usually requiring professional help to correct (Morano, 1977).

Both stress thresholds and recovery rates from stress differ from person to person. While absolute amounts of stress will influence the level of productivity, consideration should be given also to levels related to individual elastic limits and recovery rates. Figure 2-4 compares the elastic limits of three hypothetical people.

A factor related to elastic limits and responsible for negative stress outcomes is a peculiarly human phenomenon referred to here as "psychological overdrive." This involves the turning off of early warning signals of excessive stress so that the individuals expose themselves to increasingly higher levels of prolonged and uninterrupted stress in which the whole system stays "hyped" and never returns to baseline levels of activity. Unlike the normal reaction to a stress situation described in Chapter 1, this pathological reaction finds the individuals maintaining constant levels of increased activity without replenishing the body in the below baseline recovery period. As shown in Figure 2-5, the reserve level available to manage additional stress is increasingly limited. As a result, the ability to absorb new stresses diminishes.

Figure 2-4 Elastic Limits of 3 Hypothetical People

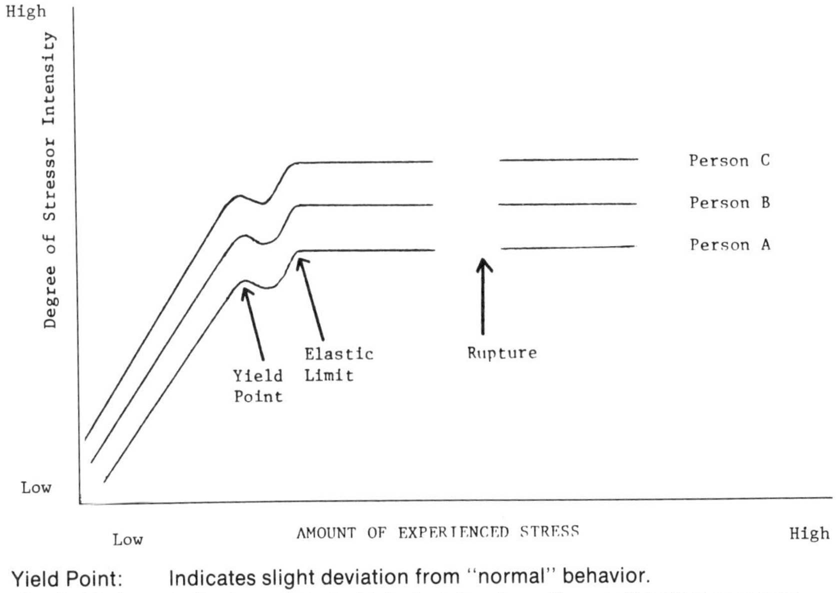

Yield Point: Indicates slight deviation from "normal" behavior.
Elastic Limit: Indicates point at which deviation from "normal" behavior occurs.
Rupture: Indicates point at which major deviation from "normal" behavior occurs.

Source: Adapted with permission of the publisher from "How to Manage Change to Reduce Stress" by Richard A. Morano, *Management Review*, p. 23. Copyright © 1977 (November) by AMACOM, a division of American Management Associations, New York. All rights reserved.

Figure 2-5 Normal and Pathological Reactions to Stress

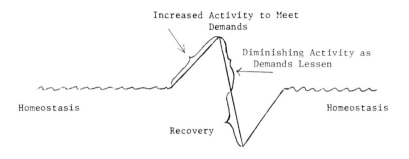

PATHOLOGICAL REACTION

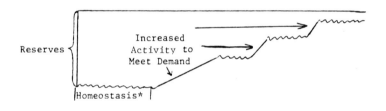

Unfortunately, there exist numerous social and organizational norms that reinforce this self-destructive behavior. The ambitious, overachieving individual, generally male and nonminority, has been presented as the model to which others climbing the corporate ladder to success should strive to emulate. To do less has led to organizational ostracism and the questions of whether or not the persons are "dedicated" and have sought to reach their "potential." To be sure, these are potential stressors in and of themselves. While there has been serious questioning of this and related ethics in organizations, their deleterious effect will continue to be felt. The negative result of such behavior is seen in a variety of stress-related physical and emotional consequences (discussed later in this chapter and Chapter 3).

SOCIOEMOTIONAL VULNERABILITY AND STRESS

The discussion of physiological and psychological causes of stress suggests that any event or the process of change itself can serve as a stressor on the human organism. It is extremely unusual, however, for any one stressor to initiate the general adaptation syndrome; rather, it is a combination of them that together work to set the stress reaction in motion. Furthermore, many physiological or psychological conditions have a chain-reaction effect. For instance, poor nutrition increases the likelihood of nutritional illness; improper posture increases fatigue and muscular tension with ripple effects of sleeplessness, lowered resistance, increased tension and fatigue, etc.

What constitutes a stressor for any given individual is highly variable across different people but the stress reaction itself, once initiated, operates in a very similar fashion. As noted earlier, differences in past experience, perception, genetic endowment, memory, and present experience ensure that no two individuals will perceive a given event in exactly the same way. The key to understanding the relevance of a stressor for a particular person depends on the nature of the event itself, the vulnerability of the individual to it at the time it occurs, and the individual's assignment of meaning to the stressor.

A number of attempts have been made to assess an individual's level of vulnerability to stress. The purpose has been to establish an individual profile of behavioral, psychological, and physical patterns that can be helpful in the early diagnosis of conditions associated with increased risk for stress-related disorders. While none of the approaches have produced truly adequate measures of reliability and validity, two such efforts bear mention because of their potential utility and some promising early research findings: (1) the McLean Self-Assessment Questionnaires (1979) and (2) the *Individual Profile of Stressors* (IPS) developed at the Stress Center, St. Louis University School of Medicine between 1980 and 1982.

The McLean Model

Alan McLean, a psychiatrist who has written numerous books on occupational stress, has developed a model that illustrates the relationship between stress event, vulnerability, and perceived meaning of the event (or context) (1979). The relationship is presented as a Venn diagram in Figure 2-6. As McLean suggests, stress occurs to the extent that there is overlap among the three factors. Each circle represents a dynamic state in some degree of flux. Each varies in context in its relationship to the two others as the flow of situational events changes over time.

McLean has devised three scales to assess personal profiles in relation to vulnerability, stressors, and context—a Coping Checklist, a Context Survey, and a Stressors Checklist. Each scale yields a rough approxima-

Figure 2-6 McLean Model of Stress

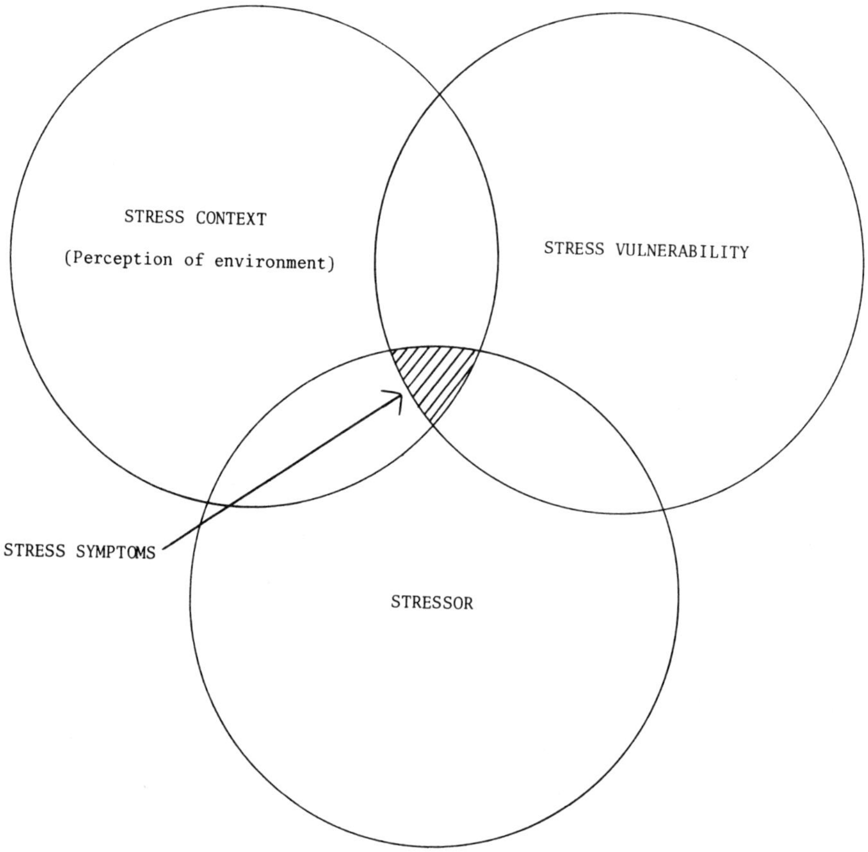

STRESS CONTEXT

(Perception of environment)

STRESS VULNERABILITY

STRESS SYMPTOMS

STRESSOR

Source: Adapted from *Work Stress* by Alan A. McLean, published by Addison-Wesley Publishing Company, Inc., Reading, Mass., p. 39. Copyright © 1979, by permission of Addison-Wesley Publishing Company, Inc.

tion that can serve as a personal guide to establishing areas of weakness and strength.

The Coping Checklist

The Coping Checklist roughly assesses work-related vulnerability by exploring how the individual copes with the job along five dimensions: self-knowledge, interest variety, reaction to stress, acceptance of others' values, and degree of activity-productivity. A cut-off figure is identified by McLean suggesting that scores above that number might indicate difficulty in coping ability, thus increasing vulnerability. McLean describes a model "ideally successful individual" to be emulated with regard to overall coping ability:

- Such an individual has effective knowledge of self, including areas of strength and weakness, capitalizes on strengths, and recognizes limitations and areas in which improvement is possible.
- Such a person has developed many interests and hobbies outside of the work setting, leading to a rounder, fuller existence.
- Such a person has an array of coping strategies that are used to respond to stressors. The individual would not always react to disappointment with withdrawal or become hyperactive under frustration.
- Such a person recognizes and accepts the fact that others have different ways of doing things and does not equate the individual's way with "right" and the alternative with "wrong."
- Such a person is active and productive at work and away from work.

The Context Survey

The Context Survey consists of 15 general items assessing satisfaction with the job, including supervision, pay, overall advancement opportunities, demands, and actual responsibilities. Scores above a cutoff point are suggestive of an overall work context that is less than satisfactory.

The Stressors Checklist

The Stressors Checklist itemizes various kinds of problems that could arise on the job, interfering with the ability to effectively carry out job-related responsibilities. The dimensions include: conflict and uncertainty, job pressure (e.g., too many demands, not enough time), job scope (lack of clarity, too little authority), and rapport with management (unpredictability, lack of clarity regarding performance). Once again, cutoff scores are suggested to indicate undesirable amounts of stress on the job.

Interrelationships among the three elements are determined by drawing three circles on a scoring sheet, based on the questionnaires' results. The degree to which the circles overlap suggests the extent to which stress is associated with the current job. If vulnerability could be reduced by changing coping strategies employed to deal with stressors, or if factors on the job could be modified, or if the effect (context) of a stressor could be lessened, stress symptoms would be alleviated.

Individual Profile of Stressors (IPS)

The IPS, developed by Dr. Kathryn D. Cramer (1981) at St. Louis University, was conceived as an overall measure of general, not specifically job-related, stress. The IPS utilizes items from measures of stress and well-being previously reported in the literature as well as from other factors shown to be related to stress. The profile consists of 20 elements, each with four items in the self-administered paper-and-pencil instrument. Each item is scored on a five-point scale of vulnerability so response figures can range from 4 to 20. Scores below 7 are considered as showing low vulnerability, those 8 to 12 as moderate, and those over 13 as high. Degree of vulnerability is believed to be directly related to the occurrence of negative stress outcomes—that is, disturbances in cognitive, emotional, and physiological functioning with subsequent implications for general well-being and interpersonal functioning.

The IPS scale elements include measures of one's physical condition, sense of belonging, adjustment, life satisfaction, interpersonal relationships, life goals, habit patterns, and attitudes toward nutrition, among others.

An initial validation study was performed comparing a group of cardiac patients who recently had experienced a myocardial infarction (N = 28) with a group of middle managers without a history of coronary disease (N = 45). It was predicted that cardiac patients would score higher than the middle managers in all of the stress scales. While all but two scales (Adjustment and Relationships) fell in the predicted direction, only four showed significant differences between the two groups (Physical Condition, Life Style, Life Satisfaction, and Aloneness).

Despite these rather weak findings, the instrument merits further testing as a device potentially useful in the early prediction of stress vulnerability. In conjunction with physiological data and measures of coping strategies, such information could be quite helpful in the prevention of negative stress outcomes. (Additional work with this instrument is reported in Chapter 4.)

It should be noted that stress vulnerability scores are similar in their interpretation to "risk factors" in disease. People with such risks have a higher likelihood of experiencing the negative effects of stress than those without the risks. As Rahe (1979) notes, risk factors with regard to disease are "notoriously nonspecific." The same must be said of stress vulnerability. In both cases, the number of those who are predicted to be vulnerable and subject to disease is greater than the number of those who actually get a disease.

LIFE EVENTS AND STRESS

One of the best-known instruments used in predicting the probability of negative stress outcomes is the *Social Readjustment Rating Scale,* also known as the *Life Change Test* (Holmes & Rahe, 1967). The scale was based on earlier research that suggested that stressful life events played an important causative role in disease by evoking neurophysiological reactions. Included in the assortment of disorders were psychosomatic diseases, traumatic illnesses, and infectious diseases. In the original, a proportionate scaling method was used to derive values representative of the average amount of change required for an individual to cope with each of the 43 life events included in the instrument.

The scale was the result of analysis of data derived from thousands of interviews with individuals admitted to a hospital with a variety of physical illnesses. The data included events that the patients reported had occurred over the year or two preceding the illness. Events were broken into categories pertaining to health, family life, work, personal life, finances, and community/social relations. The resulting scale was designed to sample from these areas of life adjustment, not to be all-inclusive.

The important premise underlying all of the events was that they necessitated a change from a previous state of adjustment (Holmes & Rahe, 1967; Rahe, Meyer, & Smith, 1964). Extremely pleasant life events (e.g., marriage) were found to require approximately the same amount of life adjustment as those of an unpleasant quality (e.g., death of a loved one). Using the physiological conception of a change in homeostasis potentially resulting in bioregulatory failure, system dysfunction, and diseases, Holmes and Rahe applied the same reasoning to abrupt changes in homeostasis brought about by psychosocial events. As discussed in Chapter 1, the interconnections of neurophysiological and psychological/cognitive processes in the brain make this an absolutely reasonable application.

As Rahe (1979) notes, there is considerable disagreement among researchers as to what constitutes an adequate array of life-change events. There is no unanimity of scientific opinion as to which events are most representative or meaningful in any given person's life. However, when Rahe (1979) compared his and Holmes's original scale with others, he concluded that their salient events were remarkably similar to those in his instrument.

Longitudinal studies have confirmed that increases in life change units increase the probability of illness (Dohrenwend, 1973; Jacobs, Prosoff, and Paykel, 1974; Myers, Lindenthal, and Pepper, 1972; Tennant and Andrews, 1978). More specifically, the work of Holmes and Rahe (1967) suggests that for people with life change units of less than 150 during the previous 12 months, there was a 30 percent probability of becoming ill (i.e., experiencing a health change) in the near future; for those with units of 150–299, a 50 percent probability; and those with units above 300, an 80 percent probability.

This is not to suggest that someone who scored more than 300 definitely would become ill or that someone who scored less than 150 definitely would not become ill. In the large groups Holmes and Rahe (1967) studied, illness occurred with much greater frequency (80 percent) in the high change group than in either the moderate (50 percent) or low change groups (30 percent). What accounts for a particular individual's experiencing a change in health status is an interaction of many factors, only one of which is life change. Similar findings have been reported by others (Dohrenwend, 1973; Jacobs, Prosoff, & Paykel, 1974; Myers, Lindenthal, & Pepper, 1972; Paykel, 1974).

Of particular interest are studies examining and confirming the relationships between life events and psychiatric disorders. In a two year longitudinal study, Myers et al. (1972) report that increases in recent life change events are associated with deterioration in mental status, regardless of whether the life changes are seen as positive (desirable) or negative (undesirable). Later analysis of these data (Eaton, 1978) elaborates on these findings: there is little relation between life events in the first year studied and in the second; thus, few persons consistently report high life change occurrences over a two-year period; symptoms follow, not precede, life changes.

Studies of depressive disorders find that persons being treated as outpatients for depression experience more recent life change events than nonpatient controls but fewer changes than inpatients being treated for depression (Jacobs et al., 1974; Paykel, 1974). Further confirmation is provided by Vinokur and Selzer (1975) who report that numerous life changes occurring close together in time (e.g. change in employment and marital status,) tend to be associated with the subsequent onset of depression. However, unlike the earlier study of Myers et al., their results suggest that the relationship between life changes and depression is accounted for primarily by the occurrence of undesirable (negative) events. Two studies (Cooper & Sylph, 1973; Tennant & Andrews, 1978) find the onset of neurotic impairment follows closely on increases in life changes.

It is apparent that a relationship exists between recent changes in an individual's life and the onset of numerous physical and emotional disorders. However, there is little relationship between the absolute number of life changes and the onset of illness. It seems that the number of events has influence only secondarily through the way in which the individual perceives them. The effect of life events also seems to be mediated by available and used social supports, psychological defense structure, coping capabilities, genetic predispositions, and history of illness (Rahe & Arthur, 1978). From a diagnostic standpoint, life change can be viewed as an increased vulnerability to stress, useful in diagnosing populations at risk for the development of physical or emotional illness.

This leaves unresolved, however, one important question, which Rahe (1979) aptly notes: what is it that makes certain individuals tolerate large amounts of recent life change and remain healthy? An investigation of that outcome would have to take into account not only the presence (or relative absence) of stressful environmental conditions but also the individuals' perceptions of these conditions, ability to cope with stressors, genetic predispositions, and personality characteristics.

Chapter 3

Sources of Stress

It has been fairly well documented that people today live in an age of anxiety, with high inflation and unemployment, almost daily reports of international crises, and the possibility of disaster in a nuclear war a bit too close for comfort. The last two decades have seen the sexual revolution, the women's revolution, the peace movement, the Vietnam war, Watergate, and the "me" generation. Divorce statistics increase yearly, which can signify either more or less stress, depending on how the data are interpreted. Since staying in a bad marriage can be worse than leaving, such figures can suggest lowered amounts of stress as a result of divorce. In any case, the figures do imply that there is less and less certainty in individuals' lives.

Obviously, stressors exist in a wide variety of places. Since the focus of this book is organizational stress, this discussion is limited to an exploration of the major areas where stressors can be found in the organization. For conceptual purposes, four major sources of job-related stress are analyzed: the physical environment, the interpersonal environment, the organizational environment, and the individual person. Before examining each of these, some general comments are in order.

STRESS: MANAGEMENT OR PERSONAL PROBLEM

Managers typically react negatively to a discussion of organizational or job-related stress. They believe that stress is not a management, but a personal, problem. This approach uses the individual differences in responses to stress reactions as a reason to adopt a philosophy of management prevalent in the 1890s. Essentially, this view translates to a form of social Darwinism, or survival of the fittest at work. Such an approach expects individuals to adapt as best they can; those meant to survive, will; those not meant to, won't.

There is another side to the coin, however. The evidence makes clear that no business can afford to ignore the impact of employee stress on the job. Some of the effects of stress on individual work performance and morale are hard to measure. Others are quite tangible. For example, people who report higher levels of perceived stress because of job dissatisfaction are more likely to experience the following problems:

- increased absenteeism (Caplan & Jones, 1975)
- higher job turnover (McKenna, Oritt, & Wolff, 1981)
- lower productivity, more accidents, greater inefficiency, mistakes on the job, possible permanent loss of job resulting from stress-related illness or death (Cooper & Marshall, 1977).

While most of the reports documenting the relationship between stress and effectiveness are anecdotal, intuitive judgment and conceptual frameworks point to the soundness of this linkage. People tend to work better when they are "up" than when they are "down," stressed, and overwhelmed.

As for turnover, stress has been reported as a significant variable in the decisions of lower level staff and managerial personnel to leave the organization (McKenna et al., 1981; Peskin, 1973). While the more recent McKenna et al. study suggests that turnover depends on an interactive effect between occupational stress and professional position (i.e., people with more professional training are more likely to experience greater amounts of organizational commitment and are less likely to leave than are lower level personnel), turnover is a problem that should be of concern to the organization, regardless of the level at which it occurs.

Turnover is an expensive part of doing business. Assuming an initial $500 per employee for unemployment taxes regardless of how long the individual stays on the payroll, the costs of recruitment, hiring, training, and integrating the person into the organization weigh significantly on the operating costs of the hospital. Increases in accidents produce a large impact by increasing workmen's compensation costs. Absence because of stress-related illness creates significant problems in terms of dollars and morale. Unlike the university setting, where classes are cancelled and rescheduled when the professor is ill, in the service-intensive health care business patients cannot be cancelled when an employee calls in sick. As a result, the institution pays sick leave and the costs of a replacement to ensure full staffing.

STRESS IN THE PHYSICAL ENVIRONMENT

Stressors in the physical environment probably are the easiest to alleviate yet often are disregarded. It is useful to think of this type of stress by way of the analogy of exposure to low-level doses of radiation. If, as with other sources of stress, there is respite from that exposure, then the person is reexposed (as with yearly dental x-rays), there are likely to be few ill effects. But if the low level of exposure continues over long periods or if there is short-term, high-level radiation, either is likely to be deadly.

Physical stressors emanate from the environment in which people work. This includes such tangibles as working space, lighting, ventilation, traffic patterns, layout of the facility, its ambience, the quality of internal and external maintenance and housekeeping, and the availability or lack of elevators. Working space among executive or administrative personnel generally is adequate and in some cases is luxurious. Given this state of affairs it is easy to forget that not all hospital employees are so privileged. A private office, carpeting, an outside window, a location away from the hustle of daily activity—all these are associated with privilege and altitude in the organizational hierarchy. Most employees do not have private places to which they can retreat during a stressful day. Continual exposure to stimuli without the availability of a quiet space is similar to constant exposure to radiation without respite. The supervisor or middle manager in such a situation is caught in a very difficult position that can have ramifications for the entire institution.

A case in point is the performance appraisal interview conducted by a head nurse. The employee is escorted to a "quiet" spot in the nurses' station where two chairs are pulled together in "closed conversation" fashion. Calls come in interrupting the discussion, distracting conversations take place in the area, irritated members of patients' families grumble that no one seems concerned about meeting their needs, and so forth. Unlikely? Another example involves a less obvious problem. Another head nurse occupies a cubbyhole that is shared by those in similar positions on other shifts. A performance appraisal/coaching session is being conducted behind closed doors. However, the evening head nurse has come in early to finish some paperwork, calls come in directly to this "office" and interrupt the flow of conversation, others knock on the door for answers to important but nonemergency questions.

The hospital executive, protected by the insulating properties of the secretary in the outer office, is likely to be unaware of these problems. It also is unlikely that the head nurse or staff will regard these occurrences as anything more than typical operating procedure.

Even where a private office is available and used for the performance appraisal session, the physical arrangement of the furniture provides a context or setting through which the communications transacted in the room are filtered. Such a context can serve to raise or lower stress associated with the appraisal interview itself. For instance, the administrator may conduct the review while seated in a large leather chair behind a rather imposing mahogany desk with the subordinate seated opposite in a lesser chair. This sets a stage associated with increased anxiety, thus adding stress to what already is a stressful situation. By contrast, the same administrator could conduct the interview seated next to the subordinate at a small round table in the same office. Physical aspects of the environment can, indeed, play a significant role in the level of stress generated by a situation and in the quality of the communications exchanged.

Meetings interrupted by telephones ringing, people walking through en route to somewhere else, beepers buzzing, etc., become less productive because of these and similar sources of stress in the physical environment. Providing employees with personal space, offices wherever possible even where they are shared, or quiet places that offer retreat for all those in need of calm is an easy means of reducing one form of environmental stressor.

Inadequately lit surroundings, whether they be too bright or too dark, constitute another form of physical stressor, as does poor ventilation. For example, there is the cafeteria or laundry that is too cold in winter and too hot in summer. Slow elevators en route to an emergency, wet floors without signs, and traffic congestion in the halls are other stress sources that can be remedied easily. For the visitor—patient, family, or outsider— the inadequacy of signs makes negotiating the maze that is the hospital a stressful ordeal it does not need to be.

One last example: in an obstetrics-gynecology department of a nationally known university medical center, the physical arrangement of the waiting room is a source of stress for patients. On Tuesdays, certain tests for infertility are performed. Once a month the waiting room is filled with men and women, usually it is dominated by women. On these Tuesdays everyone is present for the sperm count test. Appointments have been made weeks, often months, in advance. Names are called and people in the very crowded waiting room are beckoned into the inner sanctum. Men glance at their watches, hoping to be able to get back to work before noon.

Smith, Jones, Wallace, and Ford have been called in the first half hour. The others in the waiting room see Smith returning from the inner area that houses examining rooms and nurses' and doctors' offices, carrying a small brown paper bag, headed for the men's room. The men's room, of course, is located at the far end of the crowded waiting room. He enters the men's room and locks the door behind him (until two months ago the door had no lock on it).

He is followed soon by Jones, sheepishly carrying a similar small brown bag. Jones tries the door. Not realizing it is only large enough for one, he rattles it, thinking it is stuck. Unsuccessful, he sits down on a waiting room chair. Next, Wallace appears and makes a similar attempt at opening the door. Frustrated, Wallace, too, sits down in the waiting area holding his brown bag. Finally, Ford emerges from the examining area, headed for the men's room. It's surprising that no one warns him and saves him from embarrassment.

Finally, a red-faced Smith emerges from the men's room, taking his brown bag and its now-filled bottle across the waiting room to deposit it with the appropriate nurse. Hospital sensitivity to the needs of patients and spouses would have lessened the embarrassment and stress of these men.

STRESS IN THE INTERPERSONAL ENVIRONMENT

Problems in interpersonal environment also are known as social stressors. Unlike those in the physical environment, these are subject to less direct control because they involve the behavior of others. Typical interpersonal stressors include chronically angry or aggressive people with whom it is necessary to interact; passive aggressive individuals; ungrateful or demanding patients, bosses, doctors, nurses, administrators, board members, subordinates; those who have difficulty expressing their needs and leave others guessing; and those who have difficulty giving and receiving negative feedback. Differing perceptions and generally poor interpersonal communication provide a frequent source of stress at this level.

Problems in Perception

As discussed in Chapter 2, perception is an important part of the cognitive appraisal system that is influential in whether or not a given stress trigger will be experienced as stressful. Since no two people have had exactly the same experiences, the ways in which each individual selectively perceives events will be different. Because people approach situations in terms of what makes sense to them in light of earlier experiences, problems in communicating with and understanding others occur, frequently leading to stress because "they just don't understand the way things ought to be." The way a person perceives something can be as important as what the situation actually is. This has implications for decision making at all levels of the organization because perception forms one of the bases for making decisions. A few related principles are:

- People can make a decision about something only after they perceive it.

- Different people make different decisions about a situation because they perceive it differently.
- Many people together involved in making a decision about a situation will have to resolve their differences in perception before a good conclusion can be reached. In other words, everyone has to have a common understanding of the situation. To the extent the decision involves personal values and is a less than "objective" issue, consensus will be harder to reach and more stress will be encountered in the process.
- Everyone's decisions are based in part on earlier experiences and future expectations so there can be no totally unbiased outcome. Value premises must always be considered in decision making (Simon, 1976).

People who are aware of their own personal characteristics are more likely to perceive others correctly. They also are less likely to view the world in black-and-white terms and are more likely to accept differences among individuals. When individuals are unsure of themselves or are insecure, they tend to attribute their own displeasure with themselves to others or to see problems in those others. They tend to reject those who have characteristics they do not like in themselves and to like those whose traits they value in themselves. Increasing perceptual accuracy ultimately is each individual's responsibility and goes far in reducing interpersonal stress in the organization.

To the extent that perception is under an individual's control, each person can exercise a great deal of influence over this very important source of stress. For instance, the observation of what others are saying or doing (or, for that matter, not saying or doing) may precipitate differing degrees of stress in the observer. What is overlooked is that the source of stress is not in the actions of others but in the meaning attributed to them—i.e., in perception of the situation. Thus, reevaluating the meaning attributed, changing perspective, and so forth may be very helpful in monitoring and alleviating stress reactions. (Examples of such techniques, including cognitive restructuring, are discussed in Chapter 10.)

Problems in Communication

Interpersonal communication is probably the single most important aspect of management and is a contributor to organizational stress. Communication affects people constantly, often without their being aware of how. It is generally accepted that one cannot *not* communicate.

Put simply, communication is verbal and nonverbal behavior that occurs in a social context. It includes interaction or transactions between people who use a variety of symbols and clues to give and receive meaning. "Meaning" refers to a host of thoughts, words, feelings, and expectations that may operate at a conscious or unconscious level. Thus, at its most basic level, communication can be regarded as the transfer of meaning through a verbal and/or nonverbal message.

How individuals communicate indicates the level and effectiveness of their interpersonal functioning. Since communication is necessary for survival, in that it is the means through which needs are made known, the ability to communicate will determine in large part the extent to which those needs are satisfied. Perhaps most importantly, communication is the tool through which people discover the world and their relationship to it. They learn what are socially approved ways of behaving. They learn what others expect of them. They learn of others' intentions and how they react to them—how the others appear to them through what they communicate. As such, communication can be regarded as a bridge between people, enabling them to meet each others' needs and expectations through knowledge of what they are.

Communication also is the means through which people get close to each other. It is the way they validate each other's experience. To be acknowledged and recognized suggests a person is worthwhile. There is perhaps nothing more devastating as not being recognized. Nonrecognition implies that the individual does not exist. It is for this reason that some people engage in destructive behavior in order to obtain a response from others on the theory that negative attention is better than none at all.

Despite the primacy of communication, numerous difficulties exist in the process. Where meaning is not exchanged accurately or adequately between participants, needs are less likely to be met and stress is more likely to result. Part of the problem in the exchange of meaning rests in the complexity of the exchange process itself. Communicator A, for example, initiates communication with Communicator B. Communicator A thinks about the message to be sent, framing the idea in the mind so it can be transmitted. In addition, A assesses the intent of the communication and the desired impact on B. The message is then encoded (the idea and the intent are put into a form that can be transmitted). It may be encoded in an overt physical movement, such as a handshake or a pat on the back, a scowl or frown, or symbols that stand for something such as writing, speaking, or crying. The message then is transmitted by oral or written means.

Communicator B perceives the message through the senses and decodes it by putting it in a form that makes it comprehensible. B assigns meaning to the message and communicates the fact that it has been received and understood. The goal of effective communication is for B to interpret and understand the message as A intended.

The process as described appears somewhat static—Communicator A transmitting a message to Communicator B. In actuality, communication between the two takes place almost simultaneously, with B giving feedback and responding to A even before the message is complete. Thus messages are subject to modification through the influence of Communicator B's feedback.

Several barriers in the process are likely to jam the works. Noise or interference may prevent the clear transmission of the message from Communicator A to Communicator B in the same way as static interrupts transmission and receipt of a radio signal. A serious problem results from the fact that people are able to encode and decode messages only in terms of a language or frame of reference and experience that makes sense to them. The "expert" communicator, for example, may encode a message only in terms of a professional frame of reference and the decoder may lack the technical expertise to find meaning in it. Or the decoder may decode merely in terms of a personal frame of reference, deriving a meaning that runs the risk of being a distortion of what was intended. If no common, shared ground exists, communication will not be received or comprehended. The participants may feel their words are bouncing off walls, not too unlike the frustration of the American traveler in France who, not speaking a word of French, shouts louder, hoping that the receiver, who speaks not a word of English, will understand by virtue of sheer volume.

The lack of shared experience is an especially acute problem in health care. Different professionals often fail to translate their thoughts into language other professionals or lay people can use. When a psychiatrist and an occupational therapist on a psychiatric unit discuss a patient's transference and countertransference reactions, the conversation is likely to reflect their separate frames of reference and result in dysfunctional communication. The occupational therapist may not have the knowledge or experience base necessary to discuss the details of the case in psychiatric terminology. Of course, the psychiatrist may know this and use jargon deliberately in a one-upmanship ploy vis-à-vis the occupational therapist. Such displays are not limited to cross-discipline interactions. Supervisors can use their knowledge and experience advantage very effectively to get one up on subordinates. Using highly technical knowledge that is beyond the capacity of subordinates to understand and apply will lead them to perform poorly, which is, in turn, the result of communications that are not "received."

Assuming that Communicator A is not interested in increasing personal power at the expense of Communicator B, other serious obstacles to clear communication exist. The two may possess skills and capacities that are quite different from one another—a differential that could cause problems. The sender may supply ambiguous messages, disorganized statements, value-laden remarks, too much or too little information. The receiver must interpret, process, and acknowledge receipt of the message, at the same time also screening out noise. What is screened out depends upon B's selective attention, interest, and how much the person likes A.

Readiness to continue the communication is influenced by B's own past experience, present needs and attributes, and future expectations. If experience has familiarized B with the content of the message, if B is in a listening stance and expects the information to be useful in the future, the receiver is more likely to attend to the particulars of the communication than if it is new information with which the person has little experience and which he perceives to be of no value either now or in the future. The less attentive B is, the more likely it is that the communication will be distorted and result in problems.

Obviously, while verbal accessibility—the degree to which a person feels free to and is able to communicate clearly and openly with words—is important, it is not sufficient for functional communication to occur. Credibility also influences how the communication will be received. Credibility depends on such factors as expertise, trustworthiness, and intent. Knowledge and experience are important aspects of expertise. The greater an individual's expertise in areas of value and interest to the receiver, the greater the likelihood that the communication will be received favorably.

An atmosphere of trust, critically important in reducing stress associated with interpersonal communications, will enhance that likelihood further. If the intent of the communication will benefit the receiver, a favorable reception is even more likely. Personality variables offer yet another credibility dimension. To the extent that a person is arrogant, offensive, condescending, officious, and the like, that individual limits receptivity to communication. It should be noted, however, that even the positive effect of personality wears off after a time, leaving such variables as communication content and expertise to assume great importance.

Regardless of the credibility of the communicator, there are limits beyond which the receiver cannot attend to and absorb new information. Overloading or exposing a person to too many verbal demands can lead to passive compliance or a shutting out of messages. (The problem of overload is explored in the discussion of stress in the organizational environment in Chapter 9.)

Stress may result from the fact that people often communicate considerably more than they intend. Goffman (1959) refers to this as the discrepancy between what people "give," which is intentional, and what they "give off," which is unintentional. Both aspects of the communication are "received" by the receiver, who is left in a quandary regarding how to respond. Communicator A sends what was intended and what was not intended. The discrepancy has been referred to as the "arc of distortion" (Hampton, Summer, & Webber, 1978; Sullivan, 1955). The wider the arc, the greater the discrepancy between the intended and nonintended aspects of the communication. The discrepancy results in an ambiguous situation for the receiver. To what should the receiver respond—the intended or unintended communication? To the extent the relationship includes a power dynamic (Communicator B is subordinate to Communicator A) and a norm that questions cannot be asked of one's superior for clarification, the situation becomes highly stressful for B.

This discrepancy is a form of incongruent communication. Incongruence also can result from a mismatch between the verbal and nonverbal aspects of a message. For example, giving someone a compliment (verbal level) while sounding angry and wearing a frown (nonverbal level) is discrepant and stress producing insofar as it forces the receiver to make sense out of the mixed messages.

Discrepancies also occur in the gray area between explicit and implicit messages. The explicit aspect refers to what actually is stated, the implicit to what is not said but is implied. For instance, a medical records employee arrives 15 minutes late to a utilization review meeting following the director's strong request for participants to arrive promptly. The employee also has forgotten a particular chart. The director makes no comment about the lateness but politely asks the employee to get the chart in question. Upon his return, the employee hands it to the director with an apology, the director smiles and says, "Thanks. We all forget things sometimes." The meeting proceeds uneventfully. However, later that day the director is found in the medical records office berating the supervisor for irresponsibility.

Ambiguity causes somewhat different but equally problematic communication difficulties. The following situation illustrates such problems. It is midafternoon in the laboratory. Things have been hectic all day. A technician bursts out, "Damn it, the flask broke again." There are several ways this may be interpreted. There is a statement of fact that something is broken. The technician's tone demonstrates that he is irritated. Is he criticizing the supervisor indirectly for insisting on ordering these flasks? Is he criticizing himself? If so, does he want sympathy? Does he need help? How these and similar questions are answered will determine whether or how to respond to the technician. The problems could have been eliminated or reduced had the technician made an explicit direct request.

In addition to the factors identified so far, other difficulties are posed by simple verbal communications:

- Words have different denotations. For example, class refers to a room, socioeconomic status, social position, educational level, style of deportment.
- Words have different connotations. "A little late" may mean 10 minutes to one person, 40 minutes to another. "A small group" may mean three or four persons to one individual, eight or nine persons to another. "A brief report" may mean a paragraph to the employee, four pages to the boss.
- Incomplete messages require the receiver to fill in the blank: "He isn't very . . . you know what I mean."
- Pronouns may be used vaguely: "We went to the meeting and they (administration) got upset."
- Connections may be left out: "Sorry I'm late." "That's O.K." "Joe is sick."
- No message is sent but people behave as though it had been: "They never stay to clean up after meetings."
- Content and relationship aspects of messages may be confused. For example, surgeon comments on opening a new brand of sterile needles, "These needles are dull." Nurse takes that to mean the physician thinks she is incompetent. This is as "relevant" as the wife who believes she is a bad cook because her husband comments that the steak is tough.
- Fear of being disappointed if a person makes a request leads to indirect suggestions and an avoidance of responsibility. Supervisor to nurse's aide: "There's a good movie playing tonight. You would like to escort Mr. and Mrs. Jones there, wouldn't you?"

This list covers only some of the various types of communication obstacles. The area of common assumptions provides another rich source of obstacles that often block effective communications and increase interpersonal stress:

1. One instance is an example of all instances.
2. Everyone feels, thinks, acts, and likes what I do.
3. My perceptions and evaluations are complete, valid, and true.
4. My perceptions and evaluations won't ever change.
5. Evaluations are best made using black/white, either/or categories.

6. Characteristics I attribute to objects or people belong to the things or the people themselves.
7. Crystal balls are accurate.
8. Vagueness is useful.
9. Incomplete messages also are useful.
10. Osmosis is a useful method of transmitting information.

Item 1 requires that the communicator generalize. Specific information answering the basic questions—what, where, who, when, why—is avoided. Words such as none, no one, never, nowhere, nothing, everything, everyone, are used liberally. In Item 2, comments such as "How could you favor *that* course of action?" suggest that views other than those the individual holds are worthless. This is egocentrism at its best, supported by Items 3 and 4, which never require consultation or elaboration and permit no change. Item 5 suggests that the world is either for or against the communicator. Compromise under such circumstances is exceedingly unlikely.

The power of the individual becomes more apparent in Item 6. "That person is incompetent" (or grandiose, arrogant, etc.) becomes a statement of "truth," not evaluative opinion, and may become as difficult to remove as the Scarlet Letter. In Item 7, "crystal balls" are popular, especially in times of crisis. This communicator favors the mentality of "I know what you're thinking and vice versa." This way no one has to risk putting one's true perceptions on the line. The remaining items follow in kind.

Vagueness may be used as a power tactic, keeping the subordinate receiver unsure. To the extent that the subordinate requires the information in order to adequately perform a job, stress is increased and performance decreased. Osmosis as a method of transmitting information is about as productive as standing next to a bank and expecting to get rich in the process.

EVALUATION AND DEFENSIVE BEHAVIOR

Perceptual distortions are likely to occur when individuals are feeling defensive. Energy that could be directed to accomplishing a task is diminished since a portion of it is diverted to self-defense. Defensiveness occurs when an interpersonal threat is perceived or anticipated. If people perceive that they are being evaluated and judged, elements of threat will appear. In ordinary circumstances, those with extremely low self-esteem tend to be defensive. While this appears congruent with experience, the opposite situation may not be so readily apparent. That is, people with extremely high self-esteem also tend to be defensive. This is because they are likely to be highly self-critical and perfectionist in their standards. Everyone falls short of perfection but those who value or strive toward it may be defensive when they fall short. Regardless of the source, defensiveness prevents the listener from concentrating on the message.

Gibb (1961) has identified six characteristics each for defensive climates and supportive climates. These characteristics are easily placed on the continuum at the bottom of Exhibit 3-1 since no climate is totally defensive or supportive. It should be noted that the behaviors appearing in the left-hand column arouse defensiveness, those in the right-hand column reduce defensiveness. These dimensions are considered next.

Evaluation vs. Description

Evaluative statements, intonations, gestures, or expressions will ignite defensive reactions quickly, for no one appreciates another's sitting in judgment. A person's guard goes up in the face of evaluation. The individual may feel like the accused awaiting sentence. Questions typically arouse defensiveness, even when the author of the question is merely attempting to obtain information. The notorious, "Why did this happen?" or "Where were you when this occurred?" most assuredly will create a defensive climate.

What about the alternative, descriptive behavior? Descriptions of behavior, unlike evaluations, tend to arouse minimal defensiveness or uneasiness in interpersonal situations. A behavior description reports specific, observable actions rather than inferences or generalizations about an individual's motives, feelings, attitudes, or personality traits. It states what was observed but does not imply why something occurred. It also

Exhibit 3-1 Characteristics of Defensive and Supportive Climates

Evaluation	Description
Control	Problem Orientation
Strategy	Spontaneity
Neutrality	Empathy
Superiority	Equality
Certainty	Provisionalism

Most Defensive————————————————— Most Supportive

Source: Adapted from "Defense Communication" by Jack R. Gibb, by permission of *The Journal of Communication,* September 1961, 9(3), 141–148, © 1961.

does not state or imply the value of what took place. It does not impute right or wrong, good or bad.

Control vs. Problem Orientation

Resistance is a typical response when people feel that another's communication is aimed at controlling their behavior. Since much communication revolves around attempting to influence others or change their attitudes, this problem has a potentially high chance of occurring. Persons attempting to control others often harbor several hidden agendas. They believe their position is correct, or at least better than the other's or the latter would not be attempting to change it. This implies that the other is not as knowledgeable, is immature, uses faulty reasoning, or is just plain ignorant. That the listener receives this implicit communication and responds defensively as though attacked should come as no surprise to the speaker. Yet many are, indeed, taken by surprise, unaware of their implied intent.

Imposition of will over another to control behavior comes in many forms. It appears formally as detailed policies and procedures that are carefully and obsessively monitored. It also appears in the barrage of friendly "persuasions" and "suggestions" emanating from the boss. Such comments as "It would be more helpful if you could deliver lab reports by 2 p.m.," and "Why don't you place the sandwiches over there?" implicitly carry with them the expectation of compliance. Defensiveness may occur more frequently because the communications are not made explicitly. The implicitness suggests that the boss is not being straightforward and therefore cannot be trusted. Hence, the receiver should be on guard, i.e., defensive.

On the other hand, problem-oriented communications carry with them a desire for mutual collaboration on a solution to a particular problem. The communicator defines the problem and requests discussion that will result in a solution. It is made clear that the communicator has not arrived at a solution already and does not have a favored approach to impose. Such an orientation assumes that the communicator has no need to control and reduces interpersonal stress.

Strategy vs. Spontaneity

Strategies entail hidden agendas aimed at control over a long range. Motivations of the communication-initiator are ambiguous, leaving the receiver distrustful. Withholding information, feigning interest, and manipulating the listener are strategies likely to call for defensive reactions by the listener.

The straightforward and candid communicator, however, is unlikely to spark resistance. In that this behavior is spontaneous and honest, the receiver can trust where the initiator is, so to speak; thus, communications are likely to be minimally defensive.

Neutrality vs. Empathy

Neutrality may be regarded as the ultimate in "scientific objectivity." However, this is a false belief. No one is without values and opinions, including, for example, the very choice of questions that reflects a scientist's values with regard to what is important, of interest, and worthy of study. Neutrality and detachment may have their place in the scientific laboratory and the field experiment. However, the workplace is neither a laboratory in an experimental sense nor a subject of scientific investigation on a daily basis. As a result, neutral, detached relations are likely to foster rejection and the feeling that the communicators do not care and are not interested in the others' well-being, resulting in defensive behavior.

In contrast is empathic behavior that connotes understanding and warmth. Concern for another comes through the communicator's facial expressions, tone of voice, and posture, in addition to verbal remarks indicating understanding and acceptance of another's feelings.

Superiority vs. Equality

The superior, condescending attitude of the boss, in particular, will lead quickly to defensive responses. Any message implying that a person possesses superior knowledge, prestige, wealth, or personal characteristics will result in another's feeling inadequate or angry that the initiator is attempting to produce a feeling of inadequacy. The "superior" stays aloof, does not engage in joint participation in task accomplishment or decision making, and does not desire feedback.

However, the person who attempts to communicate on the basis of equality is likely to be perceived as a peer or colleague, even when real status differentials exist. The director who values the ideas of the staff and encourages feedback fosters such equality even though that individual is, administratively, more powerful and may possess greater expertise in particular areas. Equality never is absolute. No two persons are identical in all, or nearly all, respects. An attitude of equality, however, carries with it mutual respect and value. It suggests that one individual is not a "better person" than another merely because of greater wealth, position, knowledge, or prestige.

Certainty vs. Provisionalism

Certainty and self-confidence often are regarded as similar. Certainty has a tendency to become dogmatism, and nothing breeds defensiveness as quickly as dogmatic statements. The individual determined to win an argument instead of solving a problem antagonizes coworkers and subordinates as well as superiors. Certainty is associated with inflexibility and a need to control others' behavior.

A more open attitude, associated with provisionalism, suggests that no ideas and opinions are cast in concrete and that everything is open to question, to investigation. People who do not resent suggestions as they solve problems will not promote defensive reactions in those around them.

While no one is supportive 100 percent of the time, individuals can strive to eliminate defense-arousing behaviors from their communications repertoire. If an atmosphere of openness and trust is the norm, an occasional defense-arousing communication may even be ignored; at least its deleterious effect will be mitigated. For an administrator, manager, or supervisor whose survival depends on the ability to communicate clearly, a reduction in defensive climates is a must. (Techniques for handling these and similar problems are discussed in Chapters 9 and 10.)

PASSIVE-AGGRESSIVE AND AGGRESSIVE

Passive-aggressive and aggressive personalities are all too common sources of interpersonal stress in organizations. Both share a serious difficulty in the direct expression of feeling—anger, in particular. However, each expresses itself in a manner quite different from the other and leaves in its wake "victims" with very different battle scars. The passive-aggressive person communicates in an indirect manner, refusing to take responsibility for feelings and needs or for the effect that individual's behavior has on others. Self-denial, emotional dishonesty, and inhibition characterize this person. The individual is likely to feel picked on, hurt, and anxious, with a well of undefined anger lurking below the surface. Those interacting with this individual are likely to feel superior themselves and direct their pity and irritation at the passive-aggressive person.

However, the passive, nondirect person is by no means powerless. This type's indirect aggression may take the form of chronic lateness, procrastination, withholding, following the letter of the law, and failing to implement policy. Such aggression also may be seen in manipulation, sarcasm, pouting, chronic "forgetting," and continuously failing to understand directives. These behaviors may be exhibited by both men and women and are subtly reinforced at the interpersonal and organizational levels.

At the interpersonal level, the passive-aggressive individual "wins" when the recipient of the behavior loses emotional cool, getting into a tug of war and accusations with this person, who calmly denies any malevolent intent or who decides to withdraw from dialogue altogether. Directed communications techniques (discussed in Chapter 10) provide a useful mechanism for the effective handling of such individuals. Such behavior also may be reinforced by an organization that places its employees in passive-dependent roles, does not reward or even tolerate the direct, constructive expression of anger, and leaves no alternative to passive-aggressive responses.

The aggressive individual, on the other hand, is expressively honest and seemingly direct in communication. Upon a closer look, however, this person is found to be self-enhancing at the expense of the other individual in the interaction. Such expressivity therefore is properly labelled "inappropriate." The aggressive person feels self-righteous, superior, and condescending toward the other who, in turn, may feel humiliated, hurt, and not respected. The other is likely to be angry and vengeful toward the aggressor. If the recipient is in a subordinate position, the stage is set for passive-aggressive, sabotage responses with negative consequences both for the participants and the organization.

Harry Levinson (1978) accurately describes the characteristics of an all-too-common aggressive figure in the organization—the abrasive personality. This is the individual who may have reached a high-level position based on pointed and incisive comments and an ability to perform well at difficult tasks. However, the person's interpersonal style has the unfortunate effect of numbing the ideas of others. Tactless at meetings and extremely willful and persuasive, this type goes out of the way to disagreeably challenge others' positions, making them reluctant to express their views. Unfortunately for the organization, these others very often are the ones responsible for carrying out this aggressor's excellent ideas. Under these interpersonal conditions, they are unlikely to follow through effectively. Sabotage through passive-aggressive means becomes a way of getting revenge. Subordinates live in great fear, feeling standards are impossible to reach, disbelieving when a compliment does come along, notably because it is lost between words describing what is missing. At the root of the problem is such a person's need for perfection and subsequent need for control, alienating everyone else, and creating a significant amount of stress for them.

STRESS AT THE ORGANIZATIONAL LEVEL

Many stressors at the level of the organization have far-reaching effects. Senior level administration often is unaware that they exist or that they cause a problem for management. Among the most noticeable of these are the following: lack of clear managerial priorities concerning work objectives; poorly defined mission statement; unresolved conflict between units, departments, and professionals; unresolved situations within units and departments; excessive time pressures for meeting work deadlines; rigid hierarchy; ineffective communications patterns; leadership styles that impede growth and creativity; discrepancies between authority and responsibility; and rampant, unmanaged change.

Organizational stress also can be identified through inferential means by a variety of symptoms such as high absenteeism, high turnover, low morale, high degree of rigidity, uncontrolled change, crisis management, and, of course, low productivity and unionization attempts where there is no union, or union problems where one exists. Unions or union problems and good management essentially are incompatible. There is no need for a union when employees at all levels of the organization are and perceive themselves to be part of a team.

Labor-management problems that often are manifested in union difficulties have become an important source of stress for health care administrators, as will be seen in Chapter 4. It is useful to explore this issue in the context of five major areas of development and concern that have implications for the health care industry as a whole: quality of work life, the role of unions, management development, the nature of internal competition, and interhospital arrangements. All of these can be regarded as sources of stress in the environment of every health care organization.

The health care sector has experienced tremendous growth during the last two decades. Its present position can be regarded as moving to maturation. Much new growth will occur from the utilization of human resources within the system, as well as from new drugs and more advanced technologies. Other industries that have experienced similar patterns demonstrate that once they have reached a growth plateau, a substantial shakeout of the weaker competitors results. As a result, the competition among the remaining organizations becomes more intense. In health care, one element of the competition is, and will continue to be, in the quality of the service provided to patients. Patient satisfaction assessment becomes one means of determining to what extent the organization is competing well and satisfying the needs of its one group of consumers.

Patient satisfaction primarily involves whether these people like the food, the hospital is clean, the staff is friendly and fair, and they feel comfortable with the technical care provided. Many patients do not perceive themselves in a position to judge the quality of the technical care. They base their assessments on rapport and comfort with staff. Whether staff members, in turn, are perceived as friendly depends in large part on how the employees are themselves treated by the organization—whether they feel they are treated fairly and identify with the institution. What is most crucial in this competitive environment because of the intimate type of service the hospital provides (beyond technology) is the nature of the interpersonal relationship between employees and patients. The question becomes: How can administration optimize the relationship between the employees and the hospital, from janitor to housekeeping to billing to direct care?

Quality of Work Life

This sets the stage for discussion of quality of work life. It is generally believed that the values of workers in this country have shifted. Discrepancies between what organizations value and what employees within them value are sources of stress. However, it is not that this generation's parents and grandparents did not value fairness, job security, good working conditions, and so on. The differences lie essentially in the fact that for the most part, they had no choices. Workers today generally have choices and voices and they are demanding "quality of work life."

Several factors account for this change. People are less likely to be centering their lives on their jobs. They are aware that they can focus more or less energy on the job. If the former, the job should fit their personal needs for challenge, participation, growth, security, or socialization, whichever they may be. Managers may experience such demands initially as stressors. To the extent that participative management can be perceived as a quality of work life intervention, there will need to be increased attention to the appropriate use of involving employees in decisions that most immediately affect their jobs.

Obviously, this has significant implications for training of supervisory and managerial staff. This is not the way most managers in health care facilities learned; it is not the way most of them were managed. Nor is participative management a panacea for whatever ails the department or organization. It requires training the management force and the employees because it essentially entails job expansion. Other examples of quality of work life include team-building efforts, career development, and quality control circles. (These are discussed in Chapter 9.)

The Role of Unions

In other industries that have reached maturity and have seen their less viable organizations disappear, the shake-out has been found to increase the likelihood that the labor force will move toward unionization as a way of dealing with perceived job insecurity. This insecurity is exacerbated by pressure for cost containment that often has the effect of eliminating jobs. It also is aggravated by the reality of the demise of the less viable institutions. Competition for each work slot increases, further menacing job insecurity and producing a tendency to drive down compensation. Obviously these factors can be serious sources of stress for employees.

In the health care field, unionization events have followed trends in other industries. Increasingly, professionals have been turning to unions as a last-ditch attempt to redress grievances against what they perceive to be unresponsive management (Abrams & Numerof, 1982). Where compensation is perceived as equitable for the particular geographic region and the job, the most typical reasons for unionization include the absence of and desire for professional autonomy, participation in management decisions, access to management, and good supervision.

Unions are antithetical to good management and potentially create a barrier between employees and the hospital and the delivery of care to patients. In addition to reducing flexibility and increasing operating expenses, they tend to increase polarization of the groups involved. The author's discussions with labor lawyers and personnel administrators across the country suggest that organizing efforts are becoming increasingly more militant, in part because unions are becoming more aggressive in their efforts. Whether or not they succeed will depend largely on the efforts of administration in the area of management development.

Another stressor affecting the attractiveness of unions is in the fact that, for the most part, health care organizations have lagged behind the industrial sector in the application of behavioral science technology to the human resource problems they face.

Management Development

Increasingly, health care institutions are recognizing that they no longer can avoid providing adequate management training for their supervisory and managerial personnel. Two problems inherent in health care further mandate the incorporation of management development: (1) a considerable amount of internal promotion and (2) the advancement of clinically/technically competent personnel into management positions without adequate training and support for those jobs.

Unfortunately, where efforts have been made, they frequently have fallen into the "garbage pail technique" of management development. This entails a hit-or-miss approach—for example, subjects for seminars are chosen at random, often with considerable political influence, and without regard to an overall, integrated management development system.

The result sees programs looking for problems to which they can be a solution without any attention to organizational diagnosis and assessment.

Organizations finally have been turning to strategic planning. This includes clinical program areas, financial concerns, and building needs. It is ironic and rather telling that human resource development planning is not included, particularly in service-intensive industries such as health care. Failure to provide adequate development is a source of stress for management at all levels of the organization. For highly trained managers there is the chronic frustration of working with peers who are not as competent managerially. For these managers and their staffs, there is the frustration of not knowing what really is supposed to be done for the former and the frustration of inconsistency and poor supervision for the latter.

Even where management development programs are thoughtfully planned and integrated, serious problems occur in failure to implement them. Such failures often are attributed to the trainer/facilitators, to the content of the program, or to the general intransigence of the participants. While the former may, indeed, be problems in some programs, responsibility for failure to implement invariably rests with the organization and not the program. For example, programs have been shown to teach new management ideas and skills to participants who then never changed their behavior to reflect this learning.

The root of the problem is the fact that in the daily stresses of managing, those good ideas and good intentions get shelved for the day "when I have some time." Of course, as might be expected, that day just never seems to arrive. Since these managers are not expected to change—that is, no one is holding them accountable for implementing these ideas—there is little incentive to change other than their own investment in their jobs and their careers. What happens is that those who would have changed without the training do and those who needed to change do not. Hence, the status quo remains. Such organizations implement management development programs one after another with no appreciable effect.

Another reason for this failure to implement reflects a reward structure that reinforces the old ways of doing things. Thus, the organization says through management development efforts that it values managerial autonomy and input from the middle and supervisory levels. In actuality, suggestions are not recognized or followed through, feedback is not given, controls are reinforced. This is an example of pernicious incongruence, a very serious source of stress for managers in particular.

It is only when administration has developed a philosophy that says it will do more than pay lip service to good management practice and organizational development that this situation will change. Such organizations hold executives accountable not only for productivity (however that is measured) but also for managing the climate of the department or unit. These organizations also provide the structure and support necessary for managers to accomplish both.

Internal Competition

Another source of stress within the organization is internal competition, especially between professional groups over professional turf. The most dramatic conflicts will continue to be between nurses and doctors and, if unresolved, create stress throughout the hospital. These conflicts translate to the delivery of programs in the institution: for example, whether money is spent for ambulatory care or inpatient medical care, whether the emphasis is on preventive medicine and health care or on the cure of disease.

The nature of this competition puts further pressure on managers to deal effectively with interpersonal conflict and necessitates the continuing training just described. Ideally, the goal in this effort is the reduction of unit suboptimization and the encouragement of competition in the context of cooperation—building effective teams that identify with the organization and not exclusively with individual units or professional groups. (In suboptimization, subgroups put their own needs ahead of those of the institution.)

Interhospital Arrangements

Interhospital arrangements have been evolving because of the trend, noted earlier, toward the maturation of the health care industry and the fall-out of the less viable institutions. One response to such a trend is for each institution to become protective and narrow in its orientation. However, it is important not to become myopic but to look to other institutions to develop ways in which to work together for mutual advantage.

There are many ways in which institutions can share services to the betterment of all while still maintaining their own identities. For instance, hospitals have developed extensive laboratory arrangements, shared radiology specialty services, bought laundry and dietary companies, shared computerized axial tomography (CAT) scan equipment, and, perhaps most innovative, have established management development consortiums. The key to the success of these ventures is that all parties see themselves as gaining. Such effort requires an ability to move beyond "keeping up with the Joneses," an orientation in which every institution perceives itself as having to have "all services"—a totally unrealistic and stress-producing way in which to operate, particularly in an environment of limited resources.

With the top of the organization as a starting point, a picture quickly emerges as to how unresolved issues there have a cascade effect throughout. If the mission statement has not been clearly defined by the board, the chief executive officer operates without clear mandates (Numerof, 1982). For example, the executive may take control and proceed in one direction, perhaps in the direction of ambulatory services, only to meet with mixed blessings (or rejection) from the board. If factions exist on the board, a not uncommon situation, the CEO may be given the green light, only to find the rug pulled out later. Persons reporting to the CEO may describe their boss as wishy-washy, unclear about direction, unsupportive, and highly changeable. Under these conditions, commitment to any new venture is likely to be modest at best, since no one is certain when the brakes will be applied and energy expended for a new effort in a totally different direction. Morale weakens, infighting spreads, good people leave.

When responsibility is not clearly delegated by the board to the CEO in an agreed-upon mission statement, the organization is headed for serious trouble. The CEO is unable to clearly delegate responsibility to administrative staff, administrative staff is unable to clearly delegate responsibility to department heads, and they, in turn, to supervisory and first-line staff. The result is a sense described by numerous individuals at all levels of organizations where this occurs:

"No one seems to know where we're headed. A new idea comes along, people get excited, argue the merits of the case upward, then it seems to go nowhere. It's an example of physics principles' not working, that is, whatever goes up must come down. We operate by crisis, not by planning."

A similar problem, a case of risk-taking fear hidden in a cloak of vague mission, is described:

"The administration here is so afraid to try anything new. We wanted to move to expanded ambulatory care years before everyone else did. What happened? As usual, nothing. It wasn't supported; it wasn't killed. Now the same thing is happening with the wellness and employee assistance programs."

More important than risk-taking in facilitating organizational stress, particularly among managers, is the role of uncertainty. When many factors are unknown, policymaking becomes an anxiety-arousing experience. With high levels of anxiety, poor judgment is the likely result. Of course, a certain amount of uncertainty is healthy and stimulating. With rapid change, technological advancement, increased legal liability, government regulation, and so on, too much uncertainty can lead to disaster.

KEY SOURCES OF PROBLEMS

Beyond uncertainty and the stressors in the environment discussed earlier, there are numerous key sources of problems for managers, three of which merit exploration here: an unsuitable role, personality conflict, and the position of middle management itself.

The Unsuitable Role

The problem of unsuitable role is particularly common in health care organizations although it finds common ground in industrial experience where a research scientist who has been "on the bench" for ten years is promoted to management because administration feels the individual "should want to get ahead." In health care, clinicians and technically trained personnel are caught in an essentially flat or horizontal hierarchy. All too often, they find that if they are interested in advancement, they must leave their chosen fields because of the way in which rewards are structured in the organization. Clinical nurses, for example, may find that advancement opportunities reside outside the clinical area, such as in management.

Such alternatives—either advancement through management or non-advancement—produce very negative consequences for both the individual and the organization. The individual who is promoted may be in a role with inadequate preparation and perhaps does not like the post. The organization has lost a competent clinician and gained a marginally competent manager who is in the position not because of an inherent desire to manage but as a means (perhaps the only route) for personal advancement.

The solution to such problems is fairly straightforward, however, and already has been implemented in some departments in hospitals around the country. Nursing administrations have established a two-track system for advancement. One track recognizes clinical levels of expertise and the other offers promotion opportunities through the traditional management route. The clinical route often combines career development whereby nurses trained and experienced in one area but interested in developing expertise in another clinical area have the opportunity to do so.

Personality Conflicts

Personality conflict as a source of managerial stress pertains here to the discrepancy between the individual in a particular position, the person's values and goals, and the demands of the organization. Institutions often manage this problem by trying to reshape employee behavior. However, there is a limit to how much the individual can adapt. Ultimately, force-fitting an employee into a job slot is not worth the emotional cost or stress-related physical problems to which a wrong fit can subject the person. Sometimes leaving a job that is secure but untenable is less stressful than moving to a new situation in the same institution. In short, it is a lot easier to change the job than to change people to fit the job description. The challenge for the organization is twofold: How does it design jobs and how does it hire people for them?

Middle Management

In some respects everyone is a middle manager in that they all are held accountable to someone else in the final analysis, whether that be a board of directors, patients, consumer groups, or an immediate superior on the organizational chart. For the middle manager in the health care organization, life is likely to be particularly stressful for a number of reasons:

- The middle manager has considerable responsibility for worker productivity and morale.
- The middle manager is held accountable for both the quality and quantity of the work produced.
- The middle manager rarely has the authority and decision-making power to make changes in the department necessary to achieve the goals associated with the first two points.

In some sense, the problem of the middle manager is potentially the problem of everyone in an organization in which this discrepancy occurs. Lack of discretion in meeting the demands of the job and in the job itself are two of the most important elements in work strain and result in a whole array of symptoms. High job demands and low decision latitude are likely to be associated with exhaustion after work, trouble waking in the morning, depression, general anxiety and tension, and insomnia. The secondary effect of these symptoms is poor performance on the job, which exacerbates the symptoms and sets in motion a negative spiral effect.

Quantity, Quality, Ambiguity, Rigidity

Some additional general factors create stress on the job. Too much or too little to do from a quantitative or qualitative (skills and knowledge) standpoint is highly stressful, as is extreme ambiguity or rigidity relative to a person's task. Such ambiguity or rigidity may entail not having enough information to do a job because communication has not been clear, or delegation has not been clear or complete, or the information has been consciously withheld by a superior who undermines subordinates and controls through access to information in a destructive fashion. Ambiguity or rigidity also may result from a lack of information concerning the job function (i.e., lack of clarity regarding how an individual fits into the organization) or specific role definition (i.e., what does this job entail) (Katz & Kahn, 1966). Finally, ambiguity and rigidity may be the result of not getting regular feedback regarding how well the job was accomplished.

Katz and Kahn (1966) identify serious role conflict as a source of stress for managers in particular and workers in general, a topic that has been picked up by numerous other researchers (Abdel-Halim, 1981; Beehr, 1976; Caplan and Jones, 1975). Conflict such as the clinical/administrative dilemma (Levinson, 1976; Numerof, 1982) mentioned previously (and discussed in Chapter 4) is common in health care organizations. The problem is aggravated for women, whose access to management positions, while less blocked than in the industrial sector, still is limited. In addition, the much-discussed problem of women's traditional socialization experiences (i.e., passive–dependent) in conflict with the demands of management (i.e., assertive) presents them with a significant amount of stress, both for those aspiring to such positions and for those already holding them (Kanter, 1977; Numerof, 1978a).

Heavy responsibility for people's lives (explored in later chapters) is a stressor inherent in the health services delivery field. Where there is an uncomplementary mix of career factors such as professional development, opportunity, and the management style of a superior (e.g., a manager with the ''abrasive personality'' who causes employee stress and job dissatisfaction), high turnover and absenteeism, low morale, and low productivity are likely consequences.

The Suboptimization Phenomenon

Finally, negative or no competition (i.e., stagnation) are sources of organizationally based stress. The former is seen most typically in unit suboptimization, a phenomenon in which units, departments, or other subgroups within the organization perceive their needs as all-important and act without regard for their interdependence with other groups and the organization as a whole. This type of situation is manifested where there is low commitment to the organization but high loyalty to the work unit or department. It also is seen in strong professional identification, such as to laboratory research, nursing, or medicine, or to some type of the last two. It involves little or no identification with corporate goals.

Administration often colludes with this phenomenon. For example, it may orient personnel in an atomistic manner, involving unrelated elements. Little, if any, time is spent orienting people as to how their particular unit connects with others or what the impact of an employee's job and department is. Communication between departments often is discouraged. Organizational objectives may not be communicated. Worse yet, these objectives may not be defined or may change often, increasing uncertainty and stress in the environment.

Unit suboptimization becomes most serious in the case of the unteam. In group dynamics terms, this refers to "when is a group not a group." It occurs when the group consists of atomized players, each with a specific role. Each player has obtained that position by a different route and has made no commitment to other group members or to the organization itself. This situation often rears its ugly head in departments of medicine (see Chapter 5).

STRESS AT THE PERSONAL LEVEL

Personal sources of stress are probably the most common of all. Among these are the "shoulds," "oughts," and "musts" that people impose on themselves daily in one form or other. Self-imposed demands and performance expectations that are impossible to attain set in motion a destructive cycle in which individuals feel as though they cannot meet the standards they set and thus experience a sense of inadequacy and frustration that raises anxiety and tension, thereby actually blocking performance. Unfortunately, many people fall into such cycles without realizing that at the root lie their own personal and professional myths concerning expected performance. These myths have an irrational basis and include statements such as the following:

- Good doctors don't ever make mistakes.
- Good doctors should always appear sure of themselves.
- Good nurses should always be responsive to others' needs.

Another type of myth involves self-comments such as these:

- If I make a mistake, that shows I am inadequate.
- If I show my anger, that tells others that I'm losing control of myself.
- If I disagree with my boss and people in authority, then I'll lose my job.
- If I admit my weaknesses, then no one will respect me.
- If I don't live up to my potentials, then I'm a failure as a person.

Such personal and professional performance myths assume some non-existent standard of perfection as a reasonable goal. While it is important for individuals to set goals at a level above where they are currently performing, it is equally important that such objectives remain reasonable, realistic, and achievable. (Guidelines for recognizing and handling such irrational beliefs are provided in Chapter 10.)

The Impact of Type A Behavior

One of the most widely and popularly discussed personal stress patterns is that associated with Type A behavior and coronary heart disease. It is generally accepted that heart disease has been increasing over the years, particularly among women, whose rates are approaching those of men. This trend may reflect the fact that women are increasingly moving into positions similar to those held by men and responding to the stresses of those responsibilities in ways that predispose them to heart disease.

High blood pressure, poor nutrition, and cigarette smoking all are contributing factors to a progressive condition. Heart disease does not develop overnight. The heart pumps blood to the body. The more rest the heart gets, the less it has to work. With hypertension the heart constantly pumps faster, therefore receiving less rest. With people constantly under pressure, they are likely to have overworked hearts. When people are under stress, the blood also contains more fats, cholesterol, and sugar (Pelletier, 1977). If these substances are not used in a physiological response to stress, they can build up over time, contributing to arteriosclerosis.

Since no two people handle stress in exactly the same manner, who gets heart attacks and who does not?

Two cardiologists, Friedman and Rosenman (1974), are credited with being among the first researchers to suggest that a relationship exists between Type A behavior and heart disease. They do not say that stress leads to heart disease or that heart disease is a stress response. Rather, they state that Type A behavior as a style leads to a stress response that is associated with heart disease.

What do Type A characteristics include? Generally, such people are aggressive and extroverted. Kenneth Pelletier (1977) describes them as ambitious, impatient, and drive oriented, with strong personalities that tend to dominate conversations. They have a continual sense of time urgency and may be easily aroused to anger. Thus, they frequently leave a wave of stress behind them. Perhaps most importantly, these people invariably are reinforced for this behavior and held as models for others to emulate. The following are typical characteristics associated with Type A behavior:

- moving, eating, or walking hurriedly
- hurrying the ends of sentences
- feeling impatient with the rate at which most things happen
- evidencing "polyphasic" thought or performance (i.e., trying to think or do several things at once)
- feeling guilty about relaxing or doing "nothing"
- thinking constantly about business or work while on vacation
- scheduling more and more in less and less time
- having difficulty listening to others because of preoccupation with one's own thoughts
- spending so much time acquiring things that there is little time left to enjoy them
- believing that success is the result of the ability to get things done quickly, therefore being afraid to stop doing everything faster and faster.

Type A persons may be regarded as their own worst enemy in the sense that they are prone to setting unreasonable deadlines to accomplish given projects, whether the projects involve cleaning up the yard or finishing a report at work. What is accomplished invariably is measured in terms of numbers—how many patients seen in a given time period, how many lives saved. These numbers themselves frequently are translated into other numbers, such as those representing income, which are used as a standard by which worth as a person is judged.

Quality of life, self-reflection, and contemplation have little if any place in these individuals' lives. Nor do camaraderie and close friendships, partly because of the lack of time devoted to such pursuits, partly because the Type As' personality is likely to alienate others over time. Acquaintances realize these persons are self-directed and self-centered, interested in being on top and climbing over people to get there. Out of a deep-seated competitive drive, Type As will sacrifice the respect of peers and subordinates in order to win favor from superiors.

The Type B Pattern

While there is a great deal of variation in people's response styles in terms of the Type A pattern and its less competitive Type B counterpart, Friedman and Rosenman (1974) believe that everyone generally falls into one category or another to varying degrees. Contrary to popular opinion, Type A personalities are no more successful than Type Bs nor do they cluster in any specific occupations.

Type B personalities also are ambitious but their drives seem to give them confidence and security as opposed to those of Type As, which become relentless and undermining to self and others (Friedman & Rosenman, 1974). The Type B is free from the sense of continual time urgency, experiencing such pressures only under true emergencies. Leisure time can be enjoyed fully for what it is without guilt. Goals and a sense of self-worth are based on more than the achievement of numbers and the accumulation of wealth. Values are internal and clear, thus freeing the Type B from the need for continuous validation from others.

Ironically, Type Bs may be more successful on the job than their counterparts because of their decision-making styles. Type Bs will ponder various sides of a question, consider alternatives, and select a course of action that has a higher likelihood of success because of such deliberation. Type As, because of the need to make a decision quickly, may make poorer ones because they have not taken all of the relevant data into account. In addition to a more thoughtful, relaxed approach to life, Type Bs are less likely to be plagued with the hostility frequently associated with Type As. More thoughtful, patient, and creative, less hostile and abrasive, they are unlikely to be stressors in the organization's social environment.

It should be noted that Type A behavior, while associated with and a contributing factor to coronary heart disease (CHD), is not the only one involved with it. In a longitudinal study of more than 250 men, Rosenman et al. (1975) also report personal history, diabetes, smoking, blood pressure, and serum-cholesterol levels significantly associated with incidence of CHD.

Other Stress-Related Ailments

Numerous other illnesses and physiological disorders have been reported in the literature as stress-related disorders: ulcers, colitis, diarrhea, constipation, allergies, arthritis, headaches, backaches, and diabetes. To the extent that stress lowers resistance to the germs that live in and around people, stress makes individuals more susceptible to flu, colds, and virus.

One of the newer and more controversial areas of investigation concerns the relationship among personality, behavioral style, and cancer. Because of the relationship between emotional/psychological factors and physiology, it is believed that those factors influence neurophysiological functioning and depress the vital immune system, thus increasing susceptibility to viral infections in which mutant cancer cells and tumors can grow unchecked (Pelletier, 1977). While this view seems widely accepted by researchers, it is unclear as to whether or not a "cancer personality" exists and, if so, to what extent it is related to the onset of cancer. Psychological testing points to a complex of traits significantly associated with the incidence of cancer. Such patients have difficulty expressing anger and conflict directly, have experienced the loss of a significant relationship within the year before the onset of the disease, and have problems expressing their needs—dependency in particular (Achterberg & Lawlis, 1978).

Childhood experiences of loneliness, anxiety, and rejection because of parental loss, separation, or chronic friction may be compensated for by trying to please others and win affection. Further frustration in such efforts is accompanied by loneliness, hopelessness, and self-hatred, all of which are suppressed and handled through a reaction formation. Cancer patients typically are described as martyrs, kind, "too good to be true" (LeShan & Worthington, 1956). Despite successful marriages and family life these people remain dependent on others for their happiness. Thus they are very responsive to the loss of loved ones through death, separation, loss, or leaving home. A study of 250 cancer patients reports they differ from a group of controls in the following ways:

- Cancer patients experienced a loss of an important relationship before the diagnosis was made.
- Cancer patients were unable to express anger on their own behalf.
- Cancer patients experienced feelings of unworthiness and low self-esteem.
- Cancer patients experienced tension in relation to one or both parents (LeShan & Worthington, 1956).

Other studies suggest that childhood trauma resulting from loss or chronic friction among parents (Kissen, 1967; Voth, 1975 cited in Pelletier, 1977, p. 140) and significant interpersonal problems associated with work (Kissen, 1967) are significantly related to the onset and course of cancer. Obviously, not all people with a history of loss in childhood develop cancer. The important question revolves around what differentiates those who do develop the disease from those who do not. Various studies link cancer patients' inability to express emotions effectively as the significant factor. As with the life events studies, it is not so much what occurs to a particular person but how the individual handles the event that may be the telling factor.

Personality factors are to a large extent determinative of an individual's reaction. The reaction may be healthy or pathogenic; the reaction tendencies seem to form patterns with long-standing histories. Once formed, the patterns tend to persist but are reversible with psychotherapy and life style change. Prospective studies, while few in number, already have shown some promising results, particularly the Johns Hopkins one (Thomas & Duszynski, 1974), which finds distinctive personality patterns differentiating medical students who become ill from those who do not, and a study by Vaillant, Sobowale, and McArthur (1972) with similar findings. As Pelletier (1977) notes, such evidence should not be taken as a sign of despair but rather of hope. Personality factors can be changed. If identified early enough, preventive action can be taken so that degenerative disease does not emerge.

In another vein, once developed, the progress of the disease can be halted when psychological factors are treated in the course of a biochemical approach to cancer. As has been shown, emotional state can have a remarkable effect on the course of malignancy (Achterberg & Lawlis, 1978; Simonton & Simonton, 1975). Another study (Achterberg, Lawlis, Simonton, & Simonton, 1977) shows that psychological measures are better predictors of disease progress than are blood chemistries.

With more precision in professionals' understanding of the role of emotional and psychological factors in illness, it is likely that in the not-too-distant future they will have a better handle on how to help people recover from malignancies and other diseases.

Part II

The Case of the Health Care Professional

The health care field is a highly stressful environment, in part because it is a people-intensive industry whose business often is the business of life and death. Research has shown that those closest to the sources of help for handling stress often are least able to deal with it effectively (McLean, 1978). Such a statement is quite an indictment.

To a large extent this problem exists because of professional socialization norms that reinforce the "I-can-cope" model of behavior. At the base of this model is the irrational belief that "I can cope with everything," implying no limits. The model also is associated with the equally erroneous belief that asking for help signifies inadequacy.

As a result of these and related behavioral styles, health care delivery personnel are particularly vulnerable to the incipient effects of excessive stress. Chapter 4 explores research studies and case examples indicating some of the special hazards of health care environments and the vulnerabilities of certain professionals. Chapter 5 examines the stressful experience of physicians while Chapters 6 and 7 look at the stress experiences of nurses and senior administrative personnel, respectively.

Chapter 4

Stress in the Health Care Environment

While a substantial portion of the literature on organizational stress derives from the industrial sector, increasing attention has been paid to this problem in the health care sector. A study by the National Institute for Occupational Safety and Health (NIOSH) reports that among the top 30 occupations ranked in terms of incidence of mental health disorder, six are in the health delivery field: health technologists, laboratory technicians, nursing aides, health aides, registered nurses, and dental assistants.

U.S. Department of Labor statistics show that the incidence of work-related injury and illness among hospital employees is 58 percent higher than among those in other service industries (*Handbook of Labor Statistics*, 1976; Siskind, 1982). Given the relationship between stress and illness and injury, high stress levels could well be expected to account for a substantial portion of the reported differences.

AN ENVIRONMENT RIPE FOR STRESS

It should not be surprising that stress in health occupations is high. Hospitals, the arena in which most medical care is delivered, are complex, heterogeneous organizations characterized by multiple levels of authority superimposed on professional personnel who generally receive their training in professional schools and pay allegiance to professional associations. Often such an atmosphere sets the stage for various forms of internal conflict that, as Katz and Kahn (1966) identified some years ago, becomes a potential source of stress and can foster institutional-professional goal conflict (Numerof, 1982).

All of the sources of stress described in Chapter 3 are prevalent in health care organizations. Among the most serious are work overload (often from understaffing); job insecurity; mismatches between the job and the employee;

75

discrepancies between what is expected and what authority is granted; serving an anxious, ill population; unresolved interpersonal conflict; inadequate resources; rapid technological change; and unfulfilled ambition. Obviously, these difficulties are by no means unique to health care. What makes their impact more serious is that these employees are responsible for people's lives. The health care field, as a whole, has lagged behind in the effective utilization of behavioral science technology and management practices, their absence adding to high levels of work-related stress.

Regardless of the level at which stress is studied, a useful approach to understanding it is through a dynamic model. Such a model (Figure 4-1) identifies four major components in the stress response: antecedents (stressors or sources of stress), moderator variables, perception of stress and consequences.

Antecedents are located in two major places: within the organization (intraorganizational) and outside it (extraorganizational). Intraorganizational stressors are further divided into three levels according to their source: individual, group, and organizational.

Moderator variables, which actually determine whether or not a given stressor will be perceived as stressful by an individual, include demographic as well as cognitive/affective variables. As noted in the diagram, demographic variables exert an effect on cognitive/affective variables, and vice versa. Both historical and current data are included under moderator variables.

Perception of stress is broken down into three components—job, career, and life—to differentiate where an individual may be experiencing problems. For example, a person may have a perception of being on schedule with regard to career ambitions but experience excessive job-related stress specific to the current position. Conversely, an individual may enjoy a job that is perceived as relatively stress-free yet feel disquieted since it is either not supportive of longer range career needs or is off target with regard to career plans. Finally, life stress—as seen in dissatisfaction with what has been accomplished to date as compared to what a person wants to do in a lifetime, as well as lack of comfort with the individual's identity, purpose, and values—has more global implications. As Exhibit 4-1 indicates, each of these three components may affect the others and may be perceived by the individual and/or significant others.

Consequences are presented in two major categories: physiological/psychological and behavioral. Both positive and negative consequences are included in each; an interaction is indicated between them, as well. What consequence occurs will be determined primarily by the moderator variables, which also include how a person copes with a stressor once it is perceived. (Coping strategies are reflected in personality variables, use

Figure 4-1 Dynamic Model of Stress and its Consequences

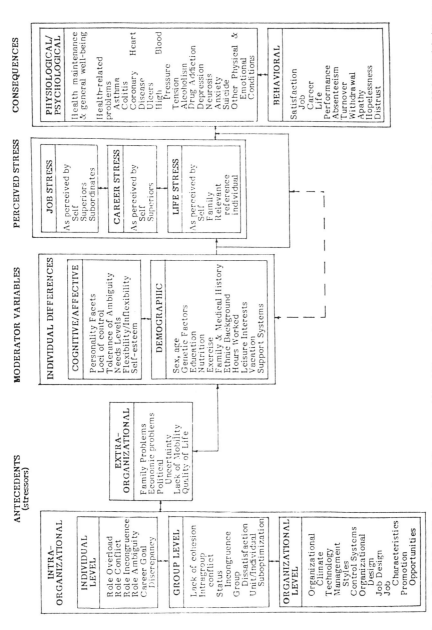

Source: Adapted from "Organizational Stressors and Heart Disease: A Research Model" by Michael T. Matteson and John M. Ivancevich, by permission of *Academy of Management Review*, 4(3), 347–357, © 1979.

of support systems, leisure, etc.) Hence, the exhibit indicates an effect by moderator variables between perceived stress and consequences. Finally, an interaction exists between moderator variables and perceived stress (as discussed in Chapter 2).

The complexity of such a model better represents the stress phenomenon than does one that suggests that stress events in and of themselves are likely to result in negative consequences. Yet a serious problem with the model and with the study of stress itself is its complexity. How does the practitioner begin to study and make sense of so many variables at once? Obviously, the answer is the incremental view, taking parts of the model and making sense out of them, then proceeding to other parts.

HASS: HEALTH ADMINISTRATORS STRESS STUDY

In an attempt to add specificity and clarity to the exploration of stress in the health care environment, the author and two colleagues in 1981 and 1982 conducted a nationwide study of stressors and coping strategies among three key management groups in health services delivery: senior level administration, medical directors, and directors of nursing in hospitals (Numerof, Shachar, and Cramer, 1983). The intent of the study was straightforward:

- to identify situations (and their magnitude) that these managers perceived as stressful regardless of whether they were positive or negative
- to identify coping strategies used by the managers in responding to stress situations
- to identify the occurrence of personal stress symptomatology
- to identify patterns of vulnerability to stress among respondents

The rest of this chapter examines the study methodology, findings, and implications for the management of stress among senior level hospital managers.

In addition to the broad points just listed, the purposes of the study were to delineate the impact of the identified stressors on mental, physical, and emotional functioning as well as on interpersonal behavior; to investigate the relationship of selected demographic, organizational (e.g., size and type of hospital), and professional (e.g., length of service, type of training) variables on perceived stress; and to analyze the relationship among stress vulnerability, sources of stress, demographic variables, and coping strategies. (Exhibit 4-1 lists the research questions that were asked.)

Exhibit 4-1 Questions Asked in the HASS Research Study

---

1. What are the sources and magnitude of stress for administrators in health care?

Hypotheses

  a. Position will be significantly related to sources of stress.
  b. Nursing administrators will report the greatest magnitude of stress, followed by chief executive officers and medical directors/chiefs of staff.

2. What is the relationship between the magnitude of stress and stress outcomes?

Hypotheses

  a. The greater the frequency and intensity of the stressors, the greater the negative stress outcomes.
  b. The greater the perceived level of stress, the greater the negative stress outcomes.

3. What is the nature of negative stress outcomes for administrators in health care?

Hypothesis

  a. Negative stress outcomes will differ by position.

4. Do stress outcomes, sources, and magnitude of stress differ as a function of demographic, organizational, and professional variables?

Hypotheses

  a. The greater the number of years in administration, the fewer the negative stress outcomes.
  b. The greater the number of years in the present position, the fewer the negative stress outcomes.
  c. The greater the number of years employed at the facility, the fewer the negative stress outcomes.
  d. Age is inversely related to perceived degree of stress.
  e. The greater the number of hours worked on a typical day, the greater the likelihood of negative stress outcomes.
  f. The fewer the number of days spent on vacation, the greater the likelihood of negative stress outcomes.
  g. Women will perceive themselves to be more stressed than men.

5. What are the types of coping strategies used by administrators in health care?

Hypothesis

  a. Position will be significantly related to type of coping strategy used.

6. What is the relationship between the frequency of use and degree of helpfulness of coping strategies and stress outcomes?

Hypothesis

  a. The greater the frequency of use and degree of helpfulness, the lesser the negative stress outcomes.

Exhibit 4-1 continued

---

7. What is the relationship between frequently used, helpful coping strategies and demographic, organizational, and professional variables?

   No hypotheses generated.

8. What is the relationship between stress vulnerability, sources and magnitude of stress, demographic variables, stress outcomes, and coping strategies?

Hypotheses

   a. Vulnerability will be directly related to the magnitude (i.e., frequency and intensity) of stressors.
   b. Vulnerability will be directly related to perceived degree of stress.
   c. Vulnerability will be directly related to negative stress outcomes.
   d. Males will have significantly higher vulnerability than females.

Source: Reprinted with permission from *The Health Administrator's Stress Study* by R.E. Numerof, K.D. Cramer, and S.A. Shachar Hendin. St. Louis: Washington University, The George Warren Brown School of Social Work, 1981–1982.

(For readers interested only in the highlights of the important findings, these are discussed in a summary at the end of the chapter.)

Before this project, no systematic study of this problem had been attempted on any large scale. In addition, no studies reported had compared these phenomena across those three key health care management groups.

The senior investigator designed a structured interview protocol to be administered by telephone with administrators in the three regions of the United States where the final study would take place. The three investigators contacted hospitals in each region requesting the voluntary participation of an administrator, medical director, and nursing director. Institutions in this phase of the project were chosen so that in each region a university, community (nonreligious), and religious-affiliated hospital would be represented.

Willingness to participate in Phase I of the study was overwhelming. Interviews were arranged to last 30 to 35 minutes but often ran for an hour as participants generally talked about stress and coping strategies considerably longer. Many respondents expressed their appreciation of the timeliness of the study and took advantage of the opportunity to talk with a professional who was a stranger. They shared intimate details and concerns about organizational stressors as a means of reducing their negative impact.

In all, 27 interviews were completed in the initial phase. The data were analyzed for content, then worked into a questionnaire. This was field tested, reexamined for content validity, and administered to a national sample of 570 subjects in 190 facilities affiliated with the American Hospital Association. The sample was composed of three regions: East Coast, Midwest, and California. The overall response rate was 40 percent (228), with 25 percent (143) of the total sample being usable.

The 89 stress-producing situations most commonly cited in the telephone surveys and the 104 most commonly mentioned coping strategies formed the major components of the survey. The questionnaire, which appears as Appendix A at the end of the book, consisted of five major sections: demographic and professional data, stress situations, coping strategies, detailed examination of specific highly stressful situations and relevant coping strategies, and the personal stress symptom assessment. The Individual Profile of Stressors (IPS) described in Chapter 2 was included as a measure of vulnerability. Respondents were asked to identify the frequency of occurrence and degree of stressfulness associated with each situation. A similar procedure was used for coping strategies, with respondents asked to identify the degree of helpfulness and frequency of use of each strategy.

THE SAMPLE

The sample consisted of 143 respondents. Of these, 34 percent (N = 48) were from the East Coast, 51 percent (N = 72) from the Midwest, and 15 percent (N = 21) from California; two were unidentified. The sample was predominantly female (57 percent) with a small percentage not identifying their sex (4 percent). The average age of the respondents was 45.3 years. A majority were married (63 percent); 22 percent were single, 9 percent divorced or separated, 4 percent widowed, and 1 percent in religious orders. Average number of children for the sample was 3.3.

Professionally, the respondents represented an interesting mix. Those with M.A. degrees accounted for 20.2 percent of the group; M.S.N., 19.2 percent; M.D., 18.2 percent; a mixed category including Ph.D., M.B.A., Ed.D., and M.S.W., 18 percent; and B.S.N., R.N., and M.A., 8 percent each. In terms of experience, the group averaged 12.3 years in administration, 7.0 years in the present position, 10.35 years with the current facility. The positions respondents held were: chief executive officer (12 percent); associate administrator (15 percent); director of nursing (44 percent); president, medical staff (4 percent); medical director (12 percent); other (13 percent). That last category included directors of education, and social services.

With regard to hospital type, university hospitals accounted for 11 percent of the sample; voluntary, religious-affiliated hospitals, 21 percent; voluntary, community, nonreligious hospitals, 45 percent; proprietary institutions, 8 percent; government hospitals, 9 percent; and "other," including HMOs and specialty clinics with beds, 6 percent. The average number of beds in the respondent's facility was 490.6.

Respondents also were asked to identify how many hours they worked in a typical day and how many vacation days they took during the year. The average number of hours worked per day was 11.1, the average number of vacation days per year, 15.7. Finally, respondents were asked to rate the degree of stress they generally experienced on a scale of 1 to 5, with 1 being almost no stress at all and 5 being high stress. The average global stress score was 3.359. This is referred to later as the perceived level of stress score.

STRESS SITUATIONS

Scores were derived for each of 89 stress situations by multiplying the frequency of occurrence by the degree of stress associated with each stressor event. (More accurate assessments of a particular event can be derived when stress is seen as a function of both frequency of occurrence and the degree of stress associated with it.) Means were derived for the computed scores and the situations were rank-ordered in terms of the amount of stress associated with each. Table 4-1 presents the rank-ordered situations with their means. The situations are grouped into high, high-moderate, low-moderate, and low stress using $+/-$ one standard deviation above and below the overall stress situation mean as the boundaries ($\sigma = 2.08$; $\overline{X} = 5.64$).

It is important to note that most of the situations were described as occurring weekly or monthly and were associated with a good deal of stress for at least a few respondents. Such a wide range in responses points to the individual nature of experienced stress, as pointed out in Chapters 1 and 2. By grouping the data as they are presented in Table 4-1 it is possible to derive a picture of what events are likely to be most stressful for the health care managers in this study. A profile derived from grouped data loses some specificity in dealing with the case of the individual but is helpful in understanding the population from which that person comes. In addition, given the broad nature of the study, it is possible to glean an understanding of stressful events for health care managers in general against which future studies might be compared.

Taken as a group, the managers in this study find the pressure of too many time demands most stressful. Interestingly, a personal stressor,

Table 4-1 Rank Order of Stress Situations

Item	Rank	Mean
High Stress Group		
61. Having too many time demands.	1	11.724
1. Meeting your own expectations for excellence.	2	9.431
63. Not having things done as quickly as I would like (waiting for others to participate).	3	9.279
44. Getting others to carry out their job responsibilities.	4	9.036
4. Seeing problems within the organization and not having the resources to correct them.	5	8.846
22. Balancing time between work and family.	6	8.694
42. Creating a well-functioning staff team.	7	8.288
14. Dealing with conflicts of needs or interests between people in the organization.	7	8.288
3. Working with administrative people who are not clear about the direction in which we need to go.	9	8.233
32. Dealing with people who do not think quickly and flexibly.	10	8.189
82. Having to meet deadlines.	11	8.128
15. Dealing with the strong personalities of staff.	12	7.726
High-Moderate Stress Group		
51. Dealing with staff incompetence.	13	7.595
37. Dealing with the stress of those who report to me.	14	7.431
83. Dealing with organizational disorganization (re policies and procedures).	15	7.410
39. Being responsible for, but not having direct control over, the quality of patient care.	16	7.395
33. Trying to be a role model for others in the institution.	17	7.362
54. Being a buffer between the staff and administration (management).	18	7.360
7. Learning that patients/families have received less than the best care/understanding from hospital staff.	19	7.355
28. Trying to get others to be committed to achieve objectives/outcomes which I feel are important.	20	7.296
65. Responding to multiple demands and not having time to see how those responses affect the department or hospital overall.	21	7.260
64. Dealing with staff complaints.	22	7.015
74. Dealing with power problems or infighting among staff.	23	6.977
88. Organizing staff to operate efficiently and effectively.	24	6.938
87. Retaining qualified staff.	25	6.932
55. Staff who have unreasonable expectations.	26	6.924
57. Giving direction and clarification to the role my profession should play in the hospital.	27	6.908
58. Having to work through a decision-making process with others rather than being able to make decisions on my own.	28	6.760

Table 4-1 continued

Item	Rank	Mean
84. Covering staff shortages.	29	6.719
76. Having to develop a power base to accomplish change.	30	6.697
71. Inability of staff to understand overall picture.	31	6.672
6. Having an active and outspoken staff which states its demands and wants action right away.	32	6.662
86. Attracting qualified staff.	33	6.631
69. Deciding what's important to get done.	34	6.612
40. Making decisions about priority expenses in times of economic constraint.	35	6.533
75. Having to resolve interdepartmental conflicts and jealousies.	36	6.500
12. Being confronted by professions/professionals fighting over turf.	37	6.419
62. Seeing ineffective treatment/procedures being used with patients.	38	6.328
66. Keeping staff informed.	39	6.221
56. Having to say no to people even though what they want is worthwhile.	40	6.168
34. Doing things others consider a high priority but I don't.	41	6.125
25. Staff resistance to innovations in clinical areas.	42	6.094
68. Having no one to talk to about the job.	43	6.085
72. Getting staff to accept new policies/procedures.	44	5.992
2. Having a lot of responsibility for projects and little authority to accomplish them.	45	5.880
35. Nursing staff seeking equal status with physicians and increased pay.	46	5.820
81. Having my words twisted around.	47	5.744
47. Miscommunication with staff.	48	5.690
80. Having to work with administrators who are insensitive to clinical issues.	49	5.667

Low-Moderate Stress Group

Item	Rank	Mean
24. Financial cutbacks.	50	5.536
67. Getting staff's participation in policy/program development.	51	5.481
36. Lack of understanding from administrative staff.	52	5.368
17. Making decisions with long-term, major implications for the institution.	53	5.331
48. Moderating committees (being prepared, keeping meetings orderly while allowing all to speak).	54	5.246
5. Attending meetings I don't want to attend.	55	5.234
79. Not having responsibility nor authority to take needed action.	56	5.216
78. Having to sacrifice/compromise professional ideals.	57	5.169
77. Having colleagues question my judgment in an area outside their expertise.	58	5.114
19. Handling patients' or families' complaints about care.	59	5.007
53. Representing clinical staff positions to administration.	60	4.876

Table 4-1 continued

Item	Rank	Mean
20. Responding to government agencies/regulations.	61	4.837
85. Delegating work.	62	4.788
60. Having inadequate opportunity to influence important, hospitalwide policies.	63	4.596
26. Conflict between line and executive staff.	64	4.475
59. Not having the support of my immediate superior or board.	65	4.152
18. Making presentations to boards or committees.	66	4.046
50. Dealing with patients for whom medical care has not been effective (e.g., chronic or traumatic problems for which medicine has no cure.)	67	3.982
30. Staff's lack of response to the quality assurance program.	68	3.965
16. Making an error in judgment with respect to a major decision for the organization.	69	3.760
13. Having to respond to demands which I cannot fulfill because of personal inadequacies (i.e., limited knowledge, attitudes, etc.)	70	3.653
10. Being given responsibility to accomplish a project and then being undercut.	71	3.625

Low Stress Group

Item	Rank	Mean
9. Being chewed out by those upon whom I depend for support.	72	3.441
70. Getting board to approve policies.	73	3.347
41. Dealing with staff reactions to the hiring of new personnel who bring new expertise or new services to the organization.	74	3.310
38. Personal experience of discrimination (e.g., minority or gender status).	75	3.010
8. Dealing with board members.	76	2.991
43. Competing demands and needs of consumers in community.	77	2.968
89. Not having the support of my subordinates.	78	2.917
31. Public expectations for more services than institution can or wants to provide.	79	2.882
46. Dealing with union problems.	80	2.759
49. Serving as resource person from hospital to the community.	81	2.622
45. Dealing with public media.	82	2.531
29. Being embarrassed or publicly criticized for the operation of the organization.	83	2.481
11. Dealing with community groups who do not feel fairly treated.	84	2.365
52. Administration done by an elected rather than appointed official.	85	2.132
23. Disagreement between board and management about the role of each.	86	1.955
21. Attempts by staff to unionize.	87	1.878
27. Trying to demonstrate community need for program to obtain HSA approval, in face of consumer activist groups which are antiprovider.	88	1.850
73. Dealing with community groups wanting staff privileges.	89	1.058

meeting the manager's own expectations for excellence, ranks second. Related to that is dissatisfaction with the rate at which others get things done. Together, these three events can be regarded as a cluster reflecting Type A characteristics and perhaps augmenting the stress these managers and those around them experience. Interpersonal stressors predominate the highest ranked events, centering on creating a team, having others do their work, handling conflict surrounding needs, interests, and personalities. Problems in balancing demands of work and home also rank high, as do lack of resources and lack of clear direction from administration, the latter two being organizational sources of stress.

STRESS AS A FUNCTION OF SEX AND POSITION

Each stress item was broken down by region, sex, and position, yielding some interesting findings. While no significant differences were obtained across regions, there were significant differences in relation to sex and position. Women rated 58 percent of the events (i.e., 52) as significantly more stressful than did men. For only two events (dealing with board members and balancing time between work and family) were men's rating higher than those of women. For the rest of the events, no significant differences were found. For all but one of the events in the high stress group (No. 15—dealing with strong staff personalities), women's ratings of the stress surrounding the event were higher than those of the men. In the low stress group of events, 44 percent of the items were associated with sexual differences.

Table 4-2 presents the results of an analysis of variance used to test differences in stress scores as a function of sex. Only the 54 (out of 89) items with significant differences are included in the table. Of particular interest are those with very high significance levels. For example, the total stress scores of women were substantially higher than those of men. In general women respondents tended to perceive problems with patient care (e.g., seeing ineffective treatment/procedures being used) as more stressful than did their male colleagues. They similarly saw interpersonal situations revolving around handling staff complaints, infighting and power problems among staff, and creating a well-functioning team as more stressful. In part this may well be a reflection of sex-role socialization.

Clinically, women typically have more difficulty with conflict since they are socialized to be harmonizers. Not surprisingly, they experienced the pressures and stress of discrimination more frequently than men. They also had greater stress in giving direction and clarification to the role their profession should play in the hospital and in serving as a role model for others.

Table 4-2 Stress Event Scores as a Function of Sex: Significant Differences

Item	$\bar{X}^a$ Male Score	$\bar{X}^a$ Female Score	F^b	Significance Level
3. Working with administrative people who are not clear about the direction in which we need to go.	5.889	10.0667	13.16	.0004
4. Seeing problems within the organization and not having the resources to correct them.	7.2264	10.507	8.447	.004
5. Attending meetings I don't want to attend.	4.0	6.2692	8.43	.004
7. Learning that patients/ families have received less than the best care/ understanding from hospital staff.	6.54	8.25	4.296	.04
8. Dealing with board members.	4.2766^c	2.1129	20.364	.0001
9. Being chewed out by those upon whom I depend for support.	2.087	4.3881	7.301	.008
12. Being confronted by professions/professionals fighting over turf.	5.463	7.4474	4.975	.03
13. Having to respond to demands which I cannot fulfill because of personal inadequacies (i.e., limited knowledge, attitudes, etc.)	2.5962	4.6818	6.474	.01
14. Dealing with conflicts of needs or interests between people in the organization.	7.1176	9.4267	6.272	.01
19. Handling patients' or families' complaints about care.	4.4906	5.6104	3.877	.05
22. Balancing time between work and family.	6.8491	10.4	11.531	.0009
23. Disagreement between board and management about the role of each.	2.9487*	1.3256	4.237	.04

Table 4-2 continued

Item	$\bar{X}^a$ Male Score	$\bar{X}^a$ Female Score	F^b	Significance Level
25. Staff resistance to innovations in clinical areas.	5.0189	7.4493	6.354	.01
28. Trying to get others to be committed to achieve objectives/outcomes which I feel are important.	5.440	9.275	19.97	.0001
29. Being embarrassed or publicly criticized for the operation of the institution.	1.8537	3.1930	4.140	.04
32. Dealing with people who do not think quickly and flexibly.	6.1321	10.0959	19.396	.0001
33. Trying to be a role model for others in the institution.	5.75	8.6329	9.678	.002
34. Doing things others consider a high priority but I don't.	4.78	7.1944	6.886	.01
35. Nursing staff seeking equal status with physicians and increased pay.	4.5217	7.1143	5.662	.02
36. Lack of understanding from administrative staff.	3.9286	6.2143	4.23	.04
37. Dealing with the stress of those who report to me.	5.9020	8.7778	12.006	.0007
38. Personal experience of discrimination (e.g., minority or gender status).	1.2121	4.0175	9.022	.004
41. Dealing with staff reactions to the hiring of new personnel who bring new expertise or new services to the organization.	2.22	4.2817	9.822	.002
42. Creating a well-functioning staff team.	6.4815	9.9494	12.232	.0006
44. Getting others to carry out their job responsibilities.	7.1132	10.7595	14.293	.0002

Table 4-2 continued

Item	$\bar{X}^a$ Male Score	$\bar{X}^a$ Female Score	F^b	Significance Level
46. Dealing with union problems.	1.5484	3.907	4.483	.04
47. Miscommunication with staff.	4.549	6.667	6.921	.01
49. Serving as resource person from hospital to the community.	2.1702	3.1067	4.217	.04
51. Dealing with staff incompetence.	6.38	8.9718	6.36	.01
54. Being a buffer between the staff and administration (management).	6.1951	8.33	4.168	.04
55. Staff who have unreasonable expectations.	5.8269	8.0	5.445	.02
56. Having to say no to people even though what they want is worthwhile.	5.434	7.1944	4.371	.04
57. Giving direction and clarification to the role my profession should play in the hospital.	5.0435	8.5286	10.469	.002
61. Having too many time demands.	10.111	13.4054	10.269	.002
62. Seeing ineffective treatment/procedures being used with patients.	4.5682	7.2857	9.0	.003
63. Not having things done as quickly as I would like (waiting for others to participate).	7.5385	10.6761	12.361	.0006
64. Dealing with staff complaints.	6.0182	7.921	7.116	.009
65. Responding to multiple demands and not having time to see how those responses affect the department or hospital overall.	5.5106	8.7183	9.428	.003
66. Keeping staff informed.	4.6364	7.275	9.9	.002
68. Having no one to talk to about the job.	4.4167	7.6481	4.828	.03

Table 4-2 continued

Item	$\bar{X}^a$ Male Score	$\bar{X}^a$ Female Score	F^b	Significance Level
71. Inability of staff to understand overall picture.	5.1176	8.1972	10.033	.002
72. Getting staff to accept new policies/procedures.	4.8302	6.8714	4.807	.03
74. Dealing with power problems or infighting among staff.	5.2745	8.1447	8.08	.005
76. Having to develop a power base to accomplish change.	5.1818	7.8732	5.86	.02
77. Having colleagues question my judgment in an area outside their expertise.	3.9184	6.2174	6.621	.01
79. Not having responsibility nor authority to take needed action.	3.7111	6.5574	7.125	.009
80. Having to work with administrators who are insensitive to clinical issues.	3.8293	7.5094	7.257	.008
81. Having my words twisted around.	4.380	7.058	6.309	.01
82. Having to meet deadlines.	6.222	9.56	12.914	.0005
83. Dealing with organizational disorganization (re policies and procedures).	5.120	9.4559	15.177	.0002
84. Covering staff shortages.	3.6383	8.8611	26.204	.00001
86. Attracting qualified staff.	4.8043	7.4	6.701	.01
87. Retaining qualified staff.	5.0	8.3377	9.73	.002
88. Organizing staff to operate efficiently and effectively.	5.9038	7.8378	4.326	.04
Total Stress Scores (54 items)	494.5	652.6173	19.446	.0001

[a] $\bar{X}$ indicates mean or average.

[b] F indicates the ratio of dispersion in the group as a whole to the dispersion of particular groups of interest.

[c] Used to highlight items for which males reported higher stress.

During the interview phase of the study one minority woman in a position as associate administrator described as a major source of stress for her the same three factors: minority status (racial and sexual); pressures from others to serve as a role model, often with very high expectations associated with that status; and internal pressures to obtain the respect and authority she believed were due her.

Women described themselves as experiencing more stress than men in relation to meeting the demands of work and family as well as to handling multiple demands in the hospital without seeing how the decisions affected overall departmental or hospital functioning. The first is understandable in terms of women's traditional responsibility for meeting family needs and of research indicating serious conflicts experienced by many women who assume full-time positions of responsibility in the work place; however, the second difference is somewhat puzzling.

It might be hypothesized that the latter difference reflects the tendency of women to hold positions of more limited responsibility in the organizational hierarchy that as a rule do not include as broad a perspective as is found at the highest levels. These women may experience stress since they want an overall perspective so they can assess the possible repercussions of their decisions but do not have the information necessary to do so. This notion would need to be examined empirically.

Insensitivity to clinical issues was more stressful for women than for men, as were staff shortages, dealing with organizational disorganization, and meeting deadlines. Ironically, frustration at not having things done quickly and dealing with people who did not think quickly and flexibly was more stressful for the women than the men. These typically Type A traits generally are associated with men. The data suggest, however, that for the women in management positions in this study, Type A tendencies in this regard were even higher than those of their male counterparts. This may reflect their actual or perceived need to be "superwomen" and more aggressive than their male counterparts to obtain and keep their positions in the hierarchy.

Stress score data also were broken down by position, yielding significant results. An analysis of variance was performed on the data, the results of which appear in Table 4-3. An analysis of variance is a statistical test to determine if there are differences in the scores across groups. More specifically, it determines if the dispersion of scores in the groups of interest (e.g. positions) are significantly different from that of the sample as a whole. On 41 percent of the 89 events (36 items), significant differences in stress scores occurred as a function of position. Total stress scores were highest for directors of nursing, with the composite group of middle managers having the next highest score. Associate administrator ranked third,

Table 4-3 Mean Stress Event Score as Function of Position: Significant Differences

Item	CEO	Assoc. Adm.	Dir. Nursing	Pres. Med. Staff	Med. Dir.	Other	F^a	Significance Level
3. Working with administrative people who are not clear about the direction in which we need to go.	4.25	8.68	10.27	6.33	4.0	8.25	3.944	.002
4. Seeing problems within the organization and not having the resources to correct them.	6.29	7.24	10.86	7.33	3.75	10.94	4.863	.0004
12. Being confronted by professions/professionals fighting over turf.	3.35	6.25	7.15	4.83	5.41	8.29	2.286	.05
16. Making an error in judgment with respect to a major decision for the organization.	2.07	3.77	4.54	1.0	2.63	4.0	2.438	.04
20. Responding to government agencies/regulations.	7.5	3.24	4.55	7.83	3.24	5.5	3.165	.01
22. Balancing time between work and family.	8.56	9.55	8.47	8.6	4.41	11.41	2.478	.04
25. Staff resistance to innovations in clinical areas.	3.06	4.56	7.91	3.0	4.5	6.75	3.589	.005
26. Conflict between line and executive staff.	2.79	2.57	5.33	1.0	2.69	7.59	3.906	.003
28. Trying to get others to be committed to achieve objectives/outcomes which I feel are important.	5.73	6.29	9.0	4.0	3.87	7.75	3.906	.003
32. Dealing with people who do not think quickly and flexibly.	6.27	7.44	9.9	5.5	5.35	8.44	3.140	.01
35. Nursing staff seeking equal status with physicians and increased pay.	4.29	3.95	7.63	6.4	2.63	4.83	2.96	.01
37. Dealing with the stress of those who report to me.	5.13	6.86	8.97	4.0	5.24	7.47	3.258	.008
39. Being responsible for, but not having direct control over, the quality of patient care.	4.95	5.62	9.1	4.8	5.2	8.69	2.299	.05
41. Dealing with staff reactions to the hiring of new personnel who bring new expertise or new services to the organization.	1.0	3.0	4.47	1.75	2.0	2.87	3.323	.008
42. Creating a well-functioning staff team.	6.12	7.41	10.85	2.75	4.24	7.59	6.219	.00001

							F	p
44. Getting others to carry out their job responsibilities.	5.75	7.19	11.73	6.4	5.69	8.56	6.516	.00001
47. Miscommunication with staff.	3.29	6.0	7.04	2.4	3.93	5.5	3.046	.01
51. Dealing with staff incompetence.	5.67	6.75	9.57	5.6	4.3	7.2	3.053	.01
53. Representing clinical staff positions to administration.	0.17	2.06	6.51	6.2	3.76	5.64	3.268	.009
54. Being a buffer between the staff and administration (management).	2.0	5.17	8.95	8.4	5.18	7.87	3.884	.003
55. Staff who have unreasonable expectations.	3.27	7.09	8.38	5.2	5.76	6.19	2.841	.02
57. Giving direction and clarification to the role my profession should play in the hospital.	3.0	5.58	9.04	6.0	3.31	7.13	4.33	.001
63. Not having things done as quickly as I would like (waiting for others to participate).	7.33	10.33	10.77	8.80	6.47	7.53	3.09	.01
64. Dealing with staff complaints.	5.18	5.77	8.55	7.83	5.65	6.29	3.4	.006
65. Responding to multiple demands and not having time to see how those responses affect the department or hospital overall.	4.36	7.16	8.72	4.0	5.06	7.54	2.361	.04
66. Keeping staff informed.	4.82	4.52	7.73	4.67	4.76	6.24	2.386	.04
71. Inability of staff to understand overall picture.	3.08	6.09	9.14	4.17	3.19	5.86	6.184	.00001
72. Getting staff to accept new policies/procedures.	3.53	6.27	7.78	3.67	4.18	5.0	2.909	.02
77. Having colleagues question my judgment in an area outside their expertise.	3.0	3.94	6.66	2.20	2.59	6.29	3.646	.004
81. Having my words twisted around.	3.29	4.15	7.63	1.80	3.56	6.53	3.152	.01
82. Having to meet deadlines.	7.0	5.80	9.49	8.17	5.69	9.41	2.473	.04
83. Dealing with organizational disorganization (re policies and procedures).	3.08	6.0	10.0	4.17	3.93	7.73	5.234	.0002
84. Covering staff shortages.	2.69	2.72	9.46	2.75	3.50	7.0	8.663	.00001
86. Attracting qualified staff.	2.93	4.71	8.29	2.67	4.44	6.40	3.994	.0022
87. Retaining qualified staff.	3.15	4.81	9.21	2.0	4.88	6.67	4.814	.0005
88. Organizing staff to operate efficiently and effectively.	5.33	4.65	8.53	6.60	5.24	7.31	2.668	.02
Total Stress Scores	460.29	508.27	641.95	479.50	385.76	606.94	5.309	.0002

[a] F indicates the ratio of dispersion in the group as a whole to the dispersion of particular groups of interest.

president of the medical staff fourth, chief executive officer fifth, and medical director sixth.

Total stress scores had a possible range of 0 to 1,780. While none of the groups' average total fell into the upper half of possible scores, the differences among the groups were highly significant and merit exploration. These findings also add support to previous studies that underscore the importance of examining differential stress and climate within the organization as a function of department, unit, or professional group (Adams, Laker, and Hulin, 1977; Charns and Beattie, 1982; Ivancevich and Matteson, 1980; Lawrence and Lorsch, 1967). An examination of position also seems warranted. The various stressor events next are explored separately in relation to the degree of stress associated with them by people in different positions.

Item 3: Working with administrative people who are not clear about the direction in which we need to go.

Data indicated that this event, ninth highest on the list in Table 4-1, was most stressful for directors of nursing, associate administrators, and other, nonmedical department heads and assistant administrators; less stressful for medical staff presidents; and least stressful for CEOs and medical directors. The results were not surprising since it is senior level administration that sets direction. Failure to do so, as noted in Chapter 3, is a source of stress for second-level administration and department heads, as these data confirmed.

Item 4: Seeing problems within the organization and not having the resources to correct them.

Those in control of and closest to the resources—medical director and CEO—were less likely to experience stress related to scarcity since they had the power to channel available resources in directions they saw fit. The data confirmed this for this fifth most stressful item listed. Nursing directors and department heads experienced the most stress with regard to this event; medical staff presidents (who were not administrators of the hospital and thus were in staff positions as opposed to medical directors) and associate administrators had somewhat less stress, CEOs and medical directors the least.

Item 12: Being confronted by professions/professionals fighting over turf.

It might be expected that positions that had direct responsibility for interdisciplinary work (e.g., education) or oversee departments where professional status was being questioned or challenged (e.g., nursing, social service, occupational therapy) would experience higher stress than those that were buffered from such conflict because of organizational position (e.g., CEO) or historically having been the seat of power (e.g., medicine). The data confirmed this. Department heads, nursing directors, and associate administrators reported more stress than medical directors, presidents of medical staffs, and CEOs.

Item 16: Making an error in judgment with respect to a major decision for the organization.

While no predictions were made regarding the role of position in understanding this type of stress, it seemed that the most vulnerable persons were not those at the very top of the organization (i.e., CEO and medical director), but those who were second in command. This might reflect a sense on the part of the latter that they had more to lose since such a mistake could have implications for impeding their career progress to higher levels of management.

Item 20: Responding to government agencies/regulations.

It would be expected that those with most direct responsibility for negotiating with government agencies (i.e., CEO) and those most likely to be directly affected by such regulations (i.e., medical staff) would experience more stress than those not so involved. As expected, the medical staff president and the CEO experienced the most stress, followed by department heads, nursing directors, and medical directors/associate administrators.

Item 22: Balancing time between work and family.

Those experiencing most stress in this category, sixth in Table 4-1, were department heads and associate administrators. Medical staff presidents, CEOs, and directors of nursing experienced less stress, with medical directors the least. It should be noted that women had substantially more stress than men in this area and were well represented among department heads, associate administrators, and directors of nursing.

Item 25: Staff resistance to innovations in clinical areas.

Managers directly responsible for the clinical work of subordinates (e.g., directors of nursing and medical directors) would be expected to experience most stress in this area. The data confirmed this. Nursing directors rated highest on this type of stress, followed by department heads, many of whom were responsible for inservice (clinical) education. Associate administrators and medical directors came next, with the least stress experienced by CEOs and medical staff presidents. (The latter generally had no responsibility for the clinical work of the medical staff. However, they were legally accountable for evidence of malpractice and/or impaired practice.) While it was not anticipated that associate administrators would rate this stress situation as high as medical directors, this finding could be understood in light of the fact that clinical departments did report to this level of administration, bringing related problems under the associates' purview.

Item 26: Conflict between line and executive staff.

The data affirmed the expectation that middle managers would be most adversely affected by this source of stress and that medical staff presidents, because they were not employees of the hospital per se, would be relatively unaffected by it. Department heads and directors of nursing reported the highest stress, medical staff presidents the lowest. There was little real difference among the three other groups, which fell close to the low end of the stress range for the item.

Item 28: Trying to get others to be committed to achieve objectives/outcomes which I feel are important.

Middle management, since its mandate is to gain commitment of staff and to attempt to influence policymakers above, would be expected to experience the most stress, followed by administration and the medical management. The data bore this out.

Item 32: Dealing with people who do not think flexibly and quickly.

While this might be expected to be more stressful to physicians, in part because of age-old stereotypes, the data for this, tenth in Table 4-1, suggested otherwise. Nursing directors and department heads, followed by associate administrators, saw this as more stressful than did the other groups even though the sample as a whole rated this as tenth among the dozen most stressful situations. It was possible that the frequency with which nursing directors and department heads must contend with this problem created the extra stress.

Item 35: Nursing staff seeking equal status with physicians and increased pay.

Nursing and medical directors and medical staff presidents might be expected to experience higher stress in this situation. The first two did, indeed, have the most stress but for some reason beyond the scope of this study, this was not particularly stressful for medical directors.

Item 37: Dealing with the stress of those who report to me.

Once again, the data indicated that people in the highest levels of the organization seemed to be buffered from this type of stress exerted by middle management. Nursing directors, department heads, and associate administrators reported the highest stress here.

Item 39: Being responsible for, but not having direct control over, the quality of patient care.

Here, too, the data suggested that nursing directors and department heads experienced the greatest stress, with few real differences among the other groups. This finding could reflect the fact that nurses ran the clinical aspects of the hospital on a daily basis yet physicians remained the dominant decision-making group.

Item 41: Dealing with staff reactions to the hiring of new personnel who bring new expertise or new services to the organization.

Nursing directors experienced by far the most stress in this category, with associate administrators and department heads next. Once again, CEOs seemed to be buffered by their administrative personnel and department heads.

Item 42: Creating a well-functioning staff team.

The data on this item, tied for seventh in Table 4-1, vividly pointed to some prevailing stereotypes concerning the nature of medical practice among hospital practitioners. Presidents of medical staffs reported the least stress, followed by medical directors. It was unclear whether this was because of a lack of concern for team functioning, given the historic trends of physician dominance, uncontested autocratic leaders, and solo practitioners. Nurses reported the most stress in this situation. Once more, it was impossible to determine whether this reflected concern for the development of teams or difficulty in bringing them about. Department heads and both levels of administration reported a fair degree of stress associated with this.

Item 44: Getting others to carry out job responsibilities.

This, the fourth most stressful item in Table 4-1, was considerably more so for directors of nursing—in fact, it was the highest for any group on any item on the list. They were followed by department heads and associate administrators, with medical directors and CEOs the least. The stress of nonsenior level management came through again.

Item 47: Miscommunication with staff.

Directors of nursing and associate administrators reported most concern with this item, followed by department heads, medical directors, CEOs, and medical staff presidents.

Item 51: Dealing with staff incompetence.

This might be expected to be most stressful for those in clinical areas. While that was true for nursing, medical staff presidents and medical directors reported somewhat lower stress levels. Whether this reflected the relatively infrequent occurrence of this problem for medical staff presidents and medical directors was unclear.

Item 53: Representing clinical staff positions to administration.

Clinical managers (i.e., directors of nursing, chiefs of staff, and medical directors) would be expected to find the most stress in this area. This was true for the first two, plus department heads. The stress reported by medical directors was substantially lower, followed by even less among administrators. Why the medical directors' stress was not higher might be understood in part by the fact that this was a "fence" position: it was regarded by the medical staff as clinical but by administration as a full-time administrative role, unlike that of chief of staff. (The problems associated with this dualism are explored in Chapter 5.)

Item 54: Being a buffer between the staff and administration (management).

As expected, nursing directors and chiefs of staff experienced the most stress, CEOs and medical directors the least. However, substantial differences did exist between medical directors and CEOs, again suggesting the stress of the "fence" position noted above.

Item 55: Staff who have unreasonable expectations.

The data confirmed that CEOs, as expected, were buffered from much of this problem and reported the lowest levels of stress. Nursing directors, associate administrators, and department heads had the highest levels of stress; presidents of medical staffs and medical directors had significantly less but still more than the CEOs.

Item 57: Giving direction and clarification to the role my profession should play in the hospital.

The expectation that nursing directors and department heads would experience the most stress in this category and chiefs of staff moderate stress, given their nonemployee voluntary status, was confirmed by the data.

Item 63: Not having things done as quickly as I would like (waiting for others to participate).

Based on stereotyped myths concerning physicians, one would expect medical directors and medical staff presidents to rate this event as more stressful than others. To the contrary, medical directors scored lowest on this item. Nursing directors and associate administrators were highest, with little difference among the three other groups. While this was rated third in the high stress group overall, differences among the positions were noteworthy.

Item 64: Dealing with staff complaints.

No predictions were made on this category. Clinical directors (nursing and chief of staff) reported the most stress, perhaps reflecting the problems in representing clinical issues to administration (Item 53). No significant differences occurred among the other positions.

Item 65: Responding to multiple demands and not having time to see how those responses affect the department or hospital overall.

Those with more circumscribed responsibility and less organizational power would be expected to express the most stress here. Nursing reported the highest stress, with department heads and associate administrators following. Medical directors, CEOs, and chiefs of staff had significantly lower scores.

Item 66: Keeping staff informed.

Nursing directors had significantly higher stress scores on this than other groups, followed by department heads with no significant differences among the other positions. Shift changes and high turnover might be involved in nurses' perceptions of difficulty in this area.

Item 71: Inability of staff to understand the overall picture.

Those highest in the organization (CEO and medical director) would be expected to have the least stress in this category and that those responsible for personnel at lower levels in the hierarchy the most stress as a function of the concerns of their position and access to information. This was confirmed by the data. Nursing directors experienced far and away the most stress, followed by associate administrators and department heads; CEOs reported the least stress, followed by medical directors and chiefs of staff. A natural question would be why nursing directors found so much more stress in this area than medical directors. One possible explanation would be the different relationships nurses and doctors tend to have with the hospital. Physicians for the most part are in independent or group practices and have staff privileges. Their status is quite different from those of nurses, who are employed directly by the hospital (except for those working through a registry or offering consultation to a number of hospitals). For nursing staff members, it is imperative that they have an understanding of hospitalwide issues likely to affect them. Experience suggests that most physicians were not as interested in such matters.

Item 72: Getting staff to accept new policies/procedures.

Once again, nursing directors experienced more stress than other groups. Associate administrators ranked next, followed by department heads. Those reporting least stress in this area were CEOs, chiefs of staff, and medical directors.

Item 77: Having colleagues question my judgment in an area outside their expertise.

Numerous war stories are related by nurses around the country complaining that physicians intrude into nursing matters. Given this, nursing directors, as expected, along with department heads, rated this as more stressful than did other groups. While there were no significant differences among the remaining groups except for associate administrators and chiefs of staff, it is important to note that those least affected by this were the physician respondents (i.e. medical directors and medical staff presidents.)

Item 81: Having my words twisted around.

While no a priori predictions were made for this item, nursing directors reported more stress than other groups, followed by department heads. Associate administrators ranked in the middle, with medical directors and CEOs a little lower. Significantly less stress was reported by chiefs of staff.

Item 82: Having to meet deadlines.

This item was 11th in the most stressful group (Table 4-1). While middle managers might be expected to report more stress than those in senior administration, this was not necessarily the case. Nursing directors again reported the most stress, with no real difference from that listed by department heads; chiefs of staff also had higher relative stress than might be expected. CEOs followed with associate administrators and medical directors reporting least relative stress.

Item 83: Dealing with organizational disorganization (re policies and procedures).

As expected, senior level administration reported the least stress since it is at that level that such disorganization emanates, sending the effects downward. Nursing directors reported the most stress, followed by department heads and associate administrators. Substantially less stress was reported by all physicians and even less by CEOs.

Item 84: Covering staff shortages.

Because of recent concern about nursing shortages, in particular, nursing service would be expected to be most affected by this issue and, to a lesser but substantial degree, department heads. This was born out by the data. All the others reported low levels of stress.

Items 86 and 87: Attracting qualified staff and retaining qualified staff.

Both problems, as expected, were of greatest concern to those directly responsible for hiring and retaining staff—nursing directors and department heads, in that order. Associate administrators and medical directors reported significantly less stress than the first two groups but more than CEOs and chiefs of staff. It is interesting to note that among all groups except chiefs of staff, the tendency was to have somewhat greater concern for retaining qualified staff members than for attracting them. This was particularly true for nursing and confirmed similar reports in the literature documenting retention as opposed to recruitment as a major problem in that profession.

Item 88: Organizing staff to operate efficiently and effectively.

As anticipated, responses on this issue paralleled those pertaining to team integration (Item 42), except for associate administrators and chiefs of staff, who switched positions. Associate administrators reported least stress on this problem, nursing directors and department heads the most.

STRESS EVENTS, OUTCOMES, AND SYMPTOMS

Respondents were requested to fill out the Personal Stress Symptom Assessment (Appendix B), which was designed to provide comprehensive data as to the degree to which they experienced negative stress outcomes. An obvious limitation of the questionnaire was that it was a self-report measure, thus subject to the accuracy and honesty of each respondent. Assuming random distribution of error, however, this report provided rich data from which to examine the relationship between coping strategies and stress symptoms, intensity of stress and stress symptoms, and so forth. The instrument was the result of a thorough review of research in stress-related illness. While it might not provide an exhaustive listing of all possible symptoms, it did offer a comprehensive selection.

Data were factor analyzed using a principle components procedure without iteration. Factors with eigen values (statistical decision for inclusion of factors in the analysis) greater than one were rotated, using a varimax rotation which assumes independence among the factors (Nie et al., 1975). The factor analysis of the stress symptoms yielded six orthogonal factors cumulatively accounting for 52.8 percent of the variance. In interpreting the factors and constructing scales, only items with a loading of 0.42 or higher were included, and only if that item did not load heavily (0.35) or more than one factor. Three items—impatience, blaming self, and blaming others—were included on two scales because of their heavy loading and importance on the two scales in question. Item-total correlations were computed to verify the homogeneity of selected items. Using these procedures, six multiple-item scales were developed (Table 4-4) as described next:

1. **Emotional:** This scale contains 14 items of a general emotional nature, primarily experienced by the individual alone as opposed to being of an interpersonal nature.
2. **Internalized Minor Somatic:** This scale consists of seven items, including stomachaches, indigestion, physical ailments, and constipation, and indicates a person's tendency toward somatic expression of stress.
3. **External behavioral:** This six-item scale reflects the individual's tendency to handle stress through behavioral means, including the use of stimulants and/or alcohol, trembling, and nervous tics. This scale represents outward behavioral expressions of stress while Scale 1 reflects internalized affect states not necessarily observable to others.
4. **Interpersonal:** The eight items in this scale reflect interpersonal behavior styles that are indicators of stress. Included are: blaming others, bossiness, irritability, agitation, and inflexibility.
5. **Unconscious:** This three-item scale contains elements of a strongly unconscious nature: nightmares, accident proneness, and major physical ailments.
6. **Depressive:** This four-item scale contains symptomatology related to clinical depression: crying, forgetfulness, blaming self, and blaming others.

Scale scores were calculated for each respondent, assuming equal weights for all items and summing responses for relevant items. An analysis of variance was performed comparing differences for each scale score and for total symptoms (i.e., the sum of all six scale scores). No significant sexual differences were found on any of the scales nor for total symptoms except for Scale 3 (External behavior). As predicted, men (mean = 10.75) tended to express stress through external means more than women (mean = 8.30). This finding reached the .05 level of significance.

An analysis of variance also was performed to determine whether stress symptom differences existed as a function of position. Here significance

Table 4-4 Personal Stress Symptom Scales and Their Loadings

Factor Loading[a]	Item #*	Item*
	Scale 1: Emotional	
.47498	6	Fatigue
.50613	9	Blaming self
.66747	16	Worrying
.71912	17	Depression
.49497	18	Agitation
.45124	19	Impatience
.65545	21	Frustration
.58965	22	Loneliness
.64420	26	General tension
.60552	32	Trouble concentrating
.64209	33	Anxiety or nervousness
.53827	38	Insomnia
.71072	48	Not feeling good about self
.69960	53	Inability to relax
	Scale 2: Internalized Minor Somatic	
.70009	2	Stomachaches
.52861	40	Frequent need to urinate
.59410	41	Diarrhea
.79353	42	Indigestion
.82118	43	Queasy stomach
.56176	49	Minor physical ailments
.47289	51	Constipation
	Scale 3: External Behavioral	
.65051	27	Drinking
.63846	28	Use of stimulant or tranquilizing drugs
.53600	31	Impulsive behavior
.57506	34	Trembling
.56900	35	Nervous tics
.63643	44	Vomiting
	Scale 4: Interpersonal	
.48717	10	Blaming others
.66171	11	Yelling
.81153	12	Bossiness
.42765	13	Irritability
.49012	18	Agitation
.48716	19	Impatience
.50332	20	Anger
.54178	23	Inflexibility

Table 4-4 continued

Factor Loading[a]	Item #*	Item*
	Scale 5: Unconscious	
.53233	46	Nightmares
.51215	47	Accident proneness
.76919	50	Major physical ailments
	Scale 6: Depressive	
.51721	7	Crying
.74028	8	Forgetfulness
.6214	9	Blaming self
.5730	10	Blaming others

[a] Factor loadings indicate the extent to which items are associated with a particular scale. For those few items that are included on more than one scale, it is expected that the loadings would be different on each scale.
* A complete list of items appears in Appendix C.

occurred for each of the six scales and for total symptoms as well. These data appear in Table 4-5.

For Scale 1 (emotional symptoms), CEOs and medical staff presidents reported the greatest number of symptoms. The possible score range on these scales was from 0 (indicating very low symptoms) to 168 (very high symptoms). Nursing directors, associate administrators, and department heads reported considerably fewer and like symptoms among themselves, with medical directors reporting the least.

Scale 2 (internalized somatic symptoms) showed substantially lower scores across all groups but with a pattern similar to that of Scale 1. Medical staff presidents and CEOs had significantly more symptoms than other groups, directors of nursing and department heads fewer, and associate administrators and medical directors the least.

Scale 3 (external behavior symptoms) reflected a similar pattern. While these scores generally were low, significant differences existed across positions. Medical staff presidents and CEOs reported more Scale 3 symptoms than did other positions, followed by department heads, associate administrators, and medical directors, with nursing directors having the fewest.

Scale 4 (interpersonal symptoms) demonstrated the same pattern: CEOs and medical staff presidents with highest relative symptomatology on this scale, medical directors the least, the other groups in between.

Scale 5 (unconscious factors) was the lowest for all positions but one where differences occur across positions. CEOs and medical staff presi-

Table 4-5 Mean Stress Symptom Scale Score as Function of Position

				Position				
Personal Stress Symptom Scale	CEO	Assoc. Admin.	Dir. of Nursing	Pres. Med. Staff	Med. Dir.	Others	F^a	Significance Level
Scale 1: Emotional	48.12	34.05	36.11	45.5	30.0	35.44	2.80	.02
Scale 2: Internalized Minor Somatic	19.12	10.95	12.35	19.67	10.59	11.22	3.25	.008
Scale 3: External Behavioral	14.29	8.95	7.98	15.67	8.88	9.33	3.10	.01
Scale 4: Interpersonal	25.88	18.73	18.41	24.5	16.59	17.67	2.73	.02
Scale 5: Unconscious	7.06	3.91	3.81	7.33	4.76	4.17	2.93	.02
Scale 6: Depressive	11.65	8.05	8.21	12.17	7.0	8.67	2.57	.03
Total Stress Symptoms	126.12	84.64	86.87	124.83	77.82	86.5	3.07	.01

[a] F indicates the ratio of dispersion in the group as a whole to the dispersion of particular groupings of interest. Larger F ratios are associated with more significant differences.

dents reported the greatest relative symptomatology, nursing directors and associate administrators the least.

Scale 6 (depressive), exhibited the same general patterning—medical staff presidents and CEOs the greatest symptomatology, medical directors the least.

Taken together, the data showed that all groups were most likely to experience emotional symptomatology, followed by interpersonal and internalized minor somatic symptomatology. Except for nursing directors, the next most frequent symptom grouping was external behavior. Nursing directors were more likely than other groups to report depressive symptomatology as opposed to external behavior symptoms. All groups were least likely to experience unconscious symptomatology.

If the total potential stress symptom scores were divided into three groupings: high (168–113), moderate (112–57), and low (56–0), it would be found that CEOs and medical staff presidents fell into the high symptom range, all other groups into the moderate range. When these results were compared with the stress situation scores discussed in the previous section, resolution of the inconsistencies proved difficult. While CEOs and medical staff presidents reported among the least situational stress, these two groups had the highest stress symptomatology. Conversely, nursing directors, with the highest situational stress, were among those reporting lesser amounts of stress symptomatology. Only medical directors reported both the lowest stress symptomatology and situational stress. It would seem reasonable to expect that high reported stress would be directly related to high reported stress symptomatology. How can these counterintuitive findings be explained?

SYMPTOMATOLOGY AND SITUATIONAL STRESS

From the data presented it appeared that those in the middle range of the organizational hierarchy—nursing directors and department heads— had the greatest amount of situational stress and those highest in the hierarchy the lowest. The latter are not subjected to the same kind of managerial stress that middle managers are.

Medical directors who reported least stress and fewest symptoms seemed to be in an unusual position, one that differentiated them from their medical staff president colleagues. Medical directors are full-time administrators hired by the hospital. They tend not to maintain clinical practices, except on a very limited basis. While they often are perceived as renegade clinicians by their staffs, they have the power vested in them by the organization. Many of these physicians have received, or are in the process of taking, management training to facilitate their successful performance as executives.

Medical staff presidents, on the other hand, hold positions akin to those of university department chairmen. The position once was considered a prestigious appointment, associated with pride and respect. During the last decade much of the prestige has been counterbalanced by rather heavy liabilities against these individuals in malpractice suits. Medical staff presidents are held accountable, along with the individual physicians, for the quality of medical care practiced in a hospital.

While the medical director also may be held responsible, the nature of that position may account for the wide differences in stress and symptomatology reported by the two groups. Medical staff presidents are elected by the organized medical staff for one to two years. The position is not compensated, so the holder of the office either simply "puts in time" for the term or expresses a sense of responsibility and dedication to the profession through many hours of service as medical staff president. There generally is no formal training associated with the office. Given these conditions, along with the demands of a busy private or group practice, it was easy to see why such an office might be associated with high symptomatology.

However, what explains the low reported situational stress? One possible explanation accounting for the inconsistencies among both medical staff presidents and CEOs lay in the psychological defense mechanism of denial. To the extent that the higher up a person is in the organization, and the more burdened with the myth of infallibility, the individual is likely to deny that situations are stressful. To the extent that acknowledging that something is stressful is a very basic stress reducer, denial serves to enhance the negative effects of the stressor, thus increasing symptomatology.

Perhaps the types of situations reported had a bearing on the level of stress symptomatology evidenced. For example, a particular situation might produce a differentially high effect (i.e. some situations might be associated with an unusually high degree of stress,) so that it would not be appropriate to weight the effect of all situations equally. When stress situations were examined separately by position, some additional points became apparent: namely, that the 10 most stressful situations showed some differences across positions.

As Table 4-6 indicates, medical staff presidents identified the following situations as most stressful while other groups did not: being a buffer between administration and management; having an inadequate opportunity to influence important, hospitalwide policies; and dealing with staff complaints. They shared with their medical director colleagues a concern

Table 4-6 Composite of the 10 Most Stressful Situations, by Position

Situation	Position					
	CEO	Assoc. Admin.	Dir. of Nursing	Pres. Med. Staff	Med. Dir.	Dept. Heads
1. Meeting your own expectations for excellence.	*	*	*		*	*
3. Working with administrative people who are not clear about the direction in which we need to go.		*	*			*
4. Seeing problems within the organization and not having the resources to correct them.	*	*	*	*		
6. Having an active and outspoken staff which states its demands and wants action right away.					*	
7. Learning that patients/families have received less than the best care/understanding from hospital staff.				*	*	
14. Dealing with conflicts of needs or interests between people in the organization.	*	*				*
15. Dealing with the strong personalities of staff.	*	*				
16. Making an error in judgment with respect to a major decision for the organization.	*	*				
20. Responding to government agencies/regulations.	*			*		
22. Balancing time between work and family.	*	*		*		
32. Dealing with people who do not think quickly and flexibly.		*	*			*
33. Trying to be a role model for others in the institution.	*	*				*
39. Being responsible for, but not having direct control over, the quality of patient care.						*
42. Creating a well-functioning staff team.			*		*	
44. Getting others to carry out their job responsibilities.			*			*

Table 4-6 continued

			Position			
Situation	CEO	Assoc. Admin.	Dir. of Nursing	Pres. Med. Staff	Med. Dir.	Dept. Heads
54. Being a buffer between the staff and administration (management).				*		
55. Staff who have unreasonable expectations.					*	
58. Having to work through a decision-making process with others rather than being able to make decisions on my own.		*				
60. Having inadequate opportunity to influence important, hospitalwide policies.				*		
61. Having too many time demands.	*	*	*	*	*	
63. Not having things done as quickly as I would like (waiting for others to participate).	*	*	*	*	*	
64. Dealing with staff complaints.				*		
74. Dealing with power problems or infighting among staff.				*	*	*
75. Having to resolve interdepartmental conflicts and jealousies.					*	
82. Having to meet deadlines.	*			*	*	*
83. Dealing with organizational disorganization (re policies and procedures).			*		*	*
84. Covering staff shortages.			*			

that patients/families might have received less than the best care/under-standing from hospital staff, having too many time demands, not having things done as quickly as they would like, and having to meet deadlines. Along with CEOs, they also reported stress associated with responding to government agencies/regulations, seeing problems within the organization and not having the resources to correct them, and balancing work between time and family.

Whether or not these situations had a substantially more negative effect than others was a question that was unanswerable at this point but certainly a fruitful avenue for pursuit in future research.

STRESS SITUATIONS AND COPING STRATEGIES

Another possible source accounting for the unexpected differences in stress situation and symptomatology scores involved the different effects of coping strategies employed by respondents in various positions. Could utilizing certain coping strategies for a given source of stress neutralize the negative effect of that stressor and reduce the level of personal stress symptomatology? The survey asked that respondents identify their coping strategies and generally how frequently they used each. The strategies are listed in Appendix C.

While the profile of most frequently used coping strategies of medical staff presidents showed some uniqueness, it did not appear to account logically for high levels of reported stress symptoms. For instance, as Table 4-7 suggests, Items 4 (I realize that some conflict is inevitable), 25 (I specify corrective action for staff to take), 28 (I spend time with family), 42 (I try to stay unemotional in conflict situations), 50 (I put things in perspective), and 76 (I develop a sense of humor) appeared only among this group's top ten—they were not rated that high by any other type of respondent. This group also was the only one that did not include Items 43 (I recognize that others have ideas which may be different from mine that are also useful) and 85 (If other people are involved, I talk the situation over with them) in the top ten list. The profile of CEOs, another group reporting high symptomatology and low situational stress, is not particu-larly outstanding relative to other groups.

Coping strategies where significant differences existed as a function of position were examined next. Table 4-8 suggests that in comparison to other groups, medical staff presidents were less likely to use the following coping strategies: Item 10, "I get the staff to participate as a team" and Item 35, "I tell staff my expectations," and were more likely than others to make lists of things needing to be done. With medical directors, there

Table 4-7 Composite of the 10 Most Frequently Used Coping Strategies, by Position

Coping Strategy		Position					
	CEO	Assoc. Adm.	Dir. Nursing	Pres. Med. Staff	Med. Dir.	Dept. Head
4. I realize that some conflict is inevitable.				*		
6. I think about alternative ways of dealing with the situation.		*	*			*
10. I get the staff to participate as a team.	*					*
12. I am sensitive to staff's needs and feelings.	*		*		*	
21. I prepare myself with as many facts as possible.		*	*			*
25. I specify corrective action for staff to take.				*		
28. I spend time with family.				*		
29. I try to keep communications channels open in the entire organization (across/up and down the formal hierarchy).	*	*	*	*	*	*
35. I tell staff my expectations.	*		*			
38. I let others air their grievances.				*	*	
42. I try to stay unemotional in conflict situations.				*		
43. I recognize that others have ideas that may be different from mine that are also useful.	*	*	*		*	*

Position

Coping Strategy	CEO	Assoc. Adm.	Dir. Nursing	Pres. Med. Staff	Med. Dir.	Dept. Head
44. I make a plan for getting things done.			*			*
48. I have open discussions with staff.					*	*
50. I put things in perspective.				*		
55. I make lists of things I need to do.		*			*	
68. I've learned to take risks and assume responsibility.	*	*			*	
70. I prioritize.	*	*	*		*	
72. I recognize and accept my limits to bring about changes alone.			*		*	
76. I develop a sense of humor.				*		
82. I use the organization's chain of command to solve problems.	*					
85. If other people are involved, I talk the situation over with them.	*	*	*		*	*
90. I look at the stresses as "part of the job."		*				
95. I talk it over with people who are directly involved.			*	*		*
103. I get support from my superior(s).		*		*		
104. I delegate responsibility downwards.	*	*		*		*

Table 4-8 Significant Differences Among Mean Coping Strategy Scores as a Function of Position

Coping Strategy	Position						F^a	Significance Level
	CEO	Assoc. Adm.	Dir. Nursing	Pres. Med. Staff	Med. Dir.	Dept. Head		
7. I think about something else during meetings.	3.67	4.0	3.65	4.33	4.41	6.46	2.628	.03
10. I get the staff to participate as a team.	12.80	12.06	12.47	8.75	9.75	13.5	2.950	.02
21. I prepare myself with as many facts as possible.	12.12	13.09	13.02	11.4	10.65	13.76	2.327	.05
32. I focus on the positive aspects of the issue.	11.31	12.0	12.58	10.4	9.0	12.29	3.452	.006
35. I tell staff my expectations.	12.41	11.89	12.77	8.50	10.31	12.41	2.842	.02
55. I make lists of things I need to do.	9.50	12.50	11.85	6.20	12.13	10.63	2.539	.03
79. I fulfill others' expectations of me.	10.46	9.11	7.49	12.0	7.69	7.69	2.285	.05
95. I talk it over with people who are directly involved.	13.0	14.0	13.47	13.20	10.71	12.88	3.832	.003
96. I look at my mistakes as learning experiences.	10.0	11.39	12.36	10.0	8.5	12.4	3.296	.008

[a] F indicates ratio of dispersion in the group as a whole to the dispersion of particular groupings of interest. Larger F ratios are associated with more significant differences.

was a tendency for these physicians not to use Item 21, "I prepare myself with as many facts as possible." Once again, these differences did not account logically for the stress situation—symptomatology difference.

An examination of the ten least frequently used coping strategies, by position, yielded an interesting profile for medical staff presidents in contrast to others. The data in Table 4-9 suggested that Item 3, negotiating to change deadlines, was one of the ten strategies least used by medical staff presidents, as were Item 62, instituting penalties for noncompliance, and Item 64, hiring extra personnel to cover shortages. However, these three were used more frequently by other positions. Whereas other groups tended not to agonize or become indifferent as coping strategies, medical staff presidents were somewhat more prone to do so. The lack of real power vested in this position, particularly with regard to the disciplining, hiring, and terminating medical personnel, who tended to be in more of a collegial than subordinate relationship to the medical staff president, might be factors making these individuals more prone to the negative effect of stress.

Table 4-9 reflects a coping pattern in which CEOs tended not to change their standards in the face of a stressor; neither did they agonize, get frustrated, lose tempers, drink, become indifferent, or report themselves developing physical symptoms. Furthermore, they characterized themselves as not ignoring problems, not becoming depressed, and not lessening demands. All this presents a picture of individuals comfortable in the face of challenge whose style was to jump in and deal directly with issues. It is conceivable that such individuals also might tend to deny being under stress, partly to maintain an image to themselves and others.

Interestingly, while CEOs reported infrequent use of somatization as a coping strategy, their personal stress symptom scores on the Internalized Minor Somatic (Table 4-4, supra) were significantly higher than all other positions except for medical staff presidents. It should be noted, however, that for all positions, somatization was reported as among the least frequently used strategies. Ironically, somatization is the third most common type of symptom reported by all positions. Denial may, indeed, be operative.

STRESS, SYMPTOMS, DEMOGRAPHICS

A number of statistical tests were performed with the data to examine relationships among demographic variables, perceived level of stress, and stress symptoms. Demographic variables examined included the following: sex, age, number of children, number of years in administration,

Table 4-9 Ten Least Used and Least Helpful Coping Strategies, by Position

Coping Strategy	Position					
	CEO	Assoc. Adm.	Dir. Nursing	Pres. Med. Staff	Med. Dir.	Dept. Head
3. I negotiate to change deadlines.				*		
8. I postpone dealing with the situation.		*			*	*
9. I change my standards.	*		*		*	*
17. I ask others involved to have different expectations of me.		*	*	*	*	*
26. I agonize.	*	*	*		*	*
27. I get frustrated.	*				*	
33. I find myself blocking things out of my mind.		*	*		*	
34. I lose my temper.	*	*	*	*	*	*
36. I drink.	*		*	*		
37. I become indifferent.	*	*	*		*	*
58. I terminate personnel.				*		
59. I develop physical symptoms (e.g., headaches, stomach problems).	*	*	*	*	*	*
62. I institute penalties for noncompliance to policy/procedure.				*		
64. I hire extra personnel to cover shortages.				*		
74. I take matters into my own hands even when they are not my responsibility.						*
80. I decrease my social life.		*		*		
91. I ignore the problem.	*	*	*			*
97. I lessen the demands on myself by changing what I expect of myself.	*		*	*		
99. I become depressed.	*	*			*	*

number of years in present position and facility, number of beds, number of hours worked daily, number of vacation days taken yearly, and perceived level of stress. Table 4-10 presents the significant correlations among these variables. Perceived level of stress is a global measure derived by asking respondents to assess the degree of stress they generally experienced on a scale of one to five, with one equal to almost no stress at all and five equal to high stress.

Perceived level of stress proved to be directly related to sex, as predicted: women reported they experienced more stress than men. Perceived level of stress was inversely related to the number of children the individual had. Thus, managers in this sample with no children or one child were more likely to report higher stress than those with larger families. Whether or not larger families might be an antidote to a stressful job is something that requires further empirical investigation.

The number of days of vacation taken during the year was inversely related to perceived stress, a finding that also was predicted. Managers who take more vacation time tended to perceive themselves as less stressed. While the number of hours worked per day also had been expected to show an inverse relationship, this figure did not reach significance, although it was in the predicted direction. It is possible that the limited variance among respondents in the number of hours worked (i.e., small differential in scores across respondents) accounted for this. Finally, total stress situation scores showed a strong positive relationship to perceived stress level, a construct validation of the global measure of stress (i.e., different measures of the same phenomenon are related, as would be expected.)

Stress symptom scores showed limited significant relationship to demographic variables. Scale 1, Emotional, demonstrated an inverse relationship to number of days of vacation, as did Scale 6, Depressive. Scale 1 also had a positive relationship to overall stress situation scores and seemed to reflect a general and fairly common response to stressors. Scale 2, Internalized Minor Somatic, showed a direct relationship to the number of years with the present facility. Scales 3 (External Behavior) and 5 (Unconscious) indicated a negative relationship to sex: women were less likely than men to exhibit Scale 3 or 5 symptomatology.

Coping strategy scores were found to be highly correlated with a number of demographic variables. Age and sex were positively related to the number of frequently used helpful strategies, indicating that women and older people used more such strategies. Number of children, years in administration, years in present position, years in present facility, number of beds, hours worked, and days vacation were inversely related.

An analysis of variance was performed on the ordinal variables using a breakdown procedure in order to examine their relationship with perceived

Table 4-10 Significant Correlations: Perceived Level of Stress, Stress Symptoms with Demographic Variables

	Sex	Age	Children	Years in Admin.	Years in Pres. Pos.	Years in Pres. Fac.	Number of Beds	Hours Worked	Days Vacation	Perceived Stress Level	Total Stress Situation Score	Total Coping Strategy Score
Sex		-.24673 p≤.02	-.18748 p≤.06				-.21662 p≤.05				.36666 p≤.01	.43572 p≤.001
Age			.25225 p≤.02				.20171 p≤.05				.20579 p≤.05	.47026 p≤.001
Children				.52683 p≤.001	.50498 p≤.0001	.49357 p≤.0001						-.61506 p≤.0001
Years in Administration									.21945 p≤.03			-.31308 p≤.01
Years in Present Position						.53509 p≤.0001		-.21892 p≤.05	.24910 p≤.03			-.48135 p≤.003
Years in Present Facility									.27565 p≤.01			-.38782 p≤.003
Number of Beds												-.50443 p≤.0001
Hours Worked Per Day												-.58068 p≤.0001
Days Vacation												-.24545 p≤.02
Perceived Stress Level	.1991 p≤.02		-.2844 p≤.001						-.1983 p≤.023		.4373 p≤.0001	
Scale 1									-.1710 p≤.049		.1799 p≤.032	
Scale 2						.1725 p≤.041						
Scale 3	-.1692 p≤.048									-.1924 p≤.022		
Scale 4												
Scale 5	-.1577 p≤.066									-.1821 p≤.030		
Scale 6									-.1612 p≤.064			

p indicates significance level.

level of stress, stress symptoms, total stress situation scores, and demographic variables (Table 4-11). No differences in any of the dependent variables occurred as a function of marital status or type of hospital. Professional degree and position both were significantly related to total stress situation scores and perceived level of stress. As a group, physicians reported the least perceived stress and the least total situational stress. R.N.s had the most of both, considerably more than nurses with B.S.N. and M.S.N. degrees. Whether these differences reflected pressures from within the field or from the organization could not be determined from these data but merit further investigation. (Among the trends in the nursing profession is the phasing out of R.N. two- and three-year degree programs in preference for four-year B.S.N.s. In many states this trend is accompanied by a strong status hierarchy, with R.N.s in a less favorable position vis-à-vis B.S.N.s.)

Table 4-11 Significant Differences: Perceived Stress Level and Total Stress as Function of Position and Degree

	Perceived Stress Level			Total Stress Situation Score		
Variable	$\overline{X}$[a]	F[b]	Significance	$\overline{X}$[a]	F[b]	Significance
Professional Degree						
M.D.	2.69			439.42		
R.N.	3.83			717.67		
B.S.N.	3.08			502.83		
M.S.N.	3.62	3.48	.002	614.15	3.38	.002
B.A.	3.18			514.0		
M.A.	3.41			572.14		
Ph.D.	3.0			615.0		
Other	3.72			674.16		
Position						
CEO	3.18			477.53		
Associate Administrator	3.09			513.32		
Director of Nursing	3.69	5.361	.0002	664.44	5.31	.0001
President, Medical Staff	2.17			493.0		
Medical Director	2.88			411.47		
Department Head	3.56			619.11		

[a] Indicates mean scores.
[b] Ratio of dispersion in the group as a whole to the dispersion of particular groupings of interest. Larger F ratios are associated with more significant differences.

Tables 4-12 to 4-16 present data from a series of stepwise regression analyses to determine what variables were able to predict scores on each of the stress symptom scales and total stress symptom scores. Multiple regression analysis is a statistical procedure that enables the analysis of the relationship between a dependent or criterion variable and a set of predictor or independent variables (Kim and Kohout, 1975). Included in this series of analyses were stress situation scores and all demographic variables (dummy variables were used in the regressions to permit inclusion of ordinal data). The regression equations for Scale 1 (Emotional) and for total stress symptom scores were not significant and are not presented in tabular form.

Table 4-12 indicated that seven demographic variables (including position that was discussed previously) were predictive of Scale 2 (Internalized Minor Somatic) symptom scores, accounting for 17.7 percent of the variance. Number of years in present position was directly related to Scale 2 symptomatology: the longer the individual has worked at the present facility, the greater the internalized minor somatic symptoms ($p \leq .001$).

Table 4-12 Regression Analysis: Stress Symptom Scale 2, Stress and Demographic Variables

Variables	Beta[a]	Multiple R[b]	F[c]
Years in Present Position	.26856	.19690	4.103***
Position	−.14868	.25825	2.608**
Children	.18422	.29478	3.394**
Age	−.24819	.31519	3.935***
Hours Worked Daily	.14609	.34120	2.455**
Perceived Stress Level	−.17870	.35594	2.803**
Total Stress Situation Score	.14550	.36774	1.818
Sex	−.07269	.37998	.527
Years in Present Facility	.15497	.38987	1.896*
Days Vacation	−.13549	.40323	1.988*
Marital Status	−.09241	.41265	.926
Years in Administration	.11458	.42048	.804
	df[d] = 12,109		
	Cumulative R^{2e} = .17681		

* $p \leq .05$
** $p \leq .01$
*** $p \leq .001$
[a] Indicates weight of a variable in explaining Stress Symptom Scale scores
[b] Indicates multiple correlation: Index of the magnitude of relationship between the dependent variable and all of the independent variables
[c] Ratio of dispersion (see note b, Table 4-11)
[d] Degrees of freedom associated with the F ratio used to assess level of significance
[e] Indicates amount of variance explained

Number of years in present facility also was directly related to these stress symptoms (p≤.05). Age was indirectly related, younger people tending to have more symptoms (p≤.001). Number of children and of hours worked showed a direct relationship: larger numbers of children and more hours worked were associated with increased symptomatology (p≤.01). This finding contrasted with the inverse relationship between number of children and perceived level of stress reported in the previous section. Number of vacation days had an inverse relationship: those taking more vacation days during the year tended to have fewer somatic symptoms (p≤.05). Contrary to what might be expected, perceived stress level was inversely related to somatic symptomatology (p≤.01). This finding, however, provided additional support for the denial hypothesis offered earlier to account for the discrepancy between stress situation scores and stress symptom scores among CEOs and medical staff presidents.

Table 4-13 presents the results of a regression analysis with five variables predicting stress symptom scores on Scale 3 (External Behavior), accounting for 18 percent of the variance at high levels of significance. Number

Table 4-13 Regression Analysis: Stress Symptom Scale 3, Stress and Demographic Variables

Variables	Beta[a]	Multiple R[b]	F[c]
Children	.23487	.17852	5.394 ***
Perceived Stress Level	−.21539	.22336	4.012 ***
Days Vacation	−.19461	.25847	3.874 ***
Years in Present Position	.23773	.28547	3.179 **
Age	−.32927	.34784	6.889 ***
Hours Worked Daily	.11863	.37297	1.557
Sex	−.12437	.39279	1.507
Years in Present Facility	.13340	.40337	1.398
Marital Status	−.08484	.41162	.775
Type Hospital	−.05049	.41625	.285
Years in Administration	.05723	.41934	.214
Total Stress Situation Score	.06756	.42204	.389
Position	−.04901	.42446	.271
	df[d] = 13,108		
	Cumulative R[2e] = .18017		

** p≤.01
*** p≤.001
[a] Indicates weight of a variable in explaining Stress Symptom Scale Scores
[b] Indicates multiple correlation: Index of the magnitude of relationship between the dependent variable and all of the independent variables
[c] Ratio of dispersion (see note b, Table 4-11)
[d] Degrees of freedom associated with the F ratio used to assess level of significance
[e] Indicates amount of variance explained

of children showed a direct relationship to external behavior symptoms ($p \leq .001$). Perceived stress level had an inverse relationship to Scale 3 symptoms ($p \leq .001$) offering additional support for the denial hypothesis. Days of vacation also were inversely related to Scale 3 ($p \leq .001$) as was age ($p \leq .001$). Finally, number of years in present position showed a direct relationship ($p \leq .01$) to external behavior symptoms.

It is possible that relatively young administrative (45 to 50 years of age) persons with considerable tenure with the facility and the position experienced a burnout phenomenon whereby they perceived themselves trapped in their jobs. They were too young for retirement and perhaps perceived themselves as too old to be seriously contemplating a change of jobs and/or careers.

As several CEOs stated, there comes a point where their knowledge of the job is so great that it ceases to be a challenge. The boredom becomes a source of great stress after so many years yet middle age, security, and inertia are stumbling blocks to something different. This problem is particularly acute for the fast-tracked administrator/manager who has advanced unusually rapidly and is not likely to be experienced by those in higher age brackets for whom retirement is a near reality.

It is important to note that position was not a significant predictor in this regression equation, in contrast to the significant score derived in an analysis of variance specifically examining the relationship between position and stress symptoms. It is possible that the addition of other variables obscured the relationship between position and symptomatology. Whereas significant sexual differences ($p \leq .05$) appeared in a correlation coefficient analysis between sex and Scale 3 scores, none were in this regression analysis.

Table 4-14 presents the results of a regression analysis with seven variables predicting stress symptom scores on Scale 4 (Interpersonal) accounting for 17.1 percent of the variance at high levels of significance. Sex was an important determinant of interpersonal symptoms ($p \leq .01$), with men being more likely than women to demonstrate the symptoms. Total stress situation score was predictive of interpersonal symptomatology ($p \leq .01$). (In fact, that was the only time total stress situation was predictive of stress symptomatology.) Perceived stress level again was inversely related to interpersonal symptoms ($p \leq .01$). Years in present position showed a strong positive relationship to interpersonal stress symptoms ($p \leq .001$) and days taken for vacation an inverse relationship to interpersonal symptomatology ($p \leq .001$) as did age ($p \leq .01$).

Table 4-15 presents the results of a regression analysis with five variables predicting stress symptom scores on Scale 5 (Unconscious), accounting for 15.3 percent of the variance. Of particular salience was the persistent

Table 4-14 Regression Analysis: Stress Symptom Scale 4, Stress and Demographic Variables

Variables	Beta[a]	Multiple R[b]	F[c]
Position	−.16510	.17446	3.231**
Sex	−.17382	.23994	2.962**
Total Stress Situation Score	.20909	.27729	3.724**
Perceived Stress Level	−.16782	.30101	2.458**
Years in Present Position	.25333	.32285	4.461***
Days Vacation	−.19638	.34737	3.963***
Age	−.19292	.36440	2.801**
Type Hospital	−.10537	.37891	1.242
Years in Present Facility	.11342	.38882	1.047
Children	.11673	.39902	1.344
Marital Status	−.09790	.40853	1.032
Hours Worked Daily	.06940	.41345	.532
	df[d] = 12,109		
	Cumulative R^{2e} = .17094		

** p≤.01
*** p≤.001
[a] Indicates weight of a variable in explaining Stress Symptom Scale scores
[b] Indicates multiple correlation: Index of the magnitude of relationship between the dependent variable and all of the independent variables
[c] Ratio of dispersion (see note b, Table 4-11)
[d] Degree of freedom associated with the F ratio used to assess level of significance
[e] Indicates amount of variance explained

inverse relationship between perceived stress level and stress symptoms (p≤.05). Years in administration showed a positive relationship to unconscious stress symptoms (p≤.05) yet years in present position and years in present facility did not yield significance. They did have a positive relationship to stress symptomatology, as discussed earlier. Age once more had a strong inverse relationship (p≤.001) as did days vacation (p≤.001). Children showed a positive relationship (p≤.001).

Table 4-16 presents the results of a regression analysis with two demographic variables predicting stress symptom scores on Scale 6 (Depressive), accounting for 7.7 percent of the variance. Days vacation were inversely related to depressive stress symptomatology (p≤.001) while years in present position were directly related (p≤.001).

Taken together, these tables indicated a number of very strong predictors of five different types of stress symptomatology. Consistently, days of vacation taken (inverse) and years in present position (direct) were consistent predictors of stress symptoms, while age (inverse), number of children (direct), and perceived stress level (inverse) generally were strong predictors. It is important to note, however, that the results accounted for

Table 4-15 Regression Analysis: Stress Symptom Scale 5, Stress and Demographic Variables

Variables	Beta[a]	Multiple R[b]	F[c]
Sex	−.12011	.17188	1.664
Days Vacation	−.21764	.20277	5.040***
Children	.19634	.24300	4.039***
Years in Present Position	.14793	.27091	1.271
Age	−.32044	.31050	6.801***
Perceived Stress Level	−.14544	.33121	2.318*
Years in Administration	.17044	.34917	1.999*
Years in Present Facility	.15009	.37026	1.761
Type Hospital	−.08739	.38331	.889
Hours Worked Daily	.08560	.39130	.811
df[d] = 10,111			
Cumulative R[2e] = .15312			

* p≤.05
** p≤.01
*** p≤.001
[a] Indicates weight of a variable in explaining Stress Symptom Scale scores
[b] Indicates multiple correlation: Index of the magnitude of relationship between the dependent variable and all of the independent variables
[c] Ratio of dispersion (see note b, Table 4-11)
[d] Degree of freedom associated with the F ratio used to assess level of significance
[e] Indicates amount of variance explained

Table 4-16 Regression Analysis: Stress Symptom Scale 6, Stress, and Demographic Variables

Variables	Beta[a]	Multiple R[b]	F[c]
Days Vacation	−.23854	.14178	6.194***
Years in Present Position	.18898	.21590	4.184**
Type Hospital	−.13399	.24692	2.177
Children	.13239	.27836	2.095
df[d] = 4,117			
Cumulative R[2e] = .07749			

** p≤.01
*** p≤.001
[a] Indicates weight of a variable in explaining Stress Symptom Scale scores
[b] Indicates multiple correlation: Index of the magnitude of relationship between the dependent variable and all of the independent variables
[c] Ratio of dispersion (see note b, Table 4-11)
[d] Degree of freedom associated with the F ratio used to assess level of significance
[e] Indicates amount of variance explained

only a relatively small percent of the variance (cumulative R^2) in stress symptom scores. This suggested that other factors not included in these analyses were very important in accounting for stress symptomatology.

A series of stepwise regression analyses investigating the relationship between coping strategies and symptomatology without accounting for stress situation data were performed, yielding insignificant results. This suggested that other factors must be considered. The results of the stress vulnerability measures and stress symptom analyses shed some light on this problem.

STRESS AND VULNERABILITY—IPS RESULTS

Vulnerability to Stress Index (GVSI)

The Global Vulnerability to Stress Index (GVSI) was calculated for each subject by summing scores across each of the 80 items on the Individual Profile of Stressors (IPS) questionnaire (Appendix D). This score was used to measure subjects' overall vulnerability or susceptibility to stress in 20 areas. As a global stress measure, then, this index score was compared to the subject's demographic variables and their reported stress situations, coping strategies, and stress symptoms.

Relationship of GVSI to Demographic Variables

The GVSI score was correlated using a Pearson R (measures the extent to which two interval-level variables are correlated with each other) with each of the subjects' demographic variables: city, sex, age, marital status, number of children, number of years in administration, number of years in present position, number of years at present facility, perceived stress level, number of hours worked daily, and number of days of vacation taken in the past year. These data are presented in Table 4-17. However, only two variables were significantly correlated with GVSI: perceived stress level ($p \le .001$) and days of vacation ($p \le .01$). The letter "p" refers to significance level: probability of the observed correlation being equal to or less than the figure noted. Two other variables—years in administration and years in present facility—demonstrated a trend toward significance ($p \le .09$ and .07, respectively). Both years in administration and days of vacation were inversely related to GVSI.

Relationship of GVSI with Stress Variables

The GVSI was correlated with the two other reported stress-related global scores—Total New Stress Situations (TNSS—the summation of

Table 4-17 Correlation of Global Vulnerability to Stress with Demographic Variables

Variable	r^a	Significance
City	.039	N.S.[b]
Sex	.063	N.S.
Age	.029	N.S.
Marital Status	.135	N.S.
Children	.052	N.S.
Professional Degree	.130	N.S.
Years in Administration	−.159	.09
Years in Present Position	−.012	N.S.
Years in Present Facility	.167	.07
Position	−.037	N.S.
Type of Hospital	.080	N.S.
Number of Beds	−.054	N.S.
Perceived Stress	.335	.001
Number Hours Worked	−.056	N.S.
Days of Vacation	−.234	.01

[a] Indicates magnitude and direction of correlation
[b] Not significant = N.S.

the products of frequency and degree of stress rated for each stress situation) and Total New Coping Strategies (TNCS—the summation of the products of frequency and degree of helpfulness for each coping strategy). The overall vulnerability to stress, GVSI, was highly positively correlated with the TNSS score ($r = .29$, $p \leq .001$) and negatively correlated with the TNCS score ($r = .20$, $p \leq .03$).

Relationship of GVSI with Personal Stress Symptoms

When correlated with each of the six Personal Stress Symptoms (PSS) factors and the Total Personal Stress Symptom Score (TPSS), the GVSI was highly positively correlated with each (Table 4-18). When a stepwise regression was computed to determine which of these factors or total score was most highly predictive of the GVSI score, the Total PSS score accounted for the greatest portion of the variance in the regression, with only minimal contributions from each of the scales. However, when simple correlations were compared (Table 4-19), both Total PSS and PSS Scale 1 had high correlations of .70, indicating that TPSS and PSS Scale 1 were similarly related to GVSI, as would be expected with a primary scale.

Table 4-18 Correlation of Global Vulnerability to Stress Index with Personal Stress Symptom Scores and Total Personal Stress Symptom Score

Scale/Score	r^a	Significance Level
Scale 1	.703	.0001
Scale 2	.488	.0001
Scale 3	.264	.005
Scale 4	.442	.0001
Scale 5	.304	.001
Scale 6	.438	.0001
Total PSS Score	.535	.0001

[a] Simple correlation between dependent variables and independent variable

Table 4-19 Regression of Global Vulnerability to Stress Index Using Personal Stress Symptom Scores and Total Score

Regression Variables	Simple R^a	Multiple R^b	R^{2c}	Beta^d
Total PSS Score	.70973	.70973	.50372	1.002
PSS Scale 1	.70266	.72444	.52482	.21260
PSS Scale 4	.44115	.73287	.53710	−.25151
PSS Scale 5	.30696	.73797	.54460	−.16283
PSS Scale 3	.27010	.74164	.55219	.14465
PSS Scale 2	.48850	.74310	.55897	−.16500
PSS Scale 6	.45818	.74833	.56000	−.04381

[a] Measures the degree of correlation between each independent variable and dependent variable separately
[b] Indicates multiple correlation: Index of the magnitude of relationship between the dependent variable and all of the independent variables
[c] Indicates additional amount of variability in the scores on the dependent variable, explained by the independent variables
[d] Indicates weight of a variable in explaining dependent variable

Discussion of Results

Lack of significant correlation between GVSI and demographic variables such as age, sex, professional training, and years in current position and in facility, is evidence that vulnerability to stressors may be independent from demographic variables. This evidence is in opposition to theories suggesting that environmental and maturational characteristics bear significantly upon vulnerability to stress and play an important part in predicting personal stress symptoms. In addition, the perceived frequency and intensity of stress situations (TNSS) was highly positively correlated with vulnerability (GVSI).

This relationship suggests that "state" aspects of the individual (i.e., characteristics that change over time and are situationally based) are more importantly associated with stress vulnerability than are demographic variables. This finding, combined with the lack of relationship between stress vulnerability and demographic (or "trait") variables (i.e., characteristics that are more stable aspects of the person, do not change over time, and are not situationally dependent), suggests that the more an individual perceives stress situations as more frequent and more intense, the greater the vulnerability to stressors, independent of age, sex, position, professional training, geographical location, etc.

In other words, vulnerability to stressors is related primarily to situational phenomena, as determined by the perception of stress, rather than upon maturational or environmental (trait) characteristics. Further evidence that overall stress vulnerability is directly associated with perception is the high correlation between vulnerability scores (GVSI) and the perceived degree of overall stress as rated in the 5-point scale.

The fact that frequently used and helpful coping strategies are associated with lower vulnerability to stress lends additional support to a situational concept of vulnerability. This finding also indicates that vulnerability to stress is in part a function of a person's ability to cope with stressors.

Global vulnerability to stress is highly correlated with both the personal stress symptom factors that emerged and with the overall personal stress symptoms. This finding is important because it indicates that overall vulnerability to stressors is highly related to symptoms that typically occur as a result of poorly managed stress. If vulnerability is manifested by the negative stress outcomes that appear in this research to depend upon a person's effectiveness in coping, it is reasonable to conclude that improving an individual's coping system can avert negative stress outcomes.

Thus, the ability to have available and to use effective coping strategies is an intervening variable between the number of stress situations and stress symptoms. If individuals report having frequent and intense stressors, and/or if they are highly vulnerable to them, effective coping systems may minimize the likelihood of negative stress outcomes.

These findings are important to the development of interventions designed to reduce vulnerability to stressors. The relationship of vulnerability to perceived number and intensity of stress situations suggests that vulnerability in and of itself is at least partly plastic, or amenable to modification, and that interventions can be developed to alter either the individuals' "perception" of stressors or actual encounter with them (i.e., stress prevention). Through interventions designed to alter perceptions and the stressors themselves, stress management techniques can modify overall vulnerability to stress (Munz & Wheeler, 1982).

Further research is needed to determine the relative contribution of state vs. trait characteristics in predicting individuals' overall vulnerability to stress. For example, it may be that trait components coexist with or are independent of state aspects whose relationship with vulnerability is more powerful and produces a "masking" effect.

Findings of this study suggest that any person's vulnerability to stressors may fluctuate over time as a function of the individual's (1) actual number and intensity of stressors present in the environment (both internal and external); (2) perception of this frequency and intensity of stressors; and (3) ability to cope with the stressors.

SUMMARY OF IMPORTANT FINDINGS

1. Position was related to sources and magnitude of stress, with nursing administrators reporting the greatest amount, followed by chief executive officers and presidents of medical staffs.

2. The top three stressors in terms of their magnitude were:

   - having too many time demands
   - meeting your own expectations for excellence
   - not having things done as quickly as I would like (waiting for others to participate).

3. The nature and magnitude of negative stress outcomes varies as a function of position (e.g., chief executive officers and presidents of medical staffs reported more negative stress symptoms than did nursing administrators and medical directors).

4. The frequency and intensity of sources of stress were inversely correlated with negative stress outcomes for all positions except medical directors. Thus, those reporting high situational stress (e.g., nursing administrators) tended to have low negative stress outcomes (i.e., stress-related symptomatology), while those with low situational stress (chief executive officers and presidents of medical staffs) tended to list high negative stress outcomes. It was hypothesized that acknowledging stress might, in and of itself, be a coping strategy that reduced the occurrence of the symptomatology. In addition, it was suggested that denial might be operative in positions reporting low stress and high stress symptomatology.

5. Perceived stress level was inversely correlated with negative outcomes.

6. Perceived stress level was directly related to the frequency of occurrence and intensity of sources of stress.

7. Demographic, organizational, and professional variables generally were unrelated to the sources and magnitude of stress and to stress outcomes with the following exceptions:

   • Sex generally was related to perceived stress level, and sources and intensity of stress situations. Women generally reported higher stress.

   • Age was inversely related to the magnitude and intensity of stress situations. Younger managers tended to report higher situational stress.

   • Number of children was inversely related to perceived stress level. (In light of an inverse relationship between days of vacation and perceived stress level and a direct relationship between number of children and days of vacation, it is possible the inverse relationship between perceived stress and children is in part a function of the fact that older people tend to have more children and more seniority and thus more vacation time.)

   • Days of vacation were inversely related to two stress symptom scales, Emotional and Depressive.

   • Years in present facility were directly related to stress symptom Scale 2 (Internalized Minor Somatic).

8. A limited number of coping strategies (nine) differed significantly as a function of position.

9. Total coping strategy score (frequency of helpful strategies used) was predictive of personal stress symptoms (regression analyses yielded significant findings). It might be thought that those with lower symptomatology scores would show higher coping strategy scores, reflecting increased competence in dealing with stress. To the contrary, however, those with low symptomatology scores tended to have low coping strategy scores, and vice versa. The reason for this finding is not clear and cannot be ascertained from these data. One possible explanation, however, may relate to specificity of strategy used with a particular stressor, thus requiring fewer strategies to derive a positive effect (i.e., stress reduction and low symptomatology). Those with more experience on the job conceivably would be in a better position to identify what those effective strategies would be.

10. Total coping strategy scores were related to a number of demographic, professional, and organizational variables:

- Sex and age were directly related to total coping strategy score.
- Number of children, years in administration, years in present position, years in present facility, number of beds, hours worked daily, and days of vacation were inversely related to total coping strategy scores.

11. Global vulnerability to stress index (GVSI) was directly related to perceived level of stress and to the total stress situation score (sources and magnitude of stress).
12. GVSI was inversely related to total coping strategy score.
13. GVSI was inversely related to days of vacation and not to any other demographic variables.
14. GVSI was directly related to total stress symptoms and to each of the six separate stress symptom scales.

BUILDING A MODEL

As noted earlier in this chapter and in preceding ones, a number of attempts have been made to build a comprehensive model of stress and its effects. The findings presented in this chapter offer further evidence suggesting useful components of such a model and their tentative relationship to each other. Figure 4-2 presents a model for examining the effects of job-related stress on the individual. The six components are: stressors, moderator variables, vulnerability, appraisal system (perceived stress), coping strategies, and personal consequences (stress symptoms).

As could be expected, stressors (frequency and intensity of stress situations) are positively related to perceived stress level and vulnerability yet show a weak positive relation to personal consequences (stress symptoms). Stressors show a positive relationship to selected moderator variables and an inverse relationship to a number of others.

Perceived stress level is positively related to stressors and vulnerability. Surprisingly, it is negatively related to personal stress symptoms and shows no significant relationship to coping strategies so a line linking those two is omitted from the model. Perceived stress level also is strongly positively related to some moderator variables, inversely to others.

Vulnerability is positively related to perceived stress level, stressors, and stress symptoms, as anticipated. It is related negatively to coping strategies and very weakly to moderator variables.

Coping strategies show no relationship to stress symptoms or appraisal system (perceived stress level) while an inverse relationship exists between coping strategies and vulnerability. Numerous moderator variables show

Figure 4-2 Model of Stress

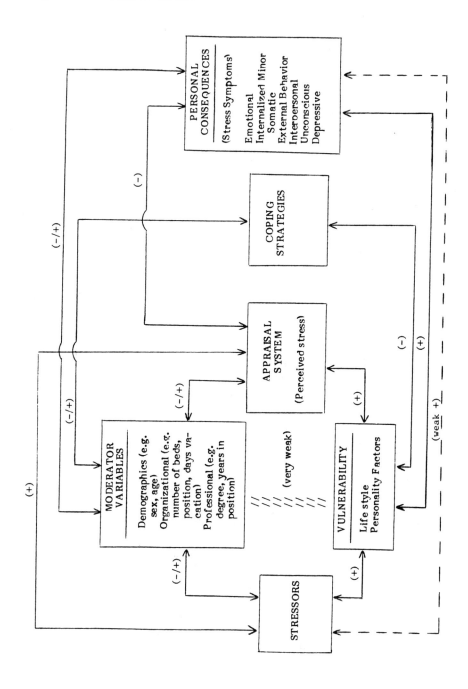

a strong inverse relationship to coping strategies while others show a positive relationship.

Personal stress symptoms surprisingly show an inverse relationship to appraisal system (perceived stress level) and a generally positive relation to moderator variables. Personal consequences (stress symptoms) are positively related to vulnerability as expected and evidence no significant relationship to coping strategies.

Chapter 5

The Physician Experience

Obviously, providers of health care are by no means immune to the effects of stress. Indeed, it could be argued that because they work in a field in which decisions often mean life or death, they are more prone to the symptoms of stress than other professionals are. While increasing attention has been paid in recent years to stress in relation to nursing service personnel, its effects on physicians generally have not been examined outside of the medical community itself. Often, those effects are not examined even by physicians themselves until they are evidenced by blatant "physician impairment" such as advanced alcoholism, drug addiction, suicide attempts, and mental disorders.

This chapter explores the physician experience, examining societal and professional expectations fostering the development of norms that tend to increase doctors' potential risks of stress. This includes the training and development of solo entrepreneurs with norms that run counter to the team approach that is being adopted increasingly in health care institutions. Defenses necessary for survival in the medical school residency experience that become key sources of later vulnerability also are identified.

Stressors evolving from the changing field of health services delivery (e.g., health maintenance vs. traditional disease models); from the expanded roles of allied health professionals, in particular nurses; from increasing regulation; and from a rapidly increasing knowledge base—all these work together to increase physician vulnerability. Finally, the inherent conflict and stress of clinical as opposed to administrative perspectives place physician managers at increased risk for the negative effects of stress.

TRAINING IN STRESS? RESIDENCY EXPERIENCE

Physician impairment has been defined as (1) incompetence, (2) maliciousness and unethical behavior, and (3) psychiatric disturbance in which competency is impaired by the doctor's failure to recognize a personal physical disability, irrational or psychotic behavior, or substance addiction. In all of these situations impairment interferes with the physician's ability to deliver quality medical care (Tokarz, Bremer, & Peters, 1979).

In recognition of the increasing incidence of resident impairment, during what have been called the most critical years in the development of doctors, the Resident Physicians Section of the American Medical Association in 1976 organized a study to develop guidelines to rehabilitate impaired physicians, in particular residents. The study soon enlarged its purview to investigate "well-being" instead of limiting itself to the failure of well-being, namely, impairment (Tokarz et al., 1979).

Those who dedicate themselves to the relief of suffering and disease also are subjected to experiences that can undermine their own well-being. For purposes of definitional clarity, well-being is defined as Sigmund Freud defined health: the ability to live and work productively, to be relatively free of excessive tension, and to be able to love and receive love fully.

What is it about the residency experience that leads not to self-fulfillment and physioemotional well-being but to life styles and the adoption of defense mechanisms that are conducive to impairment?

Residents, like other health care professionals, are not oriented to seeking help for themselves or to preventive mental health. Perhaps most importantly, they are not aware that they face increased risks of impairment and less severe negative stress effects. When help is sought it often is after a serious crisis has developed.

One source of stress lies in the nature of medical education itself. As Tokarz et al. (1979) suggest, medicine as a discipline is predominantly a cognitive enterprise that inadequately recognizes the intimate relationship between mind and body, between feelings and cognition. Residents have a long-standing history of neglecting the emotional and interpersonal aspects of their psychosocial development because of an almost total emphasis through high school and college on academic achievement to prepare for and ensure acceptance to medical school, so they are less prepared personally to deal with the challenges medical education brings (Donnelly, 1979).

With years of intimate contact with death, hopelessness, pain, and despair, physicians-to-be are likely to generate considerable emotional distress. Where educational programs have been undertaken to help these individuals turn encounters with adverse patient conditions into challenges, the outcomes in terms of professional and personal growth have been quite promising. The growth of medical school and residency programs and the increasing complexity of medical technology have been tipping the scales in favor of ever more cognitive emphasis in education.

The more human aspects of the educational experience and of medicine itself are likely to suffer because of this trend.

Overworked and feeling unappreciated, often powerless to effect change, residents are primed for increased distress and frustration. Ill equipped to cope with the very real problems they face from a developmental (e.g., young adult tasks of forming intimate relationships) and professional standpoint (e.g., consolidating their knowledge of medicine and seeing themselves as competent practitioners) they are at serious risk.

Self-Management: A Major Problem

A number of studies have revealed significantly high proportions of students in medical school unable to effectively manage their own emotions or regulate their responses to others' needs (Becker, 1961; Coombs, 1978; Donnelly, 1979; Lief, 1971; Small, 1981). Coombs (1978) notes that while most students leave medical school functioning at social and emotional levels similar to those they had when they entered, the subjective aspects of their education rarely are discussed. When the subjective aspects are handled, the approach to emotional issues generally is an intellectual one. Coombs rightly ponders the ability of physicians to provide healing and to allay others' anxieties and fears when they handle their own through suppression and denial, never fully resolving them. An earlier longitudinal study shows the development of cynicism among physicians as an adaptive response to the social and emotional demands of medical school where no structured outlets for the expression of anxieties and stress are available (Becker, 1961).

Exposure to disease, including such infections as hepatitis, viruses, and tuberculosis, obviously carries risk for physicians. Added to this is the fact that residency programs do not emphasize the importance of good nutrition and regular exercise. Chronic sleep deprivation—a common medical school and residency experience—is known to affect performance and general health. One study shows physicians' sleep deprivation reduces the ability of interns to recognize arrhythmias on electrocardiogram tests (Friedman, Bigger, & Kornfeld, 1971). In another study, sleep deprivation is associated with the onset of emotional disturbances: irritability, short-term memory loss, feelings of depression, depersonalization, and hypersensitivity to criticism (Friedman, Kornfeld, & Bigger, 1973). Chronically tired and held responsible for medical decisions they often lack the knowledge to make these young physicians find their altruism often turns to cynicism toward people in general and medicine in particular.

The problems of overwork and fatigue, resulting in sleep deprivation and its deleterious effects, seem to be unrelated to the type of program these individuals enter but are a function of the entire residency experience, particularly influenced by field of specialty. A longitudinal study (Gillanders & Heiman, 1971) shows that the similarities of three medical intern programs (county hospital, university hospital, and federal hospital) far outweigh any differences in stress among them. The study of stressors and coping strategies among hospital administrators described in Chapter 4 finds no significant differences as a function of type of hospital.

A study of job-related stress factors among a resident group in an academic medical center (Pettigrew & Raney, 1982) indicates that specialties account for the greatest differences among the stress factors while years of training and hospital play only a relatively insignificant role in accounting for stress differences. This analysis reports that obstetrics-gynecology (OB-GYN), specialty surgery, and general surgery are associated with the highest levels of stress, psychiatry and pediatrics the lowest. OB-GYN in particular is described as an environment characterized by low levels of individual autonomy evidenced by high scores on measures of nonparticipation and an authoritarian management style. Not surprisingly, low levels of job satisfaction are reported for this specialty.

The opposite characteristics are associated with psychiatry and pediatrics. (While it is tempting to generalize from this study to all residency experiences, it is important to note that these results are the outcome of a single investigation and do merit replication and elaboration before being accepted as the last word.) Of the various measures used to evaluate job stress, two are found to be the best predictors of stressful units/departments: (1) role overload (i.e., the absence of sufficient resources in time, personnel, financial, knowledge-to-perform optimally) and (2) role conflict (i.e., the presence of two or more conflicting and incompatible work demands, such as between the individual and organizational policies/procedures, etc.).

These findings concur with other research in the field. The variable most frequently associated with increased stress levels among residents is job overload. Time pressures are identified as a major source of stress by Mawardi (1979) and by Bates and Moore (1975). More specifically, Werner and Korsch (1979) and Nelson and Henry (1978) find that time pressures outside the job caused by the high work demands (i.e., not having enough time for family, friends, and personal activities) constitute a great source of stress for residents and their spouses.

Organizational Characteristics a Factor

One factor not studied specifically in the previously described research but of significance to the investigation of job-related stress among residents is that of organizational characteristics such as equipment not available when needed or a frustrating environment (Charns & Beattie, 1982). In contrast to the other studies, Charns and Beattie report no significant differences across specialty (perhaps a function of the different types of measures used to determine organizational stress). A variety of coping strategies, referred to as coordination approaches (Charns, Stoelwinder, Millen, & Schaefer, 1981), also are found useful in reducing stress. These strategies include standardization (as long as it is not used inappropriately to control behavior, when it is referred to as red tape), discussions, and meetings. Standardization is reported to be helpful in resolving ambiguity in work and in relations across departments; discussions and meetings serve the purpose of resolving problems and releasing frustration (Charns & Beattie, 1982).

To the extent that physicians are socialized to be independent (in contrast to interdependent) and are expected to act that role, an important area of human development and experience is minimized in their training. That area revolves around healthy human dependency needs that are present in various forms throughout life. Even before medical school, future physicians have been trained to develop intellectual capacities, ambitious drive, and the obsessive-compulsive personality traits associated with medical school success. In school, dependency needs are minimized by role models who epitomize the aloof, driving, intellectual physician-researcher.

There is little support for exploration and acceptance of the neglected elements of personality—the arena of dependency needs (Tokarz et al., 1979). It is the overemphasis on the independence, aloof, and driving qualities that research evidence (Thomas & Duszynski, 1974; Vaillant, Sobowale, & McArthur, 1972) suggests is the source of vulnerability for many physicians and physicians-to-be. An understanding of the dynamics of addictive disease and suicide points to the difficulties such individuals have in forming meaningful interpersonal relationships in which their dependency needs can be met. Their own denial of such needs predisposes them to avoid relationships even when they are available. Those in most need are likely to reject the relationship along with the need.

Since the mid-1970s, a number of medical schools have undertaken pilot projects for medical students and residents. These projects generally have involved support groups for students, often including their spouses, or separate programs for married students attempting to combine family and career needs. Tokarz et al. (1979) note that these programs have conveyed faculty concern for the emotional development of students but such approaches suffer from insufficient time and financial resources.

Programs for residents have become somewhat more common. Begun initially for psychiatric residents, the programs have expanded to include pediatric, internal medicine (Siegel & Donnelly, 1978), and family practice residents (Kantner & Vastyan, 1978; Werblun, Deshler, & Martin, 1977). More recently have come weekend retreats and seminars for residents, students, and spouses on stress and coping strategies. While short-term evaluations and anecdotal reports suggest that these programs are well attended and well received, there is no hard evidence documenting their effectiveness.

Given a national preoccupation with limited resources and cost containment, it is unlikely that these programs will become an integrated part of curriculum offerings unless there is research evidence documenting their effectiveness. What is needed is longitudinal research documenting the evolution of the physician; an analysis of the long-term effects of programs designed to promote well-being; an analysis of the types of coping strategies used by physicians who handle stress effectively and avoid impairment; and comparative studies examining differential stresses and coping strategies among physicians, nurses, and health administrators.

BEYOND RESIDENCY: STRESS AND IMPAIRMENT

It is generally assumed that having made it through the stressful training ritual of medical school, the physician has somehow become impervious to the detrimental effects of stress. It also is assumed that, practicing physicians, having survived that experience, find their level of stress decreases. Does the stress level really decline and are these physicians really impervious?

It could be argued that the level of stress following medical school and residency does not decline but increases. New physicians are faced with several psychological and environmental pressures:

- The medical knowledge base is expanding at an exponential rate.
- The increased reliance on technology in diagnosis leads some physicians, generalists in particular, to tend to doubt their own judgment (Reiser, 1978).
- The new physicians must contend with the real problems of establishing a practice.
- Physicians must be constantly aware of their legal liability, especially with the increase in malpractice suits—a defensive perspective that serves as a stressor.

Challenges to the professional dominance of the medical hierarchy have come from a variety of directions, bringing with them additional sources of stress. The medical community sees continuing encroachment on a territory that once was the exclusive domain of the physician as a result of the expanded roles of nursing, social work, administration, occupational therapy, physical therapy, etc. The new orientation toward holistic medicine provides another set of real challenges to traditional Western medicine and the role of the physician. Both of these challenges are explored in more detail later in the chapter.

The last and probably most important source of stress is the psychological effect of the image of physicians as omniscient beings, an idealized concept that is an integral part of every doctor's professional socialization and a myth that the health care community fosters even in light of contrary evidence.

Are physicians impervious to the negative effects of stress? Even if the medical community likes to pretend that they are, actuaries know differently. The suicide rate of women physicians is reported to be approximately four times that of the general population (Pitts, Schuller, & Rich, 1979) and the suicide rate for male physicians doubles that of males in general (Steppacker & Mausner, 1974). Divorced doctors regardless of sex have an astronomical risk: they are 13 times as likely to kill themselves as are their married colleagues (Frederick, 1979).

The effects of stress also are manifested in chronic, nonterminal but nonetheless serious problems: alcoholism, drug addiction, emotional difficulties, and marital discord. Reports suggest, for example, that narcotics abuse is more prevalent among physicians than among the general population (Anslinger, 1957; Jones, 1958; Vaillant, Brighton, & McArthur, 1970; Vaillant, Sobowale, & McArthur, 1972). In 1957 the U.S. Commissioner of Narcotics estimated that one out of 100 physicians was addicted, compared to one out of 3,000 persons in the general population (Anslinger, 1957). In 1958 the California State Board of Medical Examiners estimated that between 1 percent and 2 percent of all California doctors abused narcotics (Jones, 1958). Another study (Winick, 1961) put the incidence even higher: 100 times that of the general population. Pearson (1975) reports increasing evidence of considerable emotional disturbance among physicians. In particular, he sees alcoholism and drug addiction as ''leading occupational hazards.'' He suggests that 1 percent to 2 percent of physicians nationally are dependent on narcotics. Unfortunately, current national figures on the incidence and prevalence of these disturbances among physicians are lacking (American Medical Association, 1983). Figures that are available from state and county medical boards frequently suffer from underreporting.

The data on marital discord are inconclusive. Studies report that divorce and separation may be equal to or less prevalent among physicians in comparison to the general population (Garvey & Tuason, 1979; Rose & Rosow, 1972; Taubman, 1979). It should not be assumed, however, that physician marriages therefore are "better" or less stressful. There may be important emotional, social, and financial elements that encourage these unions to remain legally intact regardless of their quality. Large settlements and expensive court battles may represent a barrier to legal separation and divorce, as may social pressures to present a "happily married" facade. To the extent that remaining in a poor marriage is more stressful than divorce, physicians may be subject to a high degree of stress.

What about the behavioral manifestations of stress that do not fall neatly into these predetermined problem categories? More specifically, what about the brief episodes of grossly inappropriate, often aberrant behavior that are whispered about in hospital corridors, rarely reported in the literature, and increasingly are turning up in malpractice suits? In psychiatric parlance, this broad group of behaviors would be labelled acute situational reactions. For simplicity, they are referred to here as "snapping."

An increasing number of court cases suggests that snapping is a serious problem, and growing (Springer, 1980; 1982). Examples of snapping include: the proctologist who, upon finishing surgery, initials the buttocks of his young female patient; the anesthesiologist who has sexual intercourse with a patient under anesthesia; the surgeon who throws a knife in the operating room; the internist who makes rounds at unusual hours dressed in unusual clothes.

It is difficult to determine the extent of physician impairment or snapping and how it compares to that of the nonphysician population. Research on the problem, while more advanced than that of physician stress, is in its infancy. In addition, it is difficult to compare results across studies to derive any meaningful sense of the problem: terms examined have been defined imprecisely or differently and populations studied have been different, hence results cannot be generalized from one group to another. Finally, most of the studies have used small, nonrandom samples that make generalizability to the population of physicians as a whole tenuous at best, a point noted by others as well (Krakowski, 1982; Von Brauchitch, 1976).

Despite these serious problems in investigation, the research does yield two significant findings. The problem of physician impairment, regardless of its incidence in comparison to nonphysician populations, exists and must be confronted by those in medicine and in the health delivery system. It is apparent that the medical community has addressed the problem:

witness the American Medical Association's Fourth (1980) and Fifth (1982) Conferences on the Impaired Physician, a variety of treatment programs across the country, case-finding activities of state medical boards, and numerous articles in professional journals. The absence of any similar concern in the health administration community is noteworthy, especially so since physicians play such a critical role in the delivery system.

VULNERABILITY: THE PERSON OR PROFESSION?

It often is assumed that the problems of drug addiction, alcoholism, marital instability, and emotional illness are occupational hazards. This assumption, however, bears critical examination, for it provides only a partial understanding of the problem. In a longitudinal study covering 30 years, 47 physicians were compared with 79 matched controls in nonmedical occupations. Extensive interviews and survey data indicate that the presence or absence of such problems is more strongly associated with life adjustment before medical school than to the practice of medicine itself (Vaillant, Sobowale, & McArthur, 1972). These findings are not new. A study of medical students seeking psychiatric help indicates that 40 percent had histories of emotional difficulty before entering medical school (Hunter, Lohrenz, & Schwartzman, 1964). Anecdotal reports indicate similar historical data. A review of the literature suggests the existence of a "preaddictive personality" and role strain associated with becoming or being a physician as factors related to addiction (Borsay & Leff, 1977).

It may well be that the physician "virtues" become "vices" for only certain types of individuals, not for physicians in general. Vaillant et al. (1972) report that the physicians at risk appear to be those who have experienced emotionally barren childhoods. Their giving to others as professionals becomes a problem for these physicians when they find themselves giving more than they themselves have received. Compounding the difficulty is their personal inability to ask directly for help and the reluctance of many others in the health care community to give it.

THE ROLE OF THE HEALTH CARE SYSTEM

In several ways, the health care system colludes, albeit unconsciously, in setting up the conditions under which snapping is likely to occur and is likely to remain unreported. Most obvious is the perpetuation of the infallibility syndrome whereby physicians are socialized in their training to presume an air of being constantly in control and in charge. Being able to say "I don't know," "I'm not sure," or "I'm stressed and overloaded" is not acceptable in an atmosphere in which behavioral norms emphasize compulsive overachievement, low trust, and aloof interpersonal relationships (Tokarz et al., 1979). Little, if any, allowance is made for limitations on individuals' stress-handling capabilities during their training. The unspoken assumption during physician training is that those who cannot stand up under the stresses are professionally unsuited to go on. It is implicitly unacceptable to admit to limitations.

This is perhaps the critical point. Given this crucial part of the professional ethos, it is not surprising that neither the hospital organization nor anywhere in the health care system is there a formal structure or mechanism to which physicians can turn for assistance with stress management. The problem is double-edged, stemming from the professionals' reluctance to participate in such programs and the system's reluctance to involve them. How can God ask for help?

(An interesting case points to the seriousness of the problem. A group of residents at a well-known teaching hospital met informally to discuss professional and personal stress with a small group of medical school faculty. When the faculty members began sharing their own personal difficulties with the group, the residents became anxious and insisted that their elders leave and resolve their problems elsewhere.)

Residents are worked under time pressures without consideration for their psychological well-being, to say nothing of their physical well-being and the effect on their professional performance. Residents are expected to survive, and generally succeed. However, it is the very skills that enable them to survive that become the source of their vulnerabilities—skills that the health care community and physicians themselves learn to value highly. As Vaillant (1980) aptly notes, vulnerabilities among physicians do not arise because they have been so weak but rather because they have been so strong.

Four virtues prized by physicians and the health care community that make doctors vulnerable are: (1) altruism, (2) independence, (3) belief in their own judgment, and (4) emotional self-control (Vaillant et al., 1972; Vaillant, 1980). Altruism in its extreme becomes a denial of a doctor's own needs. A person who is feeling badly asks, "What can I do for someone else?" Under stress, physicians learn to care for others more assiduously and then, perhaps, write their own prescription. "Putting the patient first" is a related value. The "selfless" physicians suffer stoically, are rewarded for such behavior, and learn not to share their own need for help with colleagues.

Independence and mastering their own needs for dependence also are rewarded by patients and nonphysician colleagues who find security as their dependency needs are met by the emotionally strong and independent doctors. Despite protestations to the contrary, there is some evidence that nurses who deny their dependent status vis-à-vis physicians are fearful of independence (Numerof, 1978a). A commonly identified source of stress among nurses is *not* having physicians available to make decisions and thus being forced to act independently (Numerof & Abrams, 1983).

While independence is, indeed, a virtue, as a reaction formation to real dependency needs it can become a weapon of self-destruction if the doctors then choose to nurture themselves and calm their anxieties with alcohol and drugs. Belief in one's own judgment exacerbates the problem as the self-medicating physician says, "I can prescribe for myself. I need not question my own judgment in these matters." Physicians' ability to dissociate their feelings from their work is essential in helping them deal with contagious disease, ignoring the fact that it could happen to them. Dissociation becomes deadly when the "It can't happen to me" protection is applied to increasing alcohol and drug consumption.

The unspoken attitude toward physicians' ability to handle stress is further reflected in the reactions of administrators, peers, and nurses, in particular. In numerous instances, administrators and health care professionals have attempted to ignore and/or deny the existence of seriously impaired physicians. The implications of this are quite profound when it is realized that impaired physicians are in a critically advanced stage of difficulty. While the reasons this has not been recognized have not been investigated empirically, several hypotheses that merit testing can be generated.

For example, is there an economic incentive that increases the reluctance of hospital administrators and those under them to report physicians' aberrant behavior? In other words, do administrators fear an economic setback if stressed or impaired physicians are identified in the institution? Hospitals' fear of losing patients of such doctors may be real, yet evidence to support the belief is lacking. Ironically, anecdotal reports from the patients of some impaired (alcoholic and drug dependent) physicians suggest that these clients are supportive and understanding and want their doctor to receive help. In the final analysis, however, the risk of legal liability far outweighs any potential loss of revenue through departing patients.

Does nonreporting occur because of a misplaced belief among colleagues and other professionals that they are serving these physicians by protecting them? Does nonreporting occur because nonphysicians do not know how or are afraid to report physicians in trouble? Do such professionals share in the myth, "It doesn't happen to doctors, does it?" Finally, is the tendency to deny physician stress and impairment a manifestation of the health care community's desire to maintain the myth that someone (namely, physicians) is invulnerable?

Regardless of why, the health care community has been reluctant to report impairment, with its increased legal liability. However, administrators and health care providers are increasingly being forced to take action and remove impaired physicians from their professional responsibilities.

CHANGING VALUES AS A SOURCE OF STRESS

As discussed in Chapter 3, values play an important role in all aspects of human existence. What people value, they tend to see as how things ought to be. Values become problems when people forget that they reflect personal judgments about intrinsic worth and, instead, assign the attribute of worthwhileness to the issue or object of discussion. Thus, a discourse is likely to become heated as participants argue the "real" or inherent worth of various actions or objects as facts rather than as alternatives associated with different personal values.

Through the experience of professional socialization each person in the health community is taught, and to various degrees internalizes, professional values—that is, what this chosen profession deems important with regard to ideas, norms of behavior, attitudes, and beliefs. This professional socialization occurs on top of a base of personal socialization that influences behavior. The latter even affects how individuals interpret and use the professional experience.

A pluralistic society provides many value perspectives that create a dynamic whole. However, that very diversity also creates problems, for with it comes variation in value orientation. What A believes to be important is not necessarily what B regards highly. If what A and B each values cannot be translated into real action, then they will compete with each other in an attempt to have their own value preference realized. At times of particularly scarce resources, value conflicts are likely to become more pronounced. Unless people understand the need to give credence to the different values of others, it will be difficult to negotiate and compromise. The task of the leader, manager, or administrator is to help many As and Bs—whether they be groups or individuals—to realize their value perspectives, clarify them if necessary, and negotiate differences in an atmosphere of mutual problem solving and trust.

CLINICAL VS. ADMINISTRATIVE PERSPECTIVES

One of the most obvious conflicts over values in health care organizations involves the difference between clinical and administrative perspectives. Clinicians, regardless of their type of training, are prepared for direct service. Their personal involvement with patients is of primary importance so they must focus some attention on developing rapport with these persons. This necessitates some flexibility in their approach to individual patients. They are likely to hold values that emphasize such qualities as caring, selflessness, empathy, kindness, and warmth. They also are likely to perceive those who do not share this value system or engage in these activities as cold, uncaring, or mechanical. On the other hand, professional administrators, concerned as they must be with employee productivity, the economic viability of the organization, and the politics of managing it, are likely to value power and influence, economic decision making, and rational or procedural determinations.

Harry Levinson, a well-known management theorist, has noted these differences in orientation as well. In fact, Levinson (1976) suggests that the administrator, whether clinical or lay, must have strong economic motivations and must be prepared to take firm positions. The executive's orientation must be one of practical utility—concern with rules and procedures even though clinicians and clinically oriented personnel may be "managerially unconcerned." The flexibility and warmth of the clinicians are necessary in patient care; administrators' systematic, orderly, "tight" approach works well in the managerial role. Switching these around, however, may have undesirable consequences. The clinician's process orientation may prove disastrous for the administrator while the tightness of the executive's approach could undermine the clinician's therapeutic effectiveness.

Unfortunately, differences in value orientation generally are not understood in terms of their varying utility. When they are understood, they usually are deprecated. As Levinson notes, one group dismisses the other with character labels, a powerful and common means of putting people down in professional circles. Even in graduate schools, students with administrative training perceive those with clinical training as "soft," "unfocused," and "too concerned with the personal and social issues of patients and employees." Clinically trained students perceive their administrative counterparts as "rigid," "cold," "product oriented," and "unconcerned with human issues and preoccupied with economics."

At both the student and real world levels, many attempt to deal with such disparities in the same manner as the foreign traveler who, unable to speak the language, shouts louder in the hopes of getting needs met. Only when each participant refrains from trying to prove that a personal perspective is right and all others are wrong can they begin to understand why each has come to view the world the way that person does. With a genuine desire to understand rather than to accuse, both parties can see how their perspectives complement each other in terms of the whole system in which both are essential.

Unfortunately, the disparity in value orientations creates serious conflicts in health care organizations, mainly because people have difficulty understanding what is psychologically important to others' roles, functions, and personalities. This dilemma poses real problems for physician administrators.

ISSUES FOR THE PHYSICIAN AS MANAGER

Physicians who become medical administrators in health care organizations (predominantly hospitals) typically do so after clinical practice. Generally, they are between 40 and 60 years of age with almost no management training prior to assuming the position. Where they have had previous training, it often has involved only an isolated seminar or two that may or may not have addressed the particular management needs of this group. Like so many other clinically trained administrators, the legitimacy of physician managers as executives is based largely on their demonstrated ability at carrying out clinical tasks rather than on understanding administrative processes.

However, not all who report to physician administrators grant those persons administrative legitimacy. The doctor remaining exclusively in clinical practice is likely, in both public comments and private conversations, to view physician managers as individuals who could not make it in medicine. If not regarded as lower in status and respect among clinical colleagues, the physician administrators may be cast in the role of Benedict Arnold—traitors for having "sold out" to the organization. Given that one of the hallmarks of professional practice in medicine in the United States has been antiorganization and anticontrol, this attitude is not surprising.

Under these circumstances, physician administrators are likely to feel ambivalent in their view of the importance of the executive role as opposed to clinical practice. As a result, where role ambiguity is high and staff conflict exists, the situation often is resolved by power plays, with favor bestowed on the individual(s) who appears to hold power (e.g., the ability to bring in more patients) regardless of the legitimacy of the issue.

Given the physician administrators' clinical background and typical lack of integrated management training, their approach as executives is likely to be oriented to crisis management, as opposed to long-range and strategic planning; independent, as opposed to team directed; control-directed, authoritarian under conditions of stress and conflict, as opposed to conflict negotiator.

The individuals who hold these positions are further hampered, even when they do take advantage of recent management development offerings specifically designed for physicians, by a number of organizational factors. Unless physician managers of departments (e.g., emergency services, internal medicine, pediatrics) are socialized to view themselves as hospital executives, medical directors are likely to be isolated, lacking a critical mass of interested colleagues with whom to share knowledge and concepts. The ability to translate new knowledge into behavioral change is undermined to a large extent without the opportunity to exchange ideas with colleagues. In addition, there is the very real frustration of having to work with department heads who are less sophisticated managerially.

To the extent that spans of control are large and unwieldy, physicians' effectiveness in the administrative role is diminished. Where actual administrative time is less than 50 percent, with clinical practice maintained for the remaining 50 percent, serious role conflict continues. On the other hand, many medical directors who do not maintain any clinical role experience a reduction in personal job satisfaction because of the loss of patient contact. Still others, committed to medical administration, find themselves having to convince the nonclinical managers of the institution of their need to be included in general matters of concern to the facility as a whole and not merely consulted in matters of clinical importance. Add to this the individualistic nature of the medical staff itself and the stresses inherent in the position become all too clear.

As the data reported in Chapter 4 indicate, among the ten most stressful situations for medical directors are the challenge of having an active and outspoken staff that states its demands and wants action right away, dealing with power problems or infighting among staff members, having a staff with unreasonable expectations, and having to resolve interdepartmental conflicts and jealousies. In the words of one seasoned medical director with more than 20 years of administrative experience: "The most stressful situation in medical administration is the increasing conflict (in medicine) of vested self-interests of turf, money, privileges, and referral patterns, all affecting the quality of care delivered to the public." The ability to make the best decision for the good of the hospital and to be prepared for the ensuing uproar requires enormous self-confidence and clarity, the strength to remain firm, and an awareness of the issues and identities of the various turfs.

At the same time, the physician administrator is most concerned about clinical matters. As noted for both medical directors and medical staff presidents, learning that patients and families receive less than the best possible care ranks among their top ten sources of stress. (While this is of great concern to other hospital managers as well, it does not rank among their top ten.) When this situation does occur, it frequently is handled directly and openly with the patients and families—working not to deceive them and attempting to negotiate a reasonable settlement of the issue for the future.

The attempt in the short run is to leave those affected feeling as good about the situation as possible. In the long run there is pressure on the organization "to avoid all mistakes." Often, public expectations for more services than the institution can or wants to provide become a source of stress for the medical director. In such cases the approach that seems to work best is an open and direct one—letting the public know what is being done already, partly through a proactive stance of greater visibility in the community. Obviously, this pertains directly to marketing, a newly accepted and critically important function of the hospital but one that historically has been incompatible with clinically concerned and trained professionals, creating another potential area of stress and conflict.

To make matters even more complex, the physician manager today exists in an era of organizationally shifting values with regard to who dominates the institution. Whereas physicians' dominance was uncontested not too many years ago, their control over new programs, outpatient facilities, other professions, and administration itself no longer is total. The expanded knowledge base and training of nursing and health care administration, for example, challenge the authority of medical personnel in nonmedical areas as well as in matters of protocol.

To the extent that the medical director has staff members who still expect to be handed the day's charts immediately upon emerging from the elevator, there will be serious value conflicts to resolve. Nor will the outcome be "fire the nurse" in the case of the nurse who legitimately and appropriately questions the physician's orders. (The expanded nurse role and its implications are discussed in Chapter 6, the implications of shifting organizational dominance in Chapter 7.)

Obviously, to survive both personally and organizationally, the physician administrator (or, for that matter, any administrator) must have excellent skills in conflict resolution and a strong background in management theory and structure (Numerof, 1982). Fortunately, the American Academy of Medical Directors has been founded (in 1974), specifically to provide medical administrators with both theoretical frameworks and practical skills in such areas as strategic planning, performance appraisal, program development, decision making, communications, discipline, and conflict resolution.

HOLISTIC VS. DISEASE MODELS OF MEDICINE

One of the most important current concerns in the health care sector focuses on the values of health maintenance and the treatment of disease. The health maintenance model often is associated with the nursing profession, the disease model with the medical profession. Unfortunately, such generalizations lead to misunderstandings and a blurring of the profound implications of the two approaches to human health. Not all nurses subscribe to the health maintenance approach, nor all physicians to a purely disease model. The fact that there is controversy within each profession adds to the challenges facing both the medical director and nursing administrator. The issues from both perspectives have implications for medicine, nursing, and the institution as a whole. The dominant features of the models are explored next.

The Vitalistic Approach

In the last decade or so, health care professionals and others have described the evolution of a new model for medicine. At the 1977 Conference of the East-West Association of the Healing Arts, the new model was called "vitalistic," in contrast to the old "mechanistic" model that viewed the human system as a collection of separate, distinct parts. With the mechanistic model, physicians prescribed medicine to attack the diseased part. The patient went to an organ or disease specialist and had the part or ailment analyzed and dissected. Laboratory reports and studies were used for diagnosis and were treated as "the facts." Patient reports of subjective experience were ignored or denied.

Within the last ten years the medical profession has been rediscovering that isolating the disease from the person does not necessarily bring about a cure. The vitalistic model, in contrast with the mechanistic model, involves patients with their illness and treatment. It views the person as a living being with properties that can help reverse or dispel disease. It also recognizes the anatomic, mental, and biochemical differences among people. The point is that pathological conditions can be treated more effectively if individual differences are taken into account.

The new model has several ground rules that tend to be at odds with the current social life style and cultural norm, which emphasize the isolation and study of specific disease entities. The new model embraces five significant points:

1. Symptoms must be viewed as part of a continuing complex system of interlocking processes. Diseases are not simply the consequence

of invasion by a particular disease entity. Rather, they are the end of a long chain of events involving life style, nutrition, and psychological and environmental stress. Treatment of diseases must take all these factors into account.

2. Bodies generally attempt to heal themselves and generally succeed.
3. Denying symptoms is dangerous.
4. Patients are an excellent source of treatment and diagnosis.
5. Training, in the form of self-knowledge, care, and stimulation, is better than medical treatment.

Essentially, this vitalistic model says that suppressing symptoms of disease without examining their root causes leads to confusion, not cure. Symptoms are seen as warnings that something is amiss and needs tending. They themselves are sometimes partial solutions to the problem. If symptoms remain after medication or other treatments, they must be heeded.

People's bodies are interested in maintaining health, not disease. Being sick is a way of insisting that individuals slow down, regardless of whether or not they want to continue the relentless pursuit of career and advancement. A "cold" should not be handled through cold pills that mask symptoms. The body may then proceed to contract the flu and, if it is still ignored, pneumonia, or perhaps hepatitis. An example of this is the stereotypical Type A heart patient who anxiously taps a foot during the checkup, impatient to return to the stressful life style that caused the heart attack in the first place.

The vitalistic approach holds that when medical professionals ignore patients' perceptions of their difficulties and adhere strictly to laboratory reports, they are responding more like veterinarians than physicians and nurses. Medical personnel are "coaches," not "interveners," with regard to patients and their well-being. Ultimately, only a patient knows whether or not a given procedure will work.

In discussion with the author, physicians and administrators have predicted that within the next 50 years Western medicine will be taken off its pedestal and placed in perspective alongside Eastern medicine, with its emphasis on holism, nutrition, and prevention. A physician/administrator in a Philadelphia acute care hospital is of the opinion that Western medicine, although useful and successful in traumatic situations, reconstructive surgery, and the like, has failed abysmally in treating degenerative disorders, including cancer.

The limits to the curative value of traditional Western medicine are sharply noted by another physician: "Fully 80 percent of illness is functional, and can be effectively treated by any talented healer who displays warmth, interest, and compassion regardless of whether he has finished grammar school. Another 10 percent of illness is wholly incurable. That leaves only 10 percent in which scientific medicine—at considerable cost— has any value at all" (Fuchs, 1974).

The Holistic Approach

These physicians are not alone in taking this perspective. Nor are they alone in recognizing the caution or outright disdain with which their ideas are received in more traditional medical circles. Holistic medicine is regarded by the establishment as a threat to medicine from two perspectives:

1. The focus on prevention and health places the medical profession in a more collaborative relationship with other fields, including nursing and nutrition, that long have emphasized these concerns. Thus holism has the effect of radically restructuring the medical hierarchy by shifting concern away from disease processes and medical specialties that treat parts of people rather than the whole person.
2. The concept of holistic health necessitates a shift, not only in professional orientation but also in personal "Weltanschauung." Holism assumes more patient awareness of personal feelings and the impact of general well-being than does traditional Western medicine. Such sensitivities are not emphasized during professional, or even personal, socialization. Both changes can be seen as threatening, especially by people who have maintained a fairly high degree of status and prestige by virtue of the fact that they were perceived as having control over others' lives.

When the locus of control is seen as internal and the patient takes charge of the condition impinging on well-being, there are dramatic power shifts. No longer is the doctor imbued with power and so, in that sense, is "demoted." But being demoted from the burden of unrealistic expectations and the responsibility for others' lives may be a blessing in disguise. This burden may be a factor in the high rate of drug addiction and suicide among physicians. By making the physician a partner in holistic health care, patients in many respects assume control of their own lives while simultaneously reducing the doctor's burden.

One physician described his personal commitment to holistic medicine as the key to his awareness that he had control of his life. Faced with the news that he had terminal cancer and 24 months to live, he realized that no one but he had the power to reverse the degenerative process working on his body. It was a new awareness and one that dramatically changed his life. He then actively concerned himself with nutrition, exercise, and meditation, and continued with his work with great vigor. Faced with the news of impending death, he approached life with new energy, acting and feeling more alive in the process. It is five years later, and he is still vigorous, with an active practice.

Individuals who face the inevitability of their own death and who take personal responsibility for their life are bound to have great bearing on their physical well-being. No longer can they be content to take their bodies to someone else on whom they depend for a cure. Ultimately people are the masters of their own bodies. Physicians, trained to help people in caring for their bodies, are consultants and are the experts to whom people turn for help to fit broken bones together. It is becoming increasingly apparent and accepted that the neat and tidy boundaries of the medical profession cannot contain the health problems with which society today is forced to cope. The biomedical establishment also cannot expect sin-glehandedly to provide the resources for meeting these issues.

The replacement of the biomedical model by a sociomedical model, a health maintenance orientation, a vitalistic model, or whatever else it may be called, has important implications for the administration of health serv-ices. These range from consumer education, policy determination, and planning to the actual management of various professionals directly engaged in the delivery of health care.

The impact of the biomedical model has been profound and it has been long lasting. Since the beginning of this century it has greatly influenced the public's way of perceiving health and disease. This influence has permeated the thinking and actions not only of professionals and institu-tions but also of consumers with regard to health and disease. One of the problems associated with giving up or replacing this model is that this forces everyone to face some of the hard medical and social realities that the model has obscured from view.

Dana (1978) notes that the biomedical model has kept the public from the following facts:

- Disease is of a long-term nature, with actual or potential loss of personal freedom and control.
- Science and technology have limited capacities to control, modify, or eradicate major life-threatening illnesses.
- Illnesses are associated with personal and family problems and often have unexpected social causes (as well as social consequences).
- The needs of many "walking sick" remain unmet.
- Biomedical benefits and services are inequitably allocated and distrib-uted among various parts of the population.

Where the biomedical model provides the "security" of relying on hard statistical data from "objective" physical findings, alternatives such as the vitalistic and holistic models do not. Neither do they protect society from factors that are troublesome to quantify. Furthermore, professional boundaries were more or less clearly defined under the biomedical model but are becoming increasingly blurred under the new approaches. Obviously, this creates new challenges for health care administrators.

Perhaps most critical is that acceptance of a new "Weltanschauung" with regard to health and disease inevitably leads to changes in the distribution of power in health care delivery. It is an uncontested fact that physicians have been in power. They have controlled the health system totally and have been accepted in that role—at least until recently.

Chapter 6

The Nurse Experience

Health care is a service-intensive industry in which organizational climate and morale have significant effects on quality and costs in the institutional setting as well as on employee stress. An important determinant of morale for any professional group is its members' perception regarding their role definition and their autonomy within that role. A significant discrepancy between desired autonomy and perceived limits is likely to lead to job dissatisfaction, interpersonal friction between professionals, higher absenteeism, reduced quality of patient care, and increased stress. Nurses comprise a central component of service delivery in hospitals and their experience with these issues has far-reaching effects throughout the health care industry.

During the last dozen or so years the literature in and about this profession has reflected significant concern with the status of nurses and the evolution of their profession into new and broadened areas of competence. Perhaps seizing the opportunities presented by the women's movement, nurses, a predominantly female group, undertook to challenge their traditional role as physicians' handmaidens and their having been defined by Etzioni (1969) as a "semiprofession." Essentially, nursing's mission, role, responsibilities, and scope of practice have been questioned. Such questioning, while important, is also a significant source of stress.

With increasing frequency, professional autonomy has been recognized as an issue of importance by nurses as well as by other professional groups. Reasons typically cited for the increasing range of nurses' decision-making responsibility include cost-effectiveness, recognition of increased professional competence, and maximizing the utilization of other health care professionals, specifically physicians. Toward these ends, some institutions have taken steps through staff development programs to encourage nurses to assume broader responsibility. At the same time, and even in these same facilities, some nurses complain of institutional intransigence on this issue. This apparent discrepancy between desired and perceived limits on autonomy has quality and cost implications for the delivery of care. More pertinent to the focus here is the potential impact on perceived stress among nurses.

One explanation for the discrepancies between expressed desire for and perceived limits on professional autonomy is a consequence of two paradoxical factors: (1) nurses' increasing professionalization and concomitant desire for increased scope and recognition and (2) the fact that to a large extent they may be a self-selected group with relatively low needs for power and control. Nurses' professional expectations have perpetuated norms that foster passive dependence and organizational and interprofessional factors that subvert autonomy. Against this background is the picture of personal and professional stress despite an expanded role.

PROFESSIONAL SOCIALIZATION AND NURSES' ROLE

Historically, the role of the nurse has been one of only indirect authority and power in caring for the sick. The physician has been identified as the chief authority, with the nurse in a supportive role. The importance of the role was the nurse's ability to keep the physical environment pleasant while looking out for the comfort and emotional well-being of the patient.

Nurses have been socialized for the most part to assume the traditional feminine passive-dependent role. The negative impact of this socialization is especially significant when it is realized that it has operated at both personal and professional levels. Research has shown that the passive-dependent stance is counterproductive to nurses' self-esteem, professional integrity, and ability to perform their work effectively (Bardwick & Donovan, 1972; Bullough, 1975; Hooyman & Kaplan, 1976; Jourard, 1971; Numerof, 1978a). Furthermore, such behaviors result in poor peer relationships and intrastaff friction. These in turn foster a poor organizational climate in which patient care, particularly from a psychosocial perspective, is likely to suffer (Nuckolls, 1974). Finally, access to positions of leadership and influence has been affected negatively.

Even within the traditionally female-dominated human service fields (social work, nursing, and teaching), sex stratification exists, with women concentrated in lower level positions (Chafetz, 1972; Epstein, 1970; Scotch, 1972; Williams, Ho, & Felder, 1974). This is explained by some as reflecting the fact that the traditional sex role for women does not prepare them adequately for leadership roles (Bardwick & Donovan, 1972). The traditional qualities of dependence, passivity, fragility, nonaggression, noncompetitiveness, yielding, inability to risk, and high emotionality generally are considered poor qualities for leadership.

It often is assumed that if the opportunity were available, women would move into administrative and supervisory positions. While they have done so in increasingly greater numbers, men tend to move more rapidly into such posts even in the traditionally female-dominated occupations (Hooyman & Kaplan, 1976). In a similar vein, Lynn, Vadem, & Vadem (1975) note that nurses were uneasy with male entrants into the profession, fearing possible usurption of the higher positions. This suggests that personality and socialization issues may prevail despite nurses' opportunity to achieve and assume leadership positions. (This is discussed in more detail later in the chapter.)

Bem and Bem (1972) note that women are socialized to believe they cannot and should not make important decisions. These beliefs may become an internal barrier to entering leadership positions or to being effective after attaining a higher level of responsibility (Hooyman & Kaplan, 1976). Barnard (1971) finds that women are uncomfortable exerting authority vis-à-vis others, especially when their actions may involve significant resources or influence over people. The nurturing, soothing model of "I'll take care of everything" is counterproductive to the delegation of responsibility and enhancement of staff accountability. These factors are likely to produce stress not only for the nurse manager but for those who report to this individual as well.

The Experience of Training

As with any professional training, education in this field contributes to nurses' definitions of their functions, sphere of influence, and involvement in their work. Except for nurses educated since the mid-1970s in more progressive programs, a great majority of them received a strong indoctrination in rigid authoritarian, hierarchical relations modeled along military lines. For example, students were expected to stand up in the presence of other students with greater seniority who, in turn, stood for teachers. Teachers and students alike were expected to stand up in the presence of physicians. Questioning of instructors for clarity often was regarded as heresy. On the other hand, not knowing the answers to questions was unacceptable. Questioning the instructor's line of reasoning was unheard of. Dress codes and living regulations were enforced rigidly. Breaches frequently resulted in suspensions.

Such training has profound psychological ramifications that directly affect professionals' self-image and work. Intimidation breeds resentment and increases fear when dealing with authority figures. The rigid structure leads to and perpetuates ritualized, stereotyped, unnatural behaviors that

subvert and suppress creativity while reinforcing dependence and insecurity.

If the nurses' anger cannot be voiced directly, it will be expressed
indirectly in rebellious acting-out and passive-aggressive behaviors.
Aggressive energy can add a vital dimension to the process of living when
expressed constructively and can enlarge the depth and authenticity of
personal and interpersonal relationships and experiences. Aggression that
is prohibited from surfacing in open, personal ways becomes diverted onto
scapegoats and enemies and is expressed in stereotypes, undermining
interpersonal and interprofessional communications. A paranoid, stress-
inducing climate emerges as the blocked aggression is projected onto
others, who then become more fearsome than they really are. Nurses
thereby become more vulnerable because they lose their ability to gauge
and control their impact on others and to read the emotional messages
others transmit.

The classic outcome of this process is exemplified by the nursing administrator who, tired of having her staff beaten down by physicians, contacted
a consultant to "help arm her nurses to do battle with the docs." Under
the camouflage of the victim position, the lack of cohesion within nursing
was blurred and responsibility for serious hierarchical and communication
problems within the profession was avoided. The enemy was out there.
Only when the group was able to recognize its own role and history that
had perpetuated an untenable position could progress be made (Numerof,
1978a).

Jourard (1971) suggests that the rigid, stereotyped bedside manner learned
in school and used by nurses in an attempt to help patients feel more
relaxed actually interferes with therapeutic aims because the clients are
not likely to express their concerns. These concerns—anxiety, questions
about illnesses, and information about sensitivity to drugs and medical
procedures—are directly related to the patients' condition. If expression
of the nurse's whole self is blocked by lack of empathy, direct squelching
of expression, avoidance, or personal threat, all of which are expressed
in a rigid demeanor, then diagnostic and therapeutic endeavors will be
hampered and the professional will experience stress.

Jourard (1971) refers to such stress as self-alienation, the result of roles
and/or self-concepts that exclude too much "real self." This in turn is
reflected in vague symptoms of anxiety, depression, and boredom, often
culminating in fatigue, headache, and digestive difficulty. In short, self-
alienation has made the nurse sick. To the extent that training and subsequent job situations have taught nurses to play a role and not express
themselves constructively, they have encouraged them to be "sick."

The Expanded Nurse Role: Sources of Controversy

Largely in response to the problems of professional socialization and the expressed desire for increased autonomy, nurses have supported the concept of an expanded role as nurse clinicians, nurse practitioners, and physician's assistants. The support, however, has been far from unanimous. Conflicting value orientations within the profession itself have been significant. These reflect deeply ingrained values that were internalized during the majority of nurses' socialization as women and later through their training. These values emphasize passivity, the avoidance of responsibility, and the fear of exercising power. They represent the antithesis of professional autonomy as embodied in the expanded nurse role concept. Despite the problems inherent in passive-dependent behaviors, they do persist among some, in part a function of the status of transition that characterized the nursing profession in the early 1980s.

Any time significant changes are occurring in a profession, resulting in an atmosphere of uncertainty, the result is a situation ripe for conflict and chaos. During such times of stress, members of the profession may fall back on earlier modes of behavior and defenses. These are likely to be less productive than others but they afford security to the individuals in conflict, giving them a patterned, familiar response. In such situations people tend to fall back on entrenched routines, to reject innovation, and to protect their territory. For nurses, the movement to an expanded role and a more professional stance vis-à-vis other professions may drive some to retreat into a defensive, stereotyped, passive role if they feel threatened about their new knowledge and their assumption of responsibility and power.

Another side effect of the educational experience and existing working situation has been the hampering of the development of professional solidarity, a situation that increases the controversy over the expanded nurse role. The variety of training programs has led to competition among nurses, particularly since unclear job descriptions and compensation scales often do not reflect differences in education. Thus, nurses with B.S.N.s may perform the same job as nurses with an R.N., and for the same pay. Status associated with the baccalaureate degree at the expense of R.N. experience serves to erode support that exists among members of the profession. Unfortunately, this competitiveness also reduces the profession's credibility in relation to the other professions. In short, this diminishes the cohesion necessary for professional identification and growth.

In spite of these obstacles, or perhaps because of them, the expanded role concept for nursing forges ahead strongly. Increasing medical costs, federal policy, and nurses' concern for professional autonomy have stimulated considerable interest in broadening their role. This, in turn, has spurred research evaluating the feasibility and impact of the expanded role.

The results of this research are fairly consistent. The use of nurse clinicians and nurse practitioners for selected diagnostic and treatment procedures reduces the cost of these activities when compared with physicians offering the same service, thus lowering overall medical expenditures (Kane, Hammer, & Byrnes, 1977; Schneider & Foley, 1977). In addition, physicians are freed to devote their energies to more complex medical matters and research (Holmes & Mills, 1976; Yodfat, Fidel, & Eliakim, 1977). When they do see patients, physicians are able to spend greater amounts of time with them.

In general, the response of patients to nurse practitioners has been positive (Levine et al., 1978). Several studies highlight the positive contributions they have made and physicians' positive response toward them. These studies recommend additional training and utilization of such professionals (Connelly & Connelly, 1979; Scheffler, Weisfeld, Ruby, & Estes, 1978; Simborg, Starfield, & Horn, 1978). Despite these gains, some real and attitudinal barriers to an expanded nurse role do remain.

Additional Barriers: Organizational and Personal

For many years nurses' access to leadership positions in their profession and in the organizational structures within which they work has been limited. The limits, an important source of stress, have extended to the power of individual nurses to exercise reasonable control over their own work. Reviews of the literature and informal discussions with nurses across the country suggest that access to these positions has been blocked by either physicians or administrative personnel, or both.

Physicians, for example, frequently resist the expanded nursing role, which many of them view as an encroachment on their professional territory; they believe it threatens not only their positions but also their ability to perform their jobs effectively. Interestingly, some doctors are more willing to hire physician's assistants than nurse practitioners (Fottler, 1979). This finding may reflect sexual discrimination, since nurse practitioners tend to be female and physician's assistants to be male. Nevertheless, none of these barriers is considered to be insurmountable. Indeed, significant progress in overcoming and removing them is reported (National Commission on Nursing, 1981; Sullivan, Dachelet, Sultz, Henry, & Carrol, 1978).

In spite of these changes, a phenomenon has been observed and confirmed by nurse professionals in leadership positions in various parts of the country: Even where access to positions of leadership is available, many nurses continue to assert that barriers to such jobs and to professional autonomy exist in the form of administrators' and physicians' attitudes toward nursing. Some physicians and administrators have reacted negatively to continued criticism. Perceiving that their efforts at change have gone unnoticed, they have defensively returned to the earlier mode that circumscribes nursing autonomy and confirms these nurses' self-fulfilling prophecy.

It seems likely that a third factor, long overlooked, may severely hamper nurses' access to leadership positions and may distort their perception of access when physicians and administrators actually present few barriers. The third factor is nurses' own interpersonal needs. A preliminary study (Numerof, 1981) of a group of staff and managerial nurses suggests that their own needs for power and dominance, affection, and inclusion are related to their job functions and autonomy, with managerial nurses tending to show slightly more elevated power needs than those in supervisory and staff positions. (No differences were found as a function of length of time in the job or size of hospital.)

These early findings, which must be regarded as tentative, and the author's own consulting experience have led to the hypothesis that nurses represent a self-selected group whose low needs for power and control have been reinforced in their educational experience and work settings. An example illustrates this point.

A large metropolitan hospital in the Midwest changed its psychiatric admissions policy. As a result of a change in the state law, nonphysician persons who were suitably trained in psychiatric diagnosis and the rudiments of patient management were legally able to admit psychiatric patients without a physician's approval. The nursing staff members with psychiatric experience were informed of their expanded responsibility, and on-call schedules were initiated with nursing administration. Much to the administration's surprise, a large number of qualified nurses reacted very negatively to the change, claiming lack of expertise rather than seeing this as a growth opportunity. Ironically, most of these nurses had been persistent in their outcries against what they viewed as their limited autonomy and involvement in patient management.

In discussion with the author they revealed that underlying their reaction was a fear of enlarged professional and legal responsibility. They admitted that fears of being sued by patients were widespread. As many others have learned, calls for professional autonomy must be accompanied by a willingness to assume responsibility for decisions and to be held increasingly accountable for them.

BEYOND SOCIALIZATION: SOURCES OF STRESS

While a great deal of the literature on professional and organizational stress derives from the industrial sector, increasing attention has been paid to this problem in the health care sector. In particular there has been a growing recognition of the stress experienced by nursing staff members in hospital settings (Caldwell & Weiner, 1981; Cassem & Hackett, 1972; Hay & Oken, 1972; Ivancevich & Matteson, 1980; Jacobson, 1978). A significant proportion of the nursing stress literature, however, rests on anecdotal evidence, making it impossible to make any clear statements about the nature of the problem and its possible solutions.

A second problem is some writers' tendency to establish a priori which sources of stress are relevant to this population. Since those sources tend to be derived from industry, their applicability to nursing may be suspect. In addition, general stressors such as "role conflict," which are represented by a limited number of nonspecific items on a survey instrument, do not provide the kind of information that can be used to make meaningful recommendations to alleviate stress.

Finally, some research is conducted with sizeable samples derived from numerous institutions, with no effort to control for factors across and within these organizations that are likely to differentially influence stress. Under these conditions, knowledge of nursing stress and its effects remains nonspecific.

To achieve some clarity on the issue, the author and a colleague studied stress among nurses in a medium-sized, religious-affiliated institution located outside a major Midwestern city (Numerof & Abrams, 1983). By using one facility, institutional variation could be controlled. The demographic and personal variables that have predictive significance for experienced stress among the group studied could then be analyzed. In this study, "experienced stress" refers to the psychological state of disturbed affect that is a response to stressors (McGrath, 1970). "Stressor" refers to an external demand or stimulus perceived by the individuals as undesirable (McGrath, 1976).

Of particular importance in this investigation was an exploration of experienced stress as a function of position in the organization. While a number of reports suggest that there are high stress specialities in nursing (Caldwell & Weiner, 1981; Cassem & Hackett, 1972; Jacobson, 1978; Peterson & Cooke, 1981) none of these rests on empirical data. However, industrial research suggests that interpretations of various aspects of a system tend to be based on individuals' personal experiences within the particular area of the organization in which they function. For example, structural factors (e.g., formalization) are found to be correlated with perceived role stress (House & Rizzo, 1972; Rogers & Molnar, 1976). In another study (Schuler, 1977a) discrepancies between the nature of the task, technology required to perform it, and managerial structure are related to experienced stress.

Applied to health care settings, this suggests that where the task/technology requires a high level of skill and independent judgment by the practitioner (e.g., medical floor) and the departmental structure constrains autonomy, employees in that environment are likely to experience high degrees of stress. Research on job attitude (Adams, Laker, & Hulin, 1977; Herman, Dunkam, & Hulin, 1975; Newman, 1975) suggests that functional specialty, department, and shift assignment are useful indexes of employees' assessments of the work experience.

Related to this is the significant contribution by Lawrence and Lorsch (1967) in delineating environments in the overall climate of an organization. As a result of their work it is largely accepted that individual departments have climates that affect employees apart from and in addition to that of the organization as a whole. Thus, as a result of industrial research and descriptive reports of nursing stress in particular areas, it seemed reasonable to expect that sources of stress would not be random within an institution but would vary systematically among different roles and across different levels in the organizational hierarchy.

Another focus of attention was on intraorganizational variables that the literature indicated were potential sources of stress: interpersonal relationships within the organization, role in the institution, and factors intrinsic to the job. The third area of concern was the influence of moderating variables, in particular interpersonal needs, a dimension that encompasses personality variables, and locus of control, all of which were described in Chapter 2 as offering important insight into individual differences in experienced stress.

An Empirical Study

Concern for stressor specificity (i.e., to nursing jobs) dictated that no a priori general categories of stressors (e.g., role conflict, role overload) be employed in the study. A review of the literature did not yield any suitable instruments so one was designed for this study based on the literature and a content analysis of numerous interviews with nurses. It also was recognized that despite increasing awareness of stress among nurses and its consequences, there had been little progress toward the development of a reliable and theoretically valid instrument that would measure the frequency of the occurrence and degree of intensity of stressors among nurses. Thus, a secondary purpose of the study was to develop such an instrument. A description of the research methodology is offered in Numerof & Abrams, 1983.

The final stress instrument (the *Nursing Stress Inventory*) consists of 46 items arranged in six multiple-item scales with internal scale reliabilities (Cronbach's Alpha) ranging between .86 and .92.

- Scale 1, *Organizational environment,* includes 13 items reflecting various dimensions of conflict such as with physicians and nurse colleagues, lack of feedback regarding job performance, management inconsistencies, and meeting demands of supervisors and physicians ($\alpha = .92$).
- Scale 2, *Work demands,* consists of six items describing the physical demands of the job: meeting patients' physical needs, charting, remembering orders, and short-staffing ($\alpha = .88$).
- Scale 3, *Emotional aspects of patient care,* is a more specific eight-item scale that addresses the nurses' need to be emotionally responsive to patients and their families, helping them to verbalize their concerns ($\alpha = .89$).
- Scale 4, *Death-related issues,* is an eight-item scale describing work with the terminally ill, facing near-death emergencies, discussing death with patient and family ($\alpha = .89$).
- Scale 5, *Lack of procedural/administrative support,* consists of seven items that cover a variety of situations from developing personal attachment to a patient to an unresponsive administration regarding clinical concerns. The common theme is a lack of direction or procedure in handling a situation that is likely to be experienced as ambiguous, calling for the nurse to exercise judgment ($\alpha = .86$).
- Scale 6, *Supervisor's role,* is a four-item scale that describes vulnerability in that function: less patient contact, an important factor for clinically trained personnel; social isolation associated with the job; and added responsibility ($\alpha = .87$).

Respondents were asked to check the frequency of occurrence and degree of stress associated with each event on a five-point scale with the response options for frequency ranging from "almost never" to "almost always" and those for degree of stress ranging from "no stress" to "very much stress." Demographic data were requested of each respondent: age, sex, nursing status (i.e., R.N., L.P.N., G.N.), marital status, number of children, type of program from which they graduated, length of time since graduation, time employed at the hospital, time in present area of nursing, and time working in that area.

Participants in the study also were asked to complete the *Fundamental Interpersonal Relations Orientation Behavior* (FIRO-B) (Schutz, 1966), a reliable and valid measure (test − retest = .76; reproducibility = .94) of interpersonal needs.

FIRO-B is a measure of three basic interpersonal needs: inclusion, control, and affection, each of which occurs along two dimensions—wanted and expressed:

- The wanted dimension reflects individuals' desire to have others express that behavior to them while the expressed dimension reflects their desire to initiate the behavior in others. The need for inclusion refers to individuals' needs to interact with others in social situations: i.e., to invite others to join them in activities (expressed inclusion) or to want to be invited to join and associate with others (wanted inclusion).
- The need for control pertains to issues of power and dominance in interpersonal situations. The need for expressed control reflects the degree to which individuals desire a dominant, directive role in interpersonal relations, influencing how and what is to be done. Conversely, the need for wanted control reflects the degree to which they wish to assume a subordinate, submissive role in interpersonal relations whereby others direct what occurs.
- The need for affection refers to the amount of caring that people feel comfortable exchanging in interpersonal relations. Thus, a high need for expressed affection indicates a person with strong desires to show affectionate behaviors to others in interpersonal relations. A high need for wanted affection suggests a person with strong desires to be the recipient of the affection behavior of others.

HYPOTHESES AND DISCUSSION

Organizational Hypotheses: Roles, Functional Specialty

Hypothesis 1

It was predicted that R.N.s would experience a higher degree of stress than L.P.N.s because they had more responsibility in direct patient care and were likely to be the persons called upon by physicians. In essence, it was perceived that the L.P.N. was buffered by the R.N. and thus likely to experience less stress than the R.N. This hypothesis was confirmed through a Pearson product moment correlation and an analysis of variance (Tables 6-1 and 6-2).

Table 6-1 Significant Pearson Product Moment Correlations: Stress and Its Relation to Demographic, Personal, and Professional Variables

Stress Scale	Demographic Variables								
	Sex	Age	Children	Time Since Grad.	Time at Hospital	Time in Nursing Area	Wanted Inclusion	Wanted Affection	Wanted Control
1. Organizational Environment	(−.3435) .018	(−.2777) .033							
2. Work Demands									
3. Emotional Aspects, Patient Care	(−.2969) .043				(−.2278) .083				
4. Death-Related Issues							(−.2722) .042	(.2338) .086	(.3788) .004
5. Lack of Procedural/ Administrative Support	(−.3587) .013		(−.3513) .006	(−.3692) .004	(−.3784) .003				
6. Supervisor's Role		(−.3424) .008							
Total Stress	(−.3768) .009	(−.2358) .072		(−.2314) .078	(−.2556) .051	(.2430) .064			

Actual significance levels are reported in the table.
Numbers in parentheses are correlations.

Table 6-2 Multiple Regression of Independent Variables, Total Stress, and Six Stress Scales: Significant Values

Independent Variables	Total Stress			Scale 1			Scale 2			Scale 3		
	R^{2a}	$Beta^b$	F^c	R^{2a}	$Beta^b$	F^c	R^{2a}	$Beta^b$	F^c	R^{2a}	$Beta^b$	F^c
Age	.25375	−.81688	**	.26062	−.40781	*	.14231	−.59857	*	.07475	−.98494	***
Nursing Status										.28327	.41484	*
Time Since Graduation	.32475	.54810	*				.20215	.53397	*	.20745	.98074	***
Area of Nursing	.12794	.38211	*				.11709	.34860	*	.1330	−.35624	*
Wanted Inclusion												
Expressed Affection												
Wanted Control												

Independent Variables	Scale 4			Scale 5			Scale 6		
	R^{2a}	$Beta^b$	F^c	R^{2a}	$Beta^b$	F^c	R^{2a}	$Beta^b$	F^c
Age				.28732	−.38723	*	.13124	−.36140	*
Nursing Status									
Time Since Graduation	.34126	.73416	***						
Area of Nursing				.14185	.43185	**			
Wanted Inclusion									
Expressed Affection	.28385	.30767	*						
Wanted Control	.16071	.38743	**						

* p≤.05
** p≤.01
*** p≤.001
ᵃ Indicates amount of variance in subjects' scores explained by each independent variable
ᵇ Indicates weight of the independent variable in explaining stress scores
ᶜ Ratio of dispersion (see Note b, Table 4-11)

Specifically, R.N.s show higher overall stress but, most significantly, they report higher stress on organizational environment and in the superior's role. The latter is particularly stressful for this group in that the supervisory role takes its occupant away from clinical work and leaves the individual in what is perceived as an isolated position, experiencing little support from private physicians or staff. Organizations may unwittingly augment the supervisor's stress by failing to provide management training that will equip the person in the new role with skills required to perform the job adequately (Numerof, 1982). These skills are quite different from that of the clinician and require new knowledge, new tools, and a new way of thinking.

Failure to provide resocialization for the manager/supervisor promoted up from the ranks further accentuates the problem as this individual no longer is a peer of the work unit now being supervised and may know little, if any, personnel outside the unit. The combination of limited training for the demands of the new position and lack of a social peer group are likely to increase tension and feelings of inadequacy, and promote the expression of behaviors that are antithetical to the success of the supervisor (e.g., defensiveness, rigidity, anxiety). (The reasons for these occurrences and their effects are discussed later in the chapter.)

Hypothesis 2

It was predicted that stress would be experienced differentially as a function of clinical department. Specifically, nurses in intensive care, emergency room, and surgery were predicted to report higher levels of stress than other units, and those in pediatric and OB-GYN the lowest levels.

The first hypothesis is supported through an analysis of variance that yields significant differences on Scales 2 (Work demands), 3 (Emotional aspects of patient care), and 5 (Lack of procedural/administrative support) (Table 6-3).

However, the most stressful areas are not necessarily those predicted. Rather, psychiatry, surgery, medicine, and intensive care units (ICU) report the highest stress on Scales 2, 3, and 5. Others suggest that ICU nursing is particularly stressful because of the nature of the work. Caldwell and Weiner (1981) in their review of studies of stress and coping among ICU nurses find that work demands (understaffing and overwork), the nurses' emotional reactions to death, organizational/interpersonal environmental factors, and personal insecurity in the face of much clinical responsibility are the most important and highly significant sources of stress for this group.

Table 6-3 Significant Differences on Personality and Stress Factors as a Function of Nursing Status and Area of Nursing[1]

	Nursing Status		Area of Nursing									Significance[2]
Variable	R.N.	L.P.N.	Emerg. Room	Recov. Room	ICU	Med.	Psych.	OB-GYN	Nursery/Peds.	Surg.	Admin.	
Expressed Inclusion			2.286	4.50	4.20	2.50	4.50	2.71	5.0	2.3	4.0	p≤.02
Expressed Control			1.571	1.50	2.80	1.24	6.00	3.00	5.18	2.63	3.33	p≤.0046
Organizational Environment	130.347	101.0354										p≤.042
Work Demands			43.664	30.663	59.512	61.73	83.0	48.109	52.685	70.247	46.275	p≤.011
Emotional Aspects, Patient Care			55.006	27.934	57.284	64.07	107.50	41.145	34.625	55.604	50.00	p≤.0001
Death-related Issues												
Lack of Procedural/ Administrative Support			36.658	41.30	68.309	64.137	87.82	56.078	61.705	63.298	45.935	p≤.074
Supervisor's Role	19.548	10.559										p≤.009

[1] Numbers represent mean scores.
[2] Significance values derived from one-way analysis of variance, two-tailed test.

The present study, however, suggests that work demands may be as stressful for nurses in psychiatry, surgery, and medicine as they are for those in ICU. Death-related issues, an important factor in this study, are a source of stress for all nurses, regardless of specialty area, and are related to individuals' interpersonal needs. Similarly, organizational/interpersonal factors are differentially stressful for nurses as a function of position in the hierarchy, rather than area of nursing.

The findings suggest that different types of stress are unit specific, thus offering increased support for the thesis of Lawrence and Lorsch (1967) that different environments exist within an institution and must be considered if people in those settings, and their stress problems, are to be understood. Any attempts to alleviate stress must take such specificity into account.

Professional and Job-Related Hypotheses: Tenure and Experience

Hypothesis 3

An inverse relationship was predicted between years of experience and degree of stress for all nurses regardless of degree and functional department. Increased time in the institution was taken as a measure of greater experience, which should serve to reduce reported stress levels. Length of employment also would be expected to be inversely related to experienced stress because of attrition. The survey shows those who find the hospital environment most stressful are more likely to leave over time. This hypothesis is supported by a significant negative correlation between length of time at the hospital and overall stress and Scale 5 (Lack of procedural/administrative support), as well as a negative correlation approaching significance on Scale 3 (Emotional aspects of patient care) in the expected direction (see Table 6-1).

These findings suggest that tolerance for ambiguity that may be a function of unclear procedural/administrative support increases with experience, thus diminishing experienced stress. Similarly, more experienced nurses are likely to have learned appropriate ways of handling such situations. It is important to note that these findings hold up regardless of nursing degree status or functional area as hypothesized.

Other studies have explored the relationship between stress and turnover, the reverse of tenure. Parasuraman and Alutto (1981) report a weak-moderate positive correlation. McKenna et al. (1981) find that perceived occupational stress is instrumental in decisions to leave the place of employment. The failure to obtain stronger results with regard to this hypothesis may be a function of external circumstances. Depressed national economic conditions at the time of this study may have been a factor in not leaving the job, regardless of inherent organizational stress. Without reasonable options, people tend to remain where they are.

Hypothesis 4

The type of program from which nurses graduated was predicted to have no relationship to experienced stress. This hypothesis is supported by an analysis of variance. Despite common assumptions in nursing suggesting that R.N.s are likely to experience stress because of subtle pressures relating to their lack of an academic degree, this study finds no empirical grounds for such a conclusion in terms of work-related stress.

Hypothesis 5

Length of time since graduation was predicted to be inversely related to experienced stress with nurses who were recent graduates having more stress than those who had graduated earlier. Strong support is found for this hypothesis in relation to Scale 5 (Lack of procedural/administrative support) through a Pearson correlation (Table 6-1). However, regression analyses demonstrate a highly significant direct relationship between length of time since graduation and overall stress, Scale 2 (Work demands), Scale 3 (Emotional aspects of patient care), and Scale 4 (Death-related issues) (Table 6-2). An underlying assumption in the hypothesis was that length of time since graduation might be an indicator of experience. This appears to be an invalid assumption despite the negative correlation with Scale 5 (Lack of procedural/administrative support).

What seems likely is that nurses leave the job market, often to raise a family, and return. To the extent that this occurs, there is no direct relationship between years of experience and time since graduation. Indeed, the latter factor may be a source of stress in that new methods, taught to more recent graduates, may not be as readily available to nurses who graduated earlier, thus placing this group at a professional disadvantage. Additional research is needed to clarify the impact of time since graduation, obviously an important and generally overlooked variable in stress analysis.

Hypothesis 6

Length of time employed in the nursing area was expected to have an inverse relationship to stress for the reasons cited in Hypothesis 1. A Pearson product moment correlation approaches significance in the predicted direction in relation to overall stress (Table 6-1). Regression analysis did not yield significance.

Moderating Variables: Demographics

Hypothesis 7

Age was predicted to be inversely related to experienced stress. It was believed that as individuals grew older and increased life experience they would be likely to develop strategies to cope effectively with stressors. Strong support for this hypothesis is shown in the results of Pearson correlations with respect to Scale 1 (Organizational environment), Scale 6 (Supervisor's role), and overall stress (Table 6-1). Regression analysis (Table 6-2) indicates very strong support except for Scales 4 and 6 where age is not found to be significantly related to death-related issues or supervisor's role.

Hypothesis 8

It was predicted that married nurses would experience less stress than unmarried ones and that stress would be directly related to the number of children they had. Married nurses, in that they are in a natural support system (i.e., marriage) were predicted to have less stress than unmarried nurses. No assessment of quality of that relationship was made, nor was information obtained concerning living with, but not married to, a significant other. Given the energy required for balancing work and child care demands, it was predicted that stress would increase as a function of number of children. Neither of these predictions is supported by the data.

Moderating Variable Hypotheses: Interpersonal Needs

Hypothesis 9

It was predicted that interpersonal needs (FIRO-B) would be related to stress in the following manner:

9a. Experienced stress is inversely related to need for expressed control.

Results of a Pearson correlation and regression analysis did not support this hypothesis.

9b. Experienced stress is directly related to need for wanted control.

Strong support for this hypothesis is found by means of a Pearson correlation in relation to Scale 4 (Death-related issues). Regression analyses of need for wanted control against the stress scales yields significance on Scale 4 and generally are in the predicted direction on other factors, although nonsignificant. Hypotheses 9a and 9b find support in the general stress literature in that individuals' belief that they can influence events (i.e., that they have a strong need for expressed control and can take charge, as opposed to being wholly dependent on others) is an important coping device to lower stress (Cooley & Keesey, 1981; Lazarus, 1978; Suls & Mullen, 1981). It is likely that feelings of helplessness become accentuated in the face of patient death, highlighting these nurses' generally high needs for wanted control. While FIRO-B has not been used in previous stress-related studies, its utility bears additional examination. It is possible that Hypothesis 9a is not supported because of the subjects' overall low needs for expressed control. Additional research with nurses and nonnursing personnel seems warranted in delineating the relationship between needs for control and experienced stress.

9c. Experienced stress is inversely related to expressed need for inclusion.

To the extent that anecdotal reports suggest that social support groups may be a buffer to experienced stress, it seemed reasonable to expect that expressed and wanted needs for inclusion, which would enhance the likelihood individuals might join such a group, would be inversely related to experienced stress. Neither the Pearson correlation nor regression analysis are significant. This area also warrants further investigation. Numerous authors (Hay & Oken, 1972; Mohl, 1980; Weiner & Caldwell, 1981) cite social groups as useful for coping with stress in an ICU. It seems likely that the need for inclusion would be an important variable in that it is likely to affect whether or not, and how, nurses use the social support to reduce stress.

9d. Wanted need for inclusion is inversely related to experienced stress.

A Pearson correlation yields significant results on Scale 4 (Death-related issues) in the predicted direction. Regression analyses, however, show significance in relation to Scale 3 (Emotional aspects of patient care) in the predicted direction. Nonsignificant differences in the predicted direction are found with respect to overall stress, Scale 4 (Death-related issues), and Scale 6 (Supervisor's role). (These are not reported in the tables.) These findings suggest the need for continued investigation in this area.

9e. Need for expressed affection is not related to experienced stress.

A Pearson correlation (Table 6-1) shows no significant relationship confirming the hypothesis. However, a regression analysis (Table 6-2) yields a positive significant relationship between expressed affection and Scale 4 (Death-related issues). Expressed affection is not related to any other measure of stress. It is possible that nurses who develop closer relations with terminally and/or seriously ill patients are more stressed than those whose relations are less personal. This should not be regarded as something necessarily warranting change. Indeed, effective nursing under these circumstances may require the demonstration of warmth, caring, and affection. In such situations, then, social support groups may be very effective in helping nurses work through their stress over losing patients with whom an emotional bond has developed.

9f. Need for wanted affection is not related to experienced stress.

A Pearson correlation approaches significance suggesting a positive relationship between wanted affection and Scale 4 (Death-related issues). Regression analysis shows no significant relationship. The positive correlation may be understood in light of the findings with need for expressed affection, particularly since Schutz (1966) regards the two needs as complementary (i.e., needs for affection tend to be similar to each other in healthy personalities).

Hypothesis 10

R.N.s have higher needs for expressed control than L.P.N.s and lower needs for wanted control.

No significant differences are found between the groups (Table 6-3).

Conclusion

Five out of 10 hypotheses were confirmed, two additional hypotheses received mixed support, and three were not confirmed.

This study suggests that what an individual brings to the job situation in terms of personality and experience factors is critically important in predicting experienced stress. In addition, such stress cannot be regarded as a single phenomenon but rather is best understood in terms of fairly discrete dimensions in which the degree of frequency of occurrence of a given event (i.e., the potential stressor) and degree of stress associated with that event are taken into account. Furthermore, stress must be understood in terms of an individual's position in the organization—the role status and the unit/department in which the person is employed. Thus, any attempt to ameliorate the negative effects of stress on the individual and to reduce actual stressors must take these variables into account. For instance, stress in handling death-related issues occurs without regard to unit. Organizationwide programs to help nurses deal more effectively with this stressor could be quite helpful. Other programs necessarily would be unit specific.

While this study points to the importance of personality and experience factors in stress and offers a reliable instrument for assessing various aspects of stress, its findings must be regarded with caution. The sample size is relatively small. While it is representative of the nurses at the hospital where the study took place, it is recommended that the study be replicated and extended to strengthen the generalizability of the findings. One fruitful area might explore such macro variables as institutional size and structure. The impact of task variables on stress (Hackman & Oldham, 1976) and the managerial style of the individual's superior, would add important dimensions not explored here. Finally, the relationship between stress outcomes and coping strategies related to specific stressors needs further examination.

STRESS: NATIONAL COMMISSION ON NURSING VIEW

The National Commission on Nursing (1981) provides an interesting perspective on the challenges and problems of nursing in the health care system of this country. Established in the autumn of 1980, this commission was composed of a wide variety of leaders in the fields of nursing, management, medicine, academia, business, and government to develop action plans for the resolution of nursing-related problems, especially as they affected patient care. Through six public hearings across the country, numerous problems were identified and solutions considered.

The five major issues pinpointed, which also are highlighted in the literature, are:

1. the status and image of nursing, particularly in relation to changes in health care delivery, interprofessional relationships, and nursing's public image
2. the interface of nursing education and practice, particularly to prepare nurses for interprofessional interaction in practice

3. the effective management of nursing, including career development, personnel planning, recruitment and retention strategies, salaries, staffing, etc.
4. the management and development of interprofessional teams focused on increasing nurses' access to and involvement in organizational decision making as it pertains to nursing care
5. the maturation of the nursing profession in terms of its right and responsibility to define the nature and scope of its practice (National Commission on Nursing, 1981).

Inherent in the last issue is a need for effective nursing leadership and enhanced unity within the profession. As with other professions, there is no single professional body that speaks for and is accepted by all nurses (National Commission on Nursing, 1981).

NURSE-PHYSICIAN-ADMINISTRATOR RELATIONSHIP

There is strong evidence indicating that health care administrators and physicians all too often do not understand or value the role of nurses in patient care. (It should be noted that the overwhelming majority of nurses are staff nurses, not nurse practitioners. It is the hospital staff nurse who is the focus of attention here). Some physicians and administrators still hold outmoded views of nursing (Felch, 1976; Lewis, 1976; Kalisch & Kalisch, 1977). Many believe that nurses are overeducated for their roles and as a result they actively discourage their participation in decisions related to their practice (Lee, 1979).

However, others believe that changing health care technology and societal demands require interprofessional collaboration that includes the sharing of both knowledge and authority among professionals (Lee, 1979). The National Commission on Nursing reports that many in this group are concerned that there are not enough adequately trained nurses to perform the jobs required. Thus, nurses are confronted by those who, believing they should be in a circumscribed function under physicians, perceive them as too highly trained for that role. On the other hand, nurses are confronted by those who favor a collaborative professional role who regard most nurses as not trained sufficiently. Given the research that relates role ambiguity to job stress, these two conflicting orientations could be expected to create a real source of stress for nurses working in hospitals.

Such conflict is illustrated by the comments of a nursing service administrator in a large, university-affiliated Eastern hospital:

Often I feel really torn and frustrated. I see myself first as a manager and second as a nurse. But when I run into doctors who think they have a right to tell me how to run my department I'm aware of feeling a strong need to defend my profession [nursing]. I also have to periodically remind the CEO that we are competent to handle nursing matters and that we must be involved in decisions affecting the organization. . . . I'm also under constant pressure from my vocal nursing staff to make sure nursing is adequately represented. Some are constantly demanding more autonomy.

But I guess one of the hardest things for me to deal with, and a really big source of stress, is that group of nurses who would be a lot happier going back to the old ways. I used to think it had something to do with age. But I really question that. I think it's a lot deeper—having to do with a personal sense of security. . . . This all makes the job [of nursing administrator] a bit tougher and more stressful. It helps to talk about it to my husband and my counterparts in other hospitals.

But I think that my ability to see this not as a personal issue but as a professional one helps lower the stress and even turn it into something positive. The field is certainly changing and I feel a certain sense of satisfaction being at the cutting edge, helping to chart our direction at the crossroads.

Unfortunately, interprofessional physician-nurse communications patterns often considered relics of another age still exist, serving as another source of stress, particularly for nurses and secondarily for administrators who often find themselves caught in the middle.

The most classic physician-nurse game was described by Stein in 1967, a game still played in numerous hospital corridors. According to Stein, the primary objective of the game is to maintain role reciprocity in such a way that physicians appear to be completely in charge and nurses appear to be subservient to them. A more subtle objective of the game is for the nurse to make significant clinical recommendations to the physician without appearing to do so. Conversely, the physician is able to solicit recommendations regarding a particular patient without appearing to do so. The final play finds the nurse thanking the physician for the action the nurse initiated, making it look like it was the physician's idea all along. Obviously, the tactics required in the game require great skill and ingenuity.

For nurses in particular, such communications games breed resentment. They are deleterious to the establishment of collaboration and effective teamwork based on mutual professional respect. It should be recognized that where these games do exist, they often cause problems for medical administrators, who regard such behavior on the part of their staffs as inappropriate and unprofessional. Indeed, as described in Chapter 4, dealing with the unreasonable demands of the medical staff, some of whom are described as "prima donnas expecting their charts to be handed to them as they walk out of the elevator," becomes a primary source of stress for medical administration.

UNION BARGAINING: ISSUES AND PROSPECTS

One possible outcome of continued noncollegial physician-nurse relationships—restricted professional autonomy and limited access to and participation in organizational decision making—is the introduction of unions among nurses as an attempt to redress their real and perceived injustices. Collective bargaining in voluntary nonprofit hospitals already is having a significant impact on the industry. Since nurses comprise the largest professional group employed in hospitals, it is useful to explore unionization issues among them (Numerof & Abrams, 1982).

Compensation

Compensation often is a central issue that precipitates collective bargaining. On this issue, nursing does not appear to be atypical. At least part of the problem stems from insufficient differential compensation based on training and experience. According to the National Commission on Nursing (1981), registered nurses, despite their training, responsibility, and experience, earn on the average only a few dollars more per hour than licensed practical nurses and nurse's aides. Similarly, only 12 percent of hospitals pay nurses with baccalaureate degrees more than registered nurses with considerably less education. An analysis of wage structures by Aiken et al. (1981) over a 30-year period suggests that nursing dissatisfaction, reflected in high turnover and subsequent shortages, is at least in part a reflection of inadequate pay, a point also noted by Ellis (1980).

However, it would be a mistake to assume that salaries are the sole, or even the primary, source of dissatisfaction for most nurses. In fact, some preliminary research suggests that economic issues are not foremost in the minds even of some unionized nurses (Bloom, Parlette, & O'Reilly, 1980). Where economic issues are a factor in job dissatisfaction, the problem seems to stem from a perceived disparity in reimbursement for similar work between what nurses in one hospital receive vis-à-vis the norm for the area. Even where financial constraints have necessitated lower-than-average pay for the area, nurses have voiced dissatisfaction primarily because the rationale for the discrepancy never was made clear to them. Thus, in some situations, it is the hospital's failure to communicate directly with staff that results in unfavorable attitudes toward the organization.

Professional Issues

A review of the literature indicates that the primary sources of dissatisfaction involve nurses' limited autonomy, lack of communication with management, exclusion from participation in organizational decision making, and dissatisfaction with compensation.

To a large extent, some of these areas (e.g., limited autonomy and exclusion from decision making) have become sources of dissatisfaction as a result of changing attitudes among nurses, rather than changing conditions of work. Two changes in nursing itself can be cited as factors:

1. Nurse recruits are coming from families of higher socioeconomic background than in the past. This is especially true for graduates of baccalaureate programs (Bloom et al., 1980). The significance of this change is that children from lower class backgrounds generally have been found to be more conforming to authority while those from higher social class backgrounds are more self-directed and desirous of autonomy (Kohn, 1969). Such characteristics predispose younger nurses to conflict with a system that traditionally has reinforced nonassertive, uncritical order following (Numerof, 1978a).
2. Nursing education in the last two decades or more has seen an upgrading of the quality of training programs. For example, between 1962 and 1972, half of the traditional three-year, hospital-affiliated nursing programs were phased out in favor of collegiate nursing programs (Twaddle & Hessler, 1977). This trend has continued with current graduates more highly skilled than in the past, capable of more self-direction in complex areas than they are generally accorded. In addition, there has been an increase in the number of nurses with master's degrees.

These changes have led younger nurses to view themselves more as professionals, capable of assuming broad responsibility and acting autonomously. As noted earlier, this differs widely from the view of nurses as self-sacrificing handmaidens to the doctor that still is firmly entrenched in the health care system. Evidence of this is seen in a survey of physician attitudes (Lee, 1979) that 74.1 percent of physicians regard nurses as assistants and nothing more, 16.7 percent view them as colleagues, and only 9.2 percent accept them as independent. This divergence creates tension in the work setting and, in the absence of more effective mediating mechanisms, leads nurses to challenge administrator-designed work arrangements.

Another source of dissatisfaction is limited career advancement stemming from the organizational structures characteristic of hospitals. As pointed out by Alutto & Belasco (1974), nurses tend to have horizontal occupational structures in vertical, multileveled organizational hierarchies. Limited pay differentials related to experience reflect this flat structure. The absence of advancement opportunities forces nurses to leave their profession to advance up the administrative hierarchy. The result is the classic up-from-the-ranks syndrome in which clinical competence is rewarded by a management position. Since such administrative positions often require different characteristics for success than those that would contribute to effective nursing, the result often is confusion, frustration, and stress for the individuals occupying the positions and for the organization itself.

The final irony of this situation is that subsequent administrative problems become the rationale for maintaining nurse administrators in positions of limited autonomy. By way of illustration, an American Hospital Association survey shows that only 56 percent of nursing service administrators have full administrative responsibility for their departmental budgets (Ellis, 1980). This is just one example of the general reluctance of many hospital administrators to give nurses a decision-making role.

Bases for Stressors

Such reluctance has far-reaching implications even in situations where nurses hold formal positions of authority. The study of key management personnel in hospitals (Chapter 4) suggests that prominent sources of stress for nursing directors are administrative insensitivity to clinical issues, pressure to sacrifice or compromise professional ideals, not having responsibility to take needed action, having judgment questioned by nonnursing personnel, inability to get medical staff to accept new policies and procedures, insufficient resources, and lack of support from administration. Also cited by this group in interviews with the author are attempts by nursing staff members to unionize, to demonstrate increasingly militant dissatisfaction, and, unfortunately, to fail to understand the overall picture.

The nurse administrator's ability to participate in organizational decision making with the hospital's administrative and medical staff is recognized by the National Commission on Nursing (1981) as a key in bringing about nursing satisfaction in the institution. Testimony by administrators and managerial nurses at public hearings of the commission revealed that while self-governance was a desired end, it would not be achieved unless the profession was represented by a competent nursing administrator who reported directly to the chief executive officer. The costs of failure to change institutional practices with regard to nursing were described as including decreased quality of patient care, increased turnover, and stepped-up unionization.

This research attests to deepening staff discontent when nursing administration itself feels powerless to effect changes perceived as desirable. If nursing administration is not influential in hospital decision making and nursing staff feels that top executives are unresponsive to its needs, the climate is ripe for outside intervention.

This last factor—the exclusion of nurses from decision-making processes and general lack of communication with management—is a frequently cited factor in nurse dissatisfaction leading to union activity. The survey by Bloom et al. (1980) of a sample of unionized nurses in California also reports these issues to be highly salient and predictive of strike behavior. It should be noted that that study did take place in a public health agency—not a hospital, where hours tend to be better and salaries higher. Despite the difference in settings, concern for autonomy is a concern for nurses in both situations. Thus, these issues might be expected to have relevance for nurses in other hospitals, along with concerns for salary and general working conditions.

Unionization—the Wave of the Future?

The importance of professional issues is reflected in the frequency with which hospital contracts specify the formation of labor-management committees. These committees generally are composed of administrators and unionized R.N.s and address policies and procedures such as peer review, admissions, and medications procedures. A survey of more than 800 contracts involving professional bargaining units in hospitals shows that fully 73 percent provide for some type of joint study committee (Juris, 1977).

As Elliott (1981) aptly notes, poor management practices leading to job insecurity are another source of growing dissatisfaction among staff nurses. Such practices include inadequate performance appraisal systems that leave staff members unclear about work performance, which in turn influence promotion and salary increases. Lack of grievance procedures and of uniform administrative guidelines on disciplinary action, favoritism, and failure to address continuing education and professional development all contribute to the feeling that "no one here cares."

Given this climate, the existence of conflict with other professions (primarily physicians), short-staffing, and the use of nurse registry personnel (who often receive higher pay than employed staff members), it is not surprising that nurses increasingly regard unions as an alternative to what they perceive as the hospital's indifference or callous refusal to deal with their concerns. While unions may not be able to provide answers to serious management and staffing problems, many nurses see them as a means for negotiating with the hospital team—of which these professionals often do not feel a part.

In summary, it appears that nurses' changing self-perceptions of their professional role have led to increasing dissatisfaction with constricted, dependent job expectations, limited career opportunities, poor management, and exclusion from the decision-making processes. Given these circumstances, what extrapolations can be made about the future of collective bargaining in health care?

Such an extrapolation requires the consideration of several critical environmental influences. Perhaps the most obvious has been the shortage of nursing personnel. The growing variety of settings in which nurses are employed and the broadening scope of their services are expected to increase demand substantially. Any shortage puts increasing pressure on management to respond to nurses' dissatisfaction or face high turnover in a tight labor market, in addition to the threat of unionization.

An emerging factor in the collective bargaining picture is the impact of cost containment legislation. As the role of publicly funded programs in the health care sector continues to grow, so does the role of government regulation of costs. With increased pressure for fiscal austerity, labor costs have become a major issue. As of 1978, 15 states had enacted voluntary or mandatory containment programs. Under most such legislation, the budgets of individual facilities are reviewed by a designated state agency. While it is too early to generalize, a review of seven years' experience with the Maryland Health Service Cost Review Commission is suggestive (Wolfe, 1979). In its efforts to control costs, that commission was a natural ally of hospital management, which eagerly used its pressures to justify limited responsiveness in bargaining. Judging from this experience, the interposition of a third party into the management-nurse relationship lessens administration's incentive to find mutually agreeable terms.

Another factor having an important impact on the course of collective bargaining is hospital management's challenge to the bargaining agent role of the American Nurses' Association and its state affiliates. The conflict arises out of the fact that the ANA makes no distinction in membership between supervisory and staff nurses. Consequently, management won a 1977 court challenge to the ANA's role on the basis of conflict of interest. Fourteen similar cases followed quickly (Crooks, 1979), and there have been numerous others in the ensuing years. At the time of this writing the ANA has won all appeals (Kellett, 1983).

To forestall similar challenges that could tie up their contracts for months or years, a number of nurse bargaining units have decertified the ANA as their agent in favor of such long-established unions as the Service Employees International Union or the American Federation of Teachers, whose role as a bargaining agent is not in question (Crooks, 1979).

Despite these occurrences, the ANA's position with regard to collective bargaining remains strong. The mainstream membership of ANA continues to endorse its joint roles as a collective bargaining agent and professional organization. In order to reduce the likelihood of being disqualified as a bargaining agent by the NLRB, state affiliates have adopted conflict of interest policies. For example, collective bargaining for the Missouri Nurses Association is handled through its Economic and General Welfare Committee. The committee is structurally separate from MNA and has its own by-laws. Except for the Nominations Committee, it is the only elected committee and requires that its members be non-supervisory. Given that the MNA Board of Directors does not have direct influence over it, the chance of being disqualified is reduced greatly. At this time approximately 100,000 nurses are under labor contracts negotiated by the ANA state affiliates—reportedly more nurses than those covered by agreements through all of the industrial unions together (Kellett, 1983). Despite the precautions outlined above and its excellent track record, there will continue to be challenges by management.

The NLRB will consider such challenges on a case-by-case basis, rather than a blanket ruling based on membership by supervisory nurses. To the extent that these challenges make the collective bargaining process more difficult, they encourage the separation of the bargaining role from the professional organization and may in the future reduce the power of the ANA in favor of more industrially oriented and possibly more militant organizations. This clearly would make the course of collective bargaining more difficult.

A tight labor market; pressure for cost containment, including the 1983 Social Security amendments regaining prospective (not after-the-fact) federal payments for Medicare and Medicaid patients; and the potentially larger role of industrial unions are conditions that make a substantial expansion of collective bargaining inescapable for the health care sector. The general rate of organizing has increased in the late 1970s and early

1980s despite a dip during the economic recession of the latter period (Kellett, 1983). The scope of bargaining may include more of the professional issues mentioned earlier in this chapter such as levels of service, role definitions, autonomy, etc. (Stern, 1977). For some authors, the question is not whether organization will continue but rather how militant it will be (Bloom, Parlette, & O'Reilly, 1980).

The outcome of these predictions depends largely on how hospital managements react to the nurses' issues of sources of dissatisfaction—autonomy, career development, and participation in organizational decision making. Research suggests that many managers believe that wages and job security are the critical issues when in fact the professional factors just described have been found to be just as important (Bloom et al., 1980).

Nurses are maturing as a professional group and their changing self-image has important implications for their relationships with other health care professionals and organizations and with the system as a whole. Managers must recognize these changes and deal with them. Whether they do so as a matter of proactive managerial planning or in reaction to union demands will be a critical factor in the future of collective bargaining in health care and in the sources of stress in the field.

THE NURSE AS MANAGER: PROMOTION PROBLEMS

Most nursing managers have been trained as clinicians and enter administration from the ranks of direct service providers. A strong case could be made to support the practice. Given the complex nature and importance of clinical matters, it is essential that they be well represented to and in management. Someone without clinical expertise might be less likely to understand and appreciate these matters. However, internal promotion presents managers and organizations with a host of problems that become serious sources of stress—problems that are not common to other positions.

It is standard practice for performance excellence on the job to be rewarded with a supervisory position. While such promotions generally are intended as rewards for technical or clinical competence, they frequently are accompanied by unforeseen costs. For the person promoted, these include stress experienced through frustration, general anxiety, tension, and fear of failure (or actual failure). For the organization, stresses may be evidenced through increased absenteeism and turnover, diminished morale, and potential losses in productivity. (It should be noted that these are potential liabilities of internal promotion—not merely internal promotion of nurses.)

Such problems arise because technical competence is no guarantee of supervisory effectiveness. It generally is recognized in industry, and increasingly in health care organizations, that a person who is promoted requires training in management skills. Training now is increasingly common in such problem areas as communications, decision making, and performance appraisal and serves to diminish the occurrence of the problems noted above. However, one important problem heretofore neglected is the change in interpersonal relations associated with internal promotion.

The newly appointed manager or supervisor is called upon to redefine relationships to those who previously were peers as well as to the organization. The change in roles has several ramifications. One is the potential for the group's resistance to the new supervisor's authority. The supervisor may well be confronted with defiant and testing behaviors reminiscent of those presented to the older sibling who is left in charge when the parents go out for the evening. Once "one of us," the new supervisor now is "one of them." Previously an equal, the new supervisor now can sit in judgment on the quantity and quality of the group members' performances and can promote and give raises or withhold them. The manager inevitably earns more money and has more status.

Given these circumstances, jealousies are bound to erupt. Negative responses by department staff members to a new supervisor can be placed on a continuum ranging from slight discomfort to active or passive hostility and blatant sabotage (e.g., non-compliance). These reactions will vary depending on the nature of the promotion, the needs and styles of the group members, the style of the new supervisor and of the predecessor, and the internal dynamics of the group itself.

Many organizations compound the problem of internal promotion by failing to provide the much-needed management training base. Under these conditions, supervisor and staff experience considerable anxiety and tension. Not trained in the mechanics of performance appraisal and discipline, for example, the new manager may approach such processes, which are critical to the success of the organization, very diffidently and superficially because of anxiety. Some situations may be approached in an inappropriate manner. For example, supervisors may fail to appreciate the difference between being a friend and a supervisor, allowing behavior requiring correction to continue with the culprit's vague promise of future improvements. Or, they may respond heavy-handedly after quiet tolerance over a prolonged period. (Some guidelines for handling such organizational processes are suggested in Chapter 9.)

At another level organizations fail their newly promoted supervisors when they do not provide a formal orientation. Unlike managers brought in from the outside, those promoted from within are assumed to know everyone in the organization who has any relevance to their new positions. Unfortunately, this is a far from accurate assumption. A staff nurse directs attention to and focuses on one set of patients and one team. The nature of the job does not require a broader organizational perspective. However, as individuals move into management, their perspectives must enlarge if they are to be effective. They must know how their department relates with others and where and how departments can work together profitably.

In addition, since the job also entails gathering information from other departments (Mintzberg, 1979) it is important to be plugged in. New supervisors without a formalized orientation may feel unsure about whom to trust, of whom to ask questions. Since they do not want to appear incompetent for the job, they tend to muddle through on their own, some successfully, others less so. Ironically, nursing administrators have expressed frustration with their management staff's inability to think in a managerial fashion. Without appropriate training and support it is unlikely that they will do so. These problems are further complicated by the position of women in management (Numerof, 1982, pp. 529–550).

To the extent that women have been socialized to assume passive dependent behaviors and leadership positions require something different, the woman as manager experiences role conflict. The definition of what has been acceptable behavior is in sharp contrast to what is required by the position. In addition, those who report to the woman manager often experience conflict since she does not fit the expected image. In other words, she is not male. As Kanter (1977) has noted, the spotlight may shine brightly on these women managers exacerbating performance anxiety. Expectations for success may be higher than for their male counterparts, thus creating stress. Access to participation in the informal organization may be restricted, creating yet another source of stress.

It could be argued that it is the responsibility of the organization to identify and teach coping strategies so that those who are promoted can deal with interpersonal problems and to provide socialization experiences that will help these persons adjust to their new role. Some health care organizations have training and education departments, and such roles might conceivably fall under their domain. Training programs for supervisors in management techniques emphasizing communications skills, conflict resolution, decision making, motivation, and similar tools could provide technical skills while also offering a structure for group support and mutual problem solving.

Such an orientation would help the newly promoted manager form an important identification with management and redefine the relationship to the work group, both of which are critical to the success of the manager. By providing management skills and facilitating the resocialization process, the organization enhances the positive aspects (eustress) of the promotion: the opportunity for growth and advancement, challenge, and the conditions under which the manager can make a meaningful difference to the organization.

Chapter 7

The Administrator's Experience

From the point of view of the hospital administrator, running a hospital is like trying to drive a car when the passengers have control of the wheel and the accelerator. The most the administrator can do is occasionally jam on the brakes (Fuchs, 1974).

The health care industry has been described by many as out of control. It has been criticized for its failure to meet the public's demand for service and to respond to the specific needs of some professionals employed in it, particularly nurses. Despite the criticism, it obviously is a growth industry, as evidenced by its achievements in new technologies, clinical capabilities, and scientific knowledge. These achievements have been accompanied by rising costs and the problems associated with unprecedented expansion. While the industry grows, the gap between the public's expectations of what it can deliver and what it does deliver widens.

Attempts to narrow the gap during the last decade have been many. A great number of these have focused on advances in the technological and clinical areas. Unfortunately, these efforts have not solved the problem. As Georgopoulos (1972) suggests, solutions lie not in the technological centers but in the organization of the system, its subsystems, and its components and in the organization and management of the people engaged in the delivery of health care at all levels.

At the top of this system sits the senior administrative group: the chief executive officer and associate and assistant administrators. In the final analysis the responsibility for the coordination and well-being of this enormous complex rests squarely on the shoulders of the chief executive officer. For many incumbents and for many about to receive their passport to the field—a master of health administration degree—reflection on the stresses of the job lead them to question why any individuals interested in preserving their sanity would want to take on such responsibility. An

191

examination of the changing nature of the role of the hospital administrator can yield insight into the sources of stress and point to coping strategies that may ameliorate some of the negative consequences associated with them.

THE EVOLUTION OF THE ADMINISTRATOR

The changing nature of the administrator's role can be studied against the background of the evolution of the hospital and its shifting goals and power bases. Obviously, hospitals have changed dramatically in the last 60 years. Once a place where only the chronically ill or those not able to afford private medical care at home might go, the hospital has become the institution through which the majority of health services are delivered in this country. As with any organization, hospitals have experienced changes in what they consider their major concerns as they have evolved over time.

When the changes are extensive, such as in the type of work that is done or in the financial base, the control of the organization also shifts in accordance with the task revisions and the competencies demanded to accomplish them. The effect of these changes can be seen in the dynamic relationships among administrators, trustees, and physicians in particular and the shifts in power that occur as a result of constantly evolving goals (Elling, 1968; Fuchs, 1974; Pfeffer, 1976).

For example, the power and influence of the trustees continues in hospitals today even though their significant contributions hark back to an era when they were appointed because of their philanthropic associations and/ or personal contributions. Now, most of the revenues the hospital requires to operate derive from other sources, not from philanthropy. Yet the trustees' influence remains and often creates barriers to change. Those with personal investments in particular hospitals, emotional and otherwise, do not look kindly on proposed mergers, cutbacks in services, and closings. Many hospitals, in an attempt to use their experience more effectively, have instituted trustee-education programs that clarify their role in today's industry.

Charles Perrow (1969) identifies a control sequence believed to be typical of most organizations, including hospitals, in which leadership dominance shifts from one group to another. (It should be noted that not all organizations go through this sequence and some do so in a different order because of individual demands. Those that do follow the sequence as presented may experience considerable variation in the process.) For example, hospitals with trustee domination and a focus on obtaining capital resources and legitimization as a viable health delivery institution, move to a medical staff domination and a concern for technological knowledge and skill, and finally to an administrative domination with its emphasis on internal and external coordination.

These shifts stem from the changing developmental needs of the organization. During the initial (trustee) phase, the focus must be on gaining enough community and political support and funds to construct a facility in which to treat patients. Because of their financial and political connections, trustees carry great influence. The second stage starts once the building is begun. The hospital must attract physicians to admit and treat patients. Patients are necessary to the survival of the facility and physicians are the primary gatekeepers to admissions. Despite the challenges noted in Chapter 6, particularly by nurses for increased autonomy, physician dominance is likely. Doctors will have input into the type of services offered, input that will continue through to the next stage—maturity. At maturity there should be a stable facility that offers a variety of services. Leadership dominance now falls to the administrator, who must coordinate the various professional staffs, provide liaison to the community, market the facility's services, and plan new programs. It is in the maturity stage that the health industry is now. It is the challenge of that coordination in particular that some administrators believe to be the most stressful part of their jobs.

Changes, necessary though they may be, often do not occur smoothly. No one likes to give up a power base. Each group has a vested interest in its own specialty. Furthermore, each sees the world with a different vision, often unable to perceive the merits of alternative perceptions. There is a tendency for one group to deprecate the perceptions of others, especially when it means a potential loss of control. The administrator, once relegated to the "business" concern of the hospital, now is in a pivotal position. This executive must understand the reasons for pulls in opposite directions in order to find suitable ways to bring the conflicting groups together. Recognition that the development needs of the organization demand different skills at different times means that some groups, while remaining important, may have to play a less dominant role.

MEDIATING ACROSS VALUE SYSTEMS

The disparity in value orientations among professions creates serious conflict in health delivery organizations, as noted in the previous two chapters. Experience suggests that much of the conflict stems from participants' difficulty in understanding what is psychologically important to the others' character and role. The administrator's challenge of the future will be to understand interprofessional conflicts within a diverse value framework and to learn techniques to help bridge gaps between people who see the world differently. Unfortunately, it appears that graduates of health administration and planning programs rarely are exposed to these problems in their training. When these problems are identified, they are passed over too frequently with, "You'll learn that on the job." Some of the specific implications of values and their translation to organizational structures and programs are explored next.

The values of any system reflect those of the majority group. One of the most important and influential sources of values has been professional socialization. The impact of professionalism in health care has been strong. In most cases the opinions of lay people are subordinated to those of professionals. Indeed, historically, even the opinion of the lay administrator has been second to that of the professional. The organization of health care revolves around professional authority. As in many systems, however, not all professional authority carries equal weight. Certain professionals hold more authority than others and those others are in subordinate positions.

Physicians as an occupational group dominate the health care sector and the hospital in particular in terms of the power they wield. Consequently, physicians' values dominate the industry. The treatment of disease, an emphasis on saving lives and delivering patient care at any cost, and the role of the doctor as the uncontested ("autocratic" as opposed to "participative") leader of the work group are physician values. These values are reflected in organizational structures, policies, and practices.

Structures and policies that are consistent with the value orientation of physicians are not always in the best interest of the health facility as an organization, of the various professional groups within it, or, for that matter, of the patients. Freidson (1970) regards this "professional dominance" as the key to the inadequacy of health care delivery and as responsible for the unresponsiveness of the system to its patients, the people Freidson regards as the real consumers.

There are those in the medical profession who recognize that changes in the distribution of power need to be and will be made but that power will not be reallocated without considerable conflict and stress for all concerned. The conflict already exists; it is clearest in battles between doctors and nurses over professional turf. The administrator's role in this reallocation of power will be critical. That executive must mediate between competing concerns and orchestrate different professional groups to achieve quality patient care.

How the administrator views health and disease will greatly influence how that power is distributed. For example, the administrator's view will influence the response to the demands of different services for increased autonomy. These services might include nursing, the organized medical staff, social services, physical therapy, and a host of others. It also will influence how the administrator responds to the need for patient advocacy. Finally, it will be reflected in how the hospital departments are organized. For instance, is the nursing service under the medical staff or are nursing and social services equal to medical services in that both report directly to administration?

As Exhibit 7-1 suggests, individuals' orientation to the delivery of care depends on the model they hold dear. Each model has ramifications for the type of care patients receive, and where; for the role they play in the course of their own treatment; and for the role various professionals perform in the delivery of it.

Administrators cannot afford to be passive observers in the organization's functioning. Some administrators perceive themselves as not "interfering" in the delivery of care or clinical matters and may protest vehemently when accused of becoming involved in them but their denials belie

Exhibit 7-1 Treatment and Role Ramifications of Health Models

Effects on:	*Medical Model*	*Health Maintenance Model*
Orientation to care	Treatment of disease Specific problem	Prevention Maintenance of health Life style, whole person
Patient role	Tends to be passive, compliant Follows prescribed regimen	Tends to be active, responsible Agent in own care
Professional role	Physician dominance Hierarchical arrangement of professional groups, with each having well-defined role and status	Shifting dominance Increased importance of allied health professionals Team approach to care Task to be performed can determine which individual(s) with specific competence is best suited to handle a situation
Place of care	Inpatient facility	Ambulatory care facility

Source: Reprinted from *The Practice of Management for Health Care Professionals* by Rita E. Numerof with permission of AMACOM, a Division of American Management Associations, © 1982.

the truth. Administrators influence and often determine the type of care in a facility through their budgetary decisions. To deny this is to deny responsibility for their actions and pave the way for a relationship of questionable trust between administration and staff. It is far better to deal directly with the consequences of budgetary actions than to avoid conflict over such complex concerns as whether money should be spent on new surgical suites or wellness centers.

Administrators tend to internalize the value system of the dominant group—the physicians. Without realizing it they act in terms of doctors' values and make policies that demonstrate a bias toward physicians' wants and needs that sometimes are detrimental to the broader well-being of the hospital. This bias may be rationalized in terms of the physicians' economic power. Doctors admit patients to the hospital. To the extent that physicians act as gatekeepers to the facility, administrators are likely to direct marketing and program efforts to them.

Even if administrators are committed to "new approaches" to the delivery of health care, they simultaneously are faced with cost containment and therefore are likely to favor a traditional medical model. Because higher utilization means increased revenues for the hospital, they are likely to emphasize inpatient treatment rather than a preventive program, ambulatory care, or short-term stays. Longer stays make the job of managing the facility easier. Lower patient turnover means a more stable environment. Paperwork is decreased and administrative costs and pressures are lower. In addition, patients who are not as acutely and seriously ill, are easier to manage.

So far, the economic balance obviously has been weighted in favor of the medical model. In the short run the potential for conflict resulting from the ambiguity of the team approach health maintenance model also is reduced. But in the long run such an approach is likely to bring about the termination of the administrator. The expansion of various professional groups and their accompanying demands to be heard, as well as legitimate claims by proponents of the health maintenance model, require that new solutions be found to handle economic issues. One alternative for the administrator would be to consider new marketing strategies that would address the need to maintain the viability of the institution while simultaneously providing care based on therapeutic considerations. To do this the administrator must be willing to take a risk and innovate in a direction that may be contrary to the orientation of the dominant group.

It is apparent that a change in attitudes among all professionals is essential for the future of health care delivery. This change must include the acceptance of interprofessional interdependence as the operative value for the organization and delivery of social health services.

THE ADMINISTRATOR AS CONFLICT NEGOTIATOR

Given the changing technological and managerial character of the health care field, several developments are visible on the horizon that will significantly affect the administrator's role and function. Interorganizational and interdepartmental cooperation will become increasingly more of a necessity as institutions find that survival in an age of increasing costs and shortages of skilled personnel demand collaboration. The wise administrator will seek opportunities for such cooperation, attempting to optimize the positions of all participants. Such cooperation will bring with it new problems and sources of conflict as the dominance of certain groups is challenged and power alliances change.

One of the biggest shifts will occur in the dominance of physicians. As noted earlier, the challenge to physician dominance comes from numerous sources: from the pressures of allied health professionals' concerns about expanded roles, from an emphasis on holistic health as opposed to traditional medicine, from consumers who demand a voice in the delivery of care, and from government sources that wish to protect that public voice and monitor the quality of care.

Perhaps most importantly, the challenge for administration and management must be one of integration and orchestration. With increasing specialization, continuously advancing technology, more vocal demands, and higher expectations on the part of consumers, allied health professionals, and medical and nonmedical personnel, administrators will be expected to and must coordinate. Administrator/managers will be forced to provide a bridge to bring together the differing needs and perceptions of these actors on the health care stage. To succeed in such a position and to gain enough power to manage effectively the administrators will have to be facilitators, setting a climate for change and coordination as they control and integrate. The political nature of health care expands the role for administrators who no longer can be content merely to manage through direction and control but must feel comfortable in and assume the role of conflict negotiator.

Such a role, however necessary for the well-being of the institution, faces built-in resistance of a historical nature. This resistance is based in the traditional structure of the professional organization as a predominantly role-oriented institution (Harrison, 1981; Levinson, 1976). The role-oriented organization performs a specific social role, such as a hospital or school. Within such organizations various occupational roles are specifically defined and differentiated. In a hospital are physicians, nurses, aides, laboratory technologists, social workers, occupational therapists, and so forth, each with highly specialized training and functions. Status and power are adhered to as a function of commitment and loyalty, legal sanctions, and perceived legitimacy. Harrison notes that in role-oriented organizations behavioral predictability and stability are overriding values. As a result, change comes slowly. Perhaps most importantly, in such organizations individual autonomy, the exercise of initiative and of independent judgment, and individuals' commitment to the institution tend not to be developed or utilized fully except at the highest administrative levels. Too often, loyalty is to the profession, not to the institution.

Power Allocation and Function

In part because of the adherence to roles, rules, and social obligations, power tends to be allocated by function, the perceived social value or importance attached to that function, and its related legal responsibility. Physicians, as noted, have assumed dominance and have wielded more power than other groups, including nursing and administration. A positive side effect of the adherence to such structure is a sense of security. However, a very complicated negative side effect is that all this tends to undermine institutional loyalty. Trained professionals generally identify primarily with and are loyal to their professions and only secondarily to the organizations in which they work.

Professional loyalty tends to undermine organizational loyalty and, as a result, to undercut interprofessional collaboration and teamwork. Professional groups all too often respond to their particular interests and needs without taking into account a broader organizational perspective that places their needs alongside those of other groups. This has implications for administrators and increases stress. For example, among the top ten stressors reported by chief executive officers in the health administrators study reported in Chapter 4, a prominent factor is dealing with conflicts of needs or interests between people in the organization.

Nonclinical administrators find additional sources of conflict and potential stress in the role-oriented organization. Nonclinical, professional administrators often are not regarded as a "first among equals" (Levinson, 1976) who coordinate all roles but are perceived in a somewhat deprecatory manner. While clinical staff members are dependent on administrators for financial and managerial support, clinicians may merely tolerate the executives' existence and openly resent their scope of power. The problem is compounded when administrators are unable to relate to any one of the clinical groups vital to the functioning of the organization.

When conflicts in the role-oriented organization arise between clinical groups, as they inevitably do, they frequently are expressed indirectly, adding to the difficulty in resolving them effectively. Part of the indirectness seems to reflect a lack of training for clinicians in conflict resolution and their general belief that conflict itself is in some way harmful. In addition, clinicians are socialized in matters relating to patient care, not to negotiation of power and conflict. Many clinicians believe themselves to be "above" needs for power (Numerof, 1982), an orientation that leads to serious problems for the organization.

Competition and power struggles are expressed in terms of service preferences that may be rationalized on any number of bases. In other situations, avoidance of power results in the inability to meet goals effectively. This problem occurs even at the level of the board of trustees. For example, discussions of the institution's mission frequently include vague references to quality of patient care. Too often, trustees do not debate exactly what that means since to question the kind of care, for whom, and delivered by whom is likely to raise conflict directly. Instead, the trustees resolve the conflict by not supporting new programs in such areas as patient education or ambulatory care.

The Mediator Role and Its Stresses

The end result for the administrators is that they must be constant mediators across roles between professions and individuals, responding to direct conflict when it occurs and bringing it out into the open for resolution when it is indirect and involves passive resistance. For administrators uncomfortable with this role and in their position as "outsiders," the resultant stress is likely to be very great. For clinical administrators there is the added burden of having to deal with internal value shifts from clinical to administrative perspectives, as noted in Chapter 5. In addition, clinical administrators may be viewed as clinical failures. In medicine, in particular, there frequently is disdain for the physician who, it is presumed, could not make it in medicine and turned to administration instead. Both clinical and nonclinical administrators face the burden of working with managerially less concerned and less sophisticated managers.

Given these stumbling blocks, what can facilitate a more smoothly run, perhaps less stressful organization? Levinson (1976) suggests that the answer lies in the ability of the administrator to lead, not merely manage. Administrators who set the tone of the organization and lead find themselves in a task-oriented organization in which the approach to problems is, "How do we solve this?" as opposed to, "This is the way we'll handle this." The new approach focuses not on roles and their inherent worth but on the specific task at hand and on the person(s) whose knowledge and competence is most likely to lead to a positive outcome.

In the task-oriented organization, everyone's commitment is to the task and to the organization. When professional role divisions that offer security to some are broken down, flexibility increases, as does change. There is even greater pressure on the administrators to enhance organizational cohesion, the job is facilitated by a diminished role differentiation. The likelihood of building interprofessional trust and respect increases when individuals are recognized not merely for their professional membership but for their own contributions. In this regard the administrator's role as integrator, as organizational team facilitator, and as leader of a diverse group of professionals is critical.

At the same time that administrators must be concerned about the internal politics of the organization, they also must be attuned to various constituencies in the community. These can present conflicting demands for service. Given very real financial constraints, yet with internal and external constituencies that have valid needs, how do administrators maintain support for the institution among these groups, keep it viable financially, and chart its course proactively as opposed to reactively?

Some attention has been given to the educational needs of hospital administrators of the future in light of these circumstances, often with somewhat controversial results (Richards, 1982). Some educators believe that attention to interpersonal dynamics in the organization are less important than fiscal and technical areas and vice versa. There is no question that skills in conflict negotiation and resolution are necessary, as are specific technical abilities in such areas as marketing, finance, and planning. At the personal level, administrators must be able to tolerate ambiguity and help lead the professional staff through the murky waters of major institutional change with its shifting role and activity boundaries. Integrating the staff in order to maintain stability and cohesion are necessary in order to meet the broad objectives reflective of the organization's purpose. To succeed in this, the administrators must create alliances and develop trust among members of the staff.

ADMINISTRATORS AND BOARDS

There is no question that the administrator's role is enormously complex. It also is regarded by some as highly vulnerable. As one seasoned administrator in a large Southern hospital stated:

> The administrator's position is really precarious when you come to think of it. He's the only one who can be fired. It's unlikely that with all the care taken now in medical credentialing that a

physician will be let go. The staff is protected by unions or due process and can't be fired without cause. But if the board decides it doesn't like you, the CEO can be out when the board calls it.

The relationship between the board and CEO often is highly conflictual, particularly where the administrator's power has not been clearly defined or delegated. The resultant stress for the organization as a whole and the CEO in particular can be quite serious.

For example, one hospital board required that it approve all new programs, changes in existing programs, and expenditures of more than $1,000. The fallout from such tight control was a bureaucratic nightmare. Middle management would present ideas for review and consideration to administration. Several months might elapse without a response. When the idea was pursued, the inevitable explanation was that the program had not yet been reviewed because other matters had taken precedence. Frustration inevitably built within middle management's staff since "no response" was fairly typical in the organization. It is small wonder that the staff attempted to unionize, often with the explicit support of these managers.

Strategies for Coping with the Board

Administrators interviewed in the stress study described in Chapter 4 who identified board/management role conflict as a significant source of stress offered some interesting coping strategies. The strategy perceived to be most effective entailed direct confrontation with the board concerning conflict, the aim being clarification of roles and responsibilities. Other administrators have utilized communications techniques to keep board members regularly informed and have made compromises in order to resolve role discrepancies. They have found this has been fairly successful in solving problems.

Less successful strategies have included working with staff to gain moral support and attempting to put pressure on board members to acquire what the executive perceives to be "needed education in modern day hospital administration." The indirectness of this approach may be what makes its effect less than ideal. Another administrator has taken to wishing for additional authority through the execution of good work within the organization. The wished-for recognition and delegation of authority is, once again, not handled directly, possibly accounting for spotty results with this strategy.

It appears that keeping issues surfaced and addressing benefits and costs of various courses of action while maintaining consistent policies and procedures has the broadest success in handling the disorganization resulting from board-administration role discrepancies. Without such consistency and openness it is likely that the staff will be left to deal with an administration perceived as being unclear about the direction in which the organization needs to go. As noted in previous chapters, such confusion increases organizational stress.

Problems and issues inherent in the CEO-board relationship are sources of potential stress. Competition is almost inevitable between the parties, despite the fact that there seem to be as many types of administrator-board relationships as there are CEOs and boards (Kovner & Norville, 1979). The distribution of power lies at the heart of the competition: who has what power and how is its distribution viewed (Moore & Wood, 1979). Part of the problem reflects the powerful triumvirate of the hospital: CEO, board, and medical staff. Where power fragmentation was the rule many years ago, now there is increasing integration, overlap, and multiple responsibility, not the least of which is legal.

Questions of whether or not the CEO and medical director or medical staff president should be full voting board members are frequent, with the debate intense on both sides. To this is added debate about nursing administration's access to and participation on the board, thus further challenging traditional lines of separate power. Interestingly, the American Hospital Association position is that the CEO should be present at all board meetings and be a full member. It also recommends medical staff membership and representation from key administrative areas.

Additional problems reflect various constraints and opportunities in the reciprocal roles: CEOs' expectations of board performance and vice versa, the actual amount of time available for contact, and the manner in which meetings are conducted. CEOs' expectations of the board range from desiring a rubber stamp on all matters to wanting a strong board with a high degree of energy and commitment to the organization. Neither type is absolutely right or wrong. What works really depends upon the organization, its history, and the mutual expectations of the participants.

The CEO, the Medical Staff, and the Board

A critical factor determining CEO-board rapport is CEO-medical staff relations. Where the latter are not congruent, power problems are likely to emerge in the CEO-board domain (Kovner & Norville, 1979). Of equal importance is the way in which the CEO regards board involvement. Does the CEO respect board members or engage in shows of power through verbal attacks? Is information presented honestly or are changes made before the auditors arrive? The interpersonal nature of this important interchange sets the stage for the entire organization.

The amount of time available for personal contact also influences the CEO-board relationship. It is extremely difficult to share ideas in a large group. It is particularly important that the CEO and board chairman spend time together sharing ideas.

The reciprocal nature of CEO-board relationships is best reflected in agenda preparation when important issues reflecting concerns of both sides are discussed, with sufficient time spent, with minutes taken, and an agenda adhered to.

The more successful CEO-based relationships appear to be characterized, not surprisingly, by mutual respect and directness, by mutual and formal evaluation (Umbdenstock, 1979), and by mutual acceptance of role interdependence. Critical to such success is the ability to differentiate between what is the role and function of the board and what is to be delegated to administration. It is here that the process often breaks down.

An important question in differentiating roles is to identify what is policy (i.e., strategic planning) and the primary responsibility of the board, and what is management and the primary responsibility of administration. A criticism by many CEOs is that boards inappropriately meddle in the day-to-day operations of the hospital. The meddling often occurs because the board has not been properly educated as to its role.

Board education, more recently referred to as governing board development, is a role for the CEO. If the administrator does not take a leadership role in giving the board the tools it needs to make informed policy decisions, the board is likely to encroach on the CEO's turf. In light of this need, in January 1980 the Joint Commission on the Accreditation of Hospitals required member institutions to conduct trustee orientation and education programs (JCAH, 1980).

Where hospital trustees traditionally were selected for philanthropic and political reasons, and played a legitimizing role for the hospital in the community, their current function has been evolving to a director role in which ultimate financial and legal responsibility rests squarely on their shoulders and is reflected in the policy directions they set. Neither the trustees nor the institution can afford to have board members who are not informed about the health system as a whole and the organization in particular. Increasingly, board members must assure that the issues of medical staff credentialing (Mattern, 1979), privileges (Sloss, 1979), quality assurance (Van Vorst, 1979), and due process (Johnson, 1979) are policed. Because of the enormity of this task alone, some (Rogatz, 1979) have recommended that the hospital hire a full-time medical director, a trend that seems timely indeed. The board, of course, also must respond to community needs (Umbdenstock, 1979).

It is because of the complexity and scope of today's hospital, complicated even more with the advent of multihospital systems, that CEOs must work to engage as partners not only their managers and clinical staffs but their trustees as well. As Cunningham (1980) suggests, administrators, trustees, and physicians who have learned to work together well as an integrated team will survive the stresses of increased competition, changing regulations, and financial cutbacks. Those who have not learned this invaluable lesson are likely to perish.

'LONELINESS AT THE TOP'

Inherent in the positions of senior administration—chief executive officer in particular—is loneliness. This often is described by incumbents as the feeling of being ultimately responsible for the organization. Others talk of the sense of isolation that results from not having organizational peers, of not being truly able to confide in subordinates, of having to be a role model for others while lacking a support network for themselves. Interestingly, CEOs and senior administrators ranked being a role model for others in the institution as one of their top ten stressors in the study described in Chapter 4.

It might be argued that the loneliness at the top occurs as a function of organizational structure and the personality of the chief executive officer. For example, there is the hospital administrator who suffers from this yet whose office arrangement sets up the very conditions about which the executive complains. The office is reached through a long corridor that houses various meeting rooms, including the rather awesome board room. The office is entered through the chambers of a number of receptionists and secretaries, the last of whom is the private secretary. The message is very clear to all staff members: This CEO does not wish to be disturbed unless it is absolutely essential. A separate entrance provides private access to the office so the executive does not have to walk through the hospital corridors upon entering and leaving. Not readily accessible, this administrator has set up an aura of organizational distance.

At the other end of the spectrum is the CEO whose presence is made known throughout the institution. This type of administrator conveys a feeling of openness and availability by first-name self-introduction to employees, attending department meetings, and holding informal weekly coffees to get to know as many as possible of his 1,600 staff members and their work-related concerns.

With position and responsibility in an organization come status and the opportunity for privilege. A side effect of increased status and privilege, however, is increased distance between the privileged and the not so privileged, and it is this distance that fosters the loneliness. This is not to suggest that all symbols of status and perquisites of position be abolished but rather that the executive identify which differences based on status and position are functional and which are merely symbolic and distance enhancers. The CEO needs a secretary but is it necessary that the secretary make the administrator's phone calls? The message in having someone else arrange the call is very clear: "My time is more valuable than yours." Such a message creates distance and emphasizes the hierarchy of the organization.

When hierarchy is emphasized, people tend to see each other in terms of the roles and positions they hold, not as individuals who tend to have different, complementary, and necessary organizational functions. If communications take place as a function of hierarchical position, distance is created in the exchange with one person "up" and the other "down." The message is filtered through power dynamics and is distorted. The subordinate may, for instance, not reveal constructive criticism directly to a superior but withhold those views. It is in passive noncompliance with implementation through forgetting, procrastinating, and so forth that the criticism finally is expressed.

Distance impedes the development of trusting interprofessional relationships. Without a relationship that has been built over time, the CEOs essentially barricade themselves in their offices and set up the conditions for "loneliness at the top."

This approach does not mean, however, that no one is upstairs running the store. Rules and procedures must exist clearly in all organizations and in certain matters it is the CEO alone who must take responsibility for a decision. This decision is more likely to be effective if it has had input from various parts of the organization. Such input is possible only when the CEO is accessible, involved, and has developed relationships with employees.

An approach such as this also is more likely to make the often difficult task of performance appraisal, for instance, much smoother and more meaningful throughout the organization. To the extent that the staff members know the boss, know , the needs, strengths, and weaknesses of the department, feel informed about their work, and have a relationship characterized by trust with the CEO, they will be receptive to input that tells them their performance is lacking in some areas. In essence they will be able to hear and use constructive criticism without reacting to it as a hostile attack.

The core element in bringing this about is the development of interpersonal relationships that foster more efficient operations in the organization and protect executives against managerial isolation and the hazards of burnout (the subject of the next chapter). Ironically, many CEOs erroneously perceive the time spent on developing these relationships as inefficient.

Part III

Meeting the Challenge

This final part begins in Chapter 8 with a detailed analysis of how individuals and potentially helpful "others" can recognize and cope with four of the major stressors that have emerged from the ever-increasing pace and pressure of today's society—burnout, alcoholism, drug abuse, and emotional disturbances.

Chapter 9, noting that organizations in many direct and indirect ways produce the conditions that can create these problems, discusses how they can meet their responsibilities to help manage such stresses. It also points out that these problems seriously affect not only personnel at all levels but also the well-being, productivity, and indeed the very survival, of the organizations themselves.

Chapter 10 looks at the personal, individual response to stress; psychological, physiological, cognitive, and behavioral causative factors; and the use of professionally conducted employee assistance programs.

It will be noted that the term "employee" is used throughout. Physicians generally are not "employees" of hospitals and their situation is treated in the section on physician impairment, but all of the material discussed here is, by extension, applicable to them as well.

Chapter 8

Recognizing Signs of Stress

"Sometimes I feel that I just don't care about the patients' problems anymore. They all begin to sound alike. I think I must respond to them automatically."

"I get home at night exhausted. I take naps but then I can't get to sleep. It doesn't seem to matter, though, if I don't take naps. I'm still unable to get to sleep. My appetite is shot and I think I must have some gastrointestinal problems causing the mess."

"I find that I'm really on edge most of the time. I used to be patient with the staff but increasingly I find it impossible to tolerate their inability to think quickly so I try to avoid them. There's so much to do I come in earlier and stay later. I can't really depend on anyone else."

"Somehow the challenge, the spark, has died. I'm bored with the job and with life in general. I hate coming to work but I don't really feel much better when I'm away. I really think it's me. Something's happened that I can't seem to respond anymore."

What all of these statements share in common are symptoms of work-related stress involving any or all of the following: psychological difficulty, as in eating and sleep disturbances; cognitive difficulty, as in impaired judgment; and interpersonal difficulty, as in short frustration tolerance and isolation. On the surface such symptoms are reminiscent of clinical depression. However, these cases are not reflective of psychiatric disorder but of stress—in particular, the phenomenon referred to as burnout.

BURNOUT

As noted throughout the book, stress manifests itself in many ways. At the physical level, symptoms range from insomnia, headaches, and stomachaches through more highly developed illnesses including gastrointestinal disorders, high blood pressure, and heart conditions. At the interpersonal level are inflexibility, impatience, generalized anger, bossiness, and blaming others. At the behavioral level, stress may manifest itself through drinking, the use of stimulants or tranquilizing drugs, trembling, nervous tics, and impulsive behavior. At the emotional level stress may appear as fatigue, self-blame, worry, agitation, feelings of depression, general anxiety or tension, frustration and an inability to relax. In the study described in Chapter 4, two scales—unconscious behaviors and depressive symptoms—were important indicators of stress symptomatology. It is apparent that stress symptoms arrange themselves in clusters. One large cluster of job overload stress symptoms may be referred to as employee burnout.

The term burnout is suggestive of a flame that once flickered and has been extinguished. To burn out implies a progressive state occurring over a period of time. For instance a person who generally is cooperative and open to constructive criticism now seems hostile when a superior makes suggestions. Errors begin to creep into work that once was of consistently high quality. The employee may feel tired all the time, complain of headaches, and cannot seem to shake a cold. Feelings of low self-esteem emerge, partly a reaction to diminished job performance, partly the cause of the poorer work. Increased difficulty in making professional decisions augments the growing problems.

Burnout, as an outcome of excessive work-related stress, is characterized by exhaustion, irritability, and apathy. The burnout process typically begins when the person's expectations are frustrated by the work environment. Burnout "likelies" are people with inadequate authority and/or resources available to do the job or those who are not receiving the financial or psychological rewards they deserve for the tasks they are performing. These people are more likely than those not experiencing burnout to suffer minor mishaps and to have problems concentrating, acting, or thinking. They are more likely to take unhealthy risks or to take no risks at all and go rigidly by the book. Some find they are unable to stop working. Others find they have no energy to work, feeling lifeless and depressed.

Maslach (1976), for example, identifies three primary aspects of the burnout syndrome that are measured by a self-report scale:

1. Emotional exhaustion: characterized by feelings of frustration at work; of fatigue in the morning in the face of having to go to work; and of being used up and emotionally drained.
2. Depersonalization: pertains to the individual's attitudes toward patients and/or clients. Feelings of depersonalization are reflected in the development of a hard attitude toward patients and staff, becoming callous to people, a lack of caring about patients, and a feeling of being blamed for their problems and physical illnesses.
3. Lack of personal accomplishment and involvement: reflected in difficulty or failure in understanding how patients feel about things, a sense of being unable to influence others' lives in one's own work, a lack of feeling of achieving goals, and difficulty in maintaining emotional equanimity in the face of problems.

In short, burnout suggests that an emotional center has gone; optimism and enthusiasm have been lost, only negativism is left.

While the research utilizing this scale has yielded some fairly consistent results (Maslach, 1978; Maslach & Pines, 1977, 1978) it seems likely that other dimensions of burnout exist and must be taken into account. Others have described related phenomena as burnout. Bardo (1979), for instance, focuses on the results of burnout as evidenced in workers' low self-esteem, inability or refusal to take their jobs seriously, and a strong "abnormal" desire for vacations, perhaps reflecting a desire to escape the work situation. Reid (1977) notes dehumanization of clients, task avoidance, isolation from colleagues, compulsive complaining, loss of creativity, and difficulty in making decisions and explaining them. Block (1978) describes burnout as resulting in an attitude of cynicism and dehumanization toward clients. Others have equated burnout with alienation, as in estrangement from self (Miller, 1967) or powerlessness (Pearlin, 1962).

The Multiple Dimensions of Burnout

However, Gillespie (1979) asserts that burnout is not related to measures of alienation but seems to be a distinct phenomenon with two underlying dimensions: active burnout and passive burnout. Active burnout is evidenced by an individual's assertive stances such as negativism or hostility and passive burnout by withdrawal behavior, apathy, or exhaustion. Gillespie (1980) finds certain externally related organizational and/or social psychological variables to be correlated with active expressions of burnout. These include professional respect, status, and the ability to influence organizational activity. The more passive expressions of burnout tend to be correlated with social psychological variables of a more internal nature:

liking the type of work, a sense of accomplishment, and feeling that the persons had a chance to do their best.

Pursuing the notion that multiple dimensions of burnout exist, Numerof and Gillespie (1983), in research into the symptoms of burnout, their causes, and organizational correlates in hospitals, suggest that, in contrast to popular views, burnout is not a pathological event. Rather, it seems to come and go in individuals, particularly among those working in high-demand, labor-intensive environments with responsibility for human life yet with severely restrained resources. Under these conditions individuals periodically experience mild symptoms of burnout that are recognized, handled, and then pass.

Pathological burnout seems to occur when an individual experiences extremely intense and/or a great many feelings related to this condition. It also may occur if a person holds onto such feelings tenaciously, thus transforming an otherwise normal, possibly adaptive response into a debilitating one. This is seen in the case of feelings of isolation on the job that can be viewed as a symptom of burnout and as a healthy, coping strategy aimed in the short run at giving the individual a needed respite from the intense demands of the work. However, when these feelings of isolation and of interpersonal behavior to reinforce actual isolation continue over an extended time, they seem to lose their ameliorative effect and instead augment feelings of burnout and their associated negative consequences.

Thus, it appears that burnout is experienced as a cyclical event with several stages of severity and fairly serious consequences in the more advanced phases for the organization and the symptomatic individual. While some of the symptoms of burnout are directed primarily at individuals (e.g. headaches, depression) or the organization (e.g., finding themselves unable to respond to the needs of the staff, just getting the job done and not doing the best they can), it is not yet feasible to separate symptomatology into discrete categories because of the interconnectedness of secondary effects.

For example, while physical symptomatology does affect the individual primarily, it has secondary effects on the organization as evidenced through increased absenteeism as a result of illness and/or reduced ability to function on the job. Similarly, individuals' disengagement from the work and not doing their best obviously affects the organization from the standpoint of reduced quality. These persons are likely to suffer through diminished self-esteem, which in turn increases disengagement.

Another conceptualization of the burnout process is offered by Edelwich and Brodsky (1980), who regard it as a cyclical five-stage process of disillusionment that includes enthusiasm, stagnation, frustration, apathy, and intervention:

Stage 1—Enthusiasm: This pertains to one initial period of excitement and high energy on the job but characterized by unrealistic expectations as well, an attitude making individuals vulnerable. People may view a job as the fulfillment of their life at this point, giving meaning to existence. Overwork, overidentification with patients, and a fervent sense of idealism are pitfalls of this stage. (This is akin to the idealism described in Chapter 5 in medical students who view themselves and their profession as offering more than they can hope to deliver—an idealism frequently turned into cynicism over time.)

Stage 2—Stagnation: This places individuals' emphasis on nonwork-related elements such as family, friends, and leisure activities. Career development and personal needs become more important than the job itself.

Stage 3—Frustration: This focuses on whether or not people are effective in what they do and on whether the organization in which they work serves to undermine what they are trying to accomplish.

Stage 4—Apathy: This occurs in response to frustration where individuals choose to remain on the job or lack realistic alternatives to it and thus are forced to stay. There they "put in time," exerting minimal effort and avoiding challenge and growth.

Stage 5—Intervention: This is an attempt to break the burnout cycle through any one of a number of actions. Intervention may occur in response to any previous stage. Frequently, it occurs once the first four stages have run their course. Interventions may include changing jobs within the organization, going to another employer, or leaving the particular field altogether. If the person remains on the job, intervention could involve modification of job responsibilities or of relationships with peers, subordinates, superiors, and/or patients. Attention to other aspects of life such as taking a vacation or pursuing a leisure interest also may help to change people's perspective and reduce the burnout cycle.

Interestingly, the causes of burnout seem to stem from a limited number of organizational factors relating to the nature of the work itself and to management practices. Organizational factors relating to management practices include:

• undefined or unrealistic job expectations from superiors
• poor interpersonal communication

- lack of trust within the organization
- management by exception
- inconsistent and changing policies.

The impact of each of these is discussed separately, then the factors stemming from the nature of the work.

Job Expectations

Undefined or unrealistic job expectations from superiors result in confusion for subordinates and is referred to in the literature on work-related climate as low job clarity (the study reported in Chapter 4 also identified such lack of definition as a source of organizational stress). Lack of definition also sets the stage for the development of unrealistic, add-on, or "creeping" job expectations. Under these circumstances management rewards competence and successful performance with challenge, increased work demands, and high expectations. Some employees have described what they perceive to be an effective coping strategy for these situations: faced with add-on jobs, they claim it pays to look confused, perform only adequately competent work, and above all to not appear too bright (on an assembly line these behaviors might be referred to as a work slowdown).

These employee protective strategies have obvious negative consequences for the organization in that achievement is reduced and managerial/subordinate trust is eroded. However, there also are less obvious negative consequences for the individuals as well. Their professional integrity and personal self-esteem are likely to be diminished. While they may feel professionally abused in the sense of being taken advantage of, they also are aware of their own professional "dishonesty" and lack of directness with management, resulting in a confused mixture of anger, guilt, disgust, and self-imposed pressure for not doing enough. Unrealistic expectations also lead them to feel trapped and increase the likelihood that they will miss deadlines because they have become overcommitted in an attempt to meet them.

Interpersonal Communication

To the extent that management is unresponsive to communication from subordinates aimed at clarifying job expectations and modifying those that are unrealistic, interpersonal communications within the organization are likely to be eroded. Thus the first organizational factor linked to burnout is related to the second. Poor communication results when people assume and/or have learned from experience that their perspectives will not be given a fair hearing or judicious consideration, so they begin to not communicate. Assumptions not necessarily based on fact can run rampant through the organization, with employees at all levels becoming angry when others do not meet their unspoken expectations.

An example is the case of the manager of the engineering department of a fairly large hospital. Having spent the last 24 hours resolving a serious matter, he is confronted by the impatient and annoyed head nurse complaining about his department's failure to fix several air conditioners that have been acting peculiarly for several days. Her request for service already was 48 hours old and she was angered by what she perceived as inefficiency. The engineering manager chose not to explain his problem (which more accurately was really the hospital's) nor identify with her perception of having been overlooked and forgotten. Instead, his response was an equally impatient, "We'll get around to it when we can."

Had the engineer chosen to communicate to the head nurse that there would be a further delay because of an emergency or that the current lag had been caused by such reasons and that her concerns would be attended to quickly, it is likely that her annoyance would have subsided quickly. Under the actual circumstances, however, the nurse went away angrier and the engineer was upset by the demands and lack of appreciation his department received from others. Insufficient understanding caused by poor communications set the stage for burnout. So much for assumptions.

Where understanding is missing from human interaction, people are likely to feel in the dark, irritated, and unappreciated. A frequent comment is, "Others aren't interested in what I'm doing." Where communication channels are not available, particularly across departments and up and down the hierarchy, anger and frustration are likely to be misplaced, including inward. Anger that is turned inward produces a variety of symptoms: insomnia, changes in eating habits, generalized fatigue, and irritability. Self-blame also may occur, lowering self-esteem and self-respect. In an attempt to overcome negative feelings about themselves, people may take on extra work, extending themselves beyond reasonable expectations, or they may lose perspective on what reasonable priorities are.

Lack of Trust

In situations where poor communications exist, the third organizational factor in burnout—lack of trust—also is evident. In part the consequence of insufficient understanding, lack of trust works as a negative feedback loop, eroding communications further. Individuals who do not trust their superiors or colleagues are likely to be reticent in communicating, thus increasing the problem of understanding. The communications-trust issue is particularly important with regard to individuals' ability to say no to unreasonable work demands. If requested to chair a committee, for instance, can they say no, with a rationale, and be assured that failure to "volunteer" for the chairmanship will not be translated into a negative performance appraisal or less than expected merit increase?

To the extent that women have been socialized to meet others' needs and not say no without seeing themselves as inadequate or a failure, the problem may be more serious for them and more conducive to burnout. However, it should not be assumed that the problem is limited to women. One senior level male administrator commented, "I've never had a problem having things turned back on me during a performance review . . . of course, I've never said no."

Management by Exception

Under management by exception, good or excellent performance is seen as not meriting comment or recognition. Only errors or less than acceptable performance evoke comment. The stage is set for burnout in the form of feelings of unappreciation and lack of recognition. These feelings are reflected in such comments as, "I put myself out for this place and no one seems to notice or care" and "People expect us to do good work but they only let us know when we screw up or do less than what's expected."

These feelings, when recurrent, breed resentment, frustration, and apathy that, in turn, may be reflected in work, culminating in the behavior expressed by: "I don't care if things don't get done, someone else will do it," or "I work just to get the job done. I don't put myself out anymore." Where management by exception is operative and individuals express feelings of being taken advantage of, there also is likely to be low organizational commitment. The latter decreases the likelihood that internal sources of support will be found, since the prevailing norm may have become: "No one here cares. Look out for yourself."

Policy Inconsistencies

Finally, inconsistent and changing policies facilitate burnout by creating poorly defined job expectations. As one manager described the situation, "We are left in turmoil over the job, constantly asking if what we are doing is right and how that is going to affect our performance review if it's not."

With regard to the nature of the job itself, the seeds of burnout can be found in repetitive, routine work that has become boring, as well as in conflicting demands inherent in a position. The former is straightforward in itself but the latter merits discussion. In hospitals, the challenge of switching gears arises if an individual functions as a manager with clinical responsibilities or has been promoted to management from a clinical position. As described in Chapters 5 and 6, the differences in values required in the two roles (i.e., clinician and manager) when coupled with insufficient training in management practices, create stress for incumbents and subordinates. Where the stress is recurrent and associated with feelings of exhaustion, in particular, burnout is likely to ensue.

Obviously, the next question pertains to remedies to the problems burnout poses. Responses to burnout in particular, and job-related stress more generally, are the focus of Chapters 9 and 10. Consideration turns now to two very serious symptoms of stress-related behavior—problems of alcohol and drug addiction.

PROBLEMS OF ADDICTION: ALCOHOL

Alcohol, in that it is a mood-altering drug, can be regarded in much the same way as others—marijuana, cocaine, heroin, amphetamines, and barbiturates. In the case of alcoholism, addiction is present. Impaired individuals have developed a physiological craving for the substance that demands satisfaction so increasing amounts become necessary to satisfy that need and produce the desired effect. The alcoholic uses alcohol as a drug addict uses drugs.

The National Council on Alcoholism estimates that approximately 10 percent of the labor force is alcoholic and another 10 percent borderline alcoholic. Others have estimated that the actual figures are higher—in the range of 20 to 25 percent (CompCare, 1976). The actual rates or prevalence of alcoholism are hard to obtain. Prevalence tests base their projections on the number of alcohol-related deaths, incidence of cirrhosis of the liver, insurance claims for alcoholism treatment, and the like. Alcoholism has been designated as the nation's leading health problem, affecting approximately seven million people. If half that many were to develop a serious disease, an epidemic certainly would be declared and the country would be put in a state of emergency. Ironically, abuse of hard drugs and marijuana has not reached anywhere near the rate for alcohol yet concern for alcoholism generally has been substantially less than that for drugs.

The costs of alcoholism have reached staggering proportions. Industrial losses have been estimated at more than $50 billion yearly ("Battling Employee Alcoholism," 1982; Milam & Ketcham, 1981; National Council on Alcoholism, 1982) with the average problem drinker missing 22 days of work a year, incurring more accidents than the nonproblem drinker, using more medical benefits than nonimpaired colleagues, and causing substantial productivity losses because of diminished quantity and quality of output. When it is considered that every problem drinker adversely affects approximately four others in the family as well as numerous business and social associates in the community, an even greater number of people is affected by alcoholism. The total cost to the nation in productivity and human loss probably is incalculable.

The Disease Concept Debate

Despite the fact that the American Medical Association, the American Hospital Association, and the American Federation of Labor-Congress of Industrial Organizations recognize alcoholism as a disease, acceptance of the disease approach to alcoholism has been less than unanimous. Since Jellinek in 1960 wrote *"The Disease Concept of Alcoholism,"* a controversy has raged in clinical circles about the nature of alcoholism and its treatment (i.e., whether it is a matter of will, symptomatic of other psychological difficulty, or whether it is an illness). Those who follow the disease model of alcoholism point to the fact that alcoholism is primarily a physiological condition resulting from the inability of those affected by it to process alcohol normally (Milam & Ketcham, 1981). Thus, for a certain group of individuals, any amount of alcohol can lead to physiological addiction. Under the disease concept, psychological or emotional problems are seen as aggravated by the addiction to alcohol since the drug undermines the addict's ability to cope with the normal problems of living.

There is widespread agreement on a number of points, however. Its major manifestation is seen in behavior. Alcoholics' drinking is repetitive and they generally are unable to control it. The results are serious dysfunction and disability, including physical addiction. It also is widely accepted that the course of alcoholism is progressive.

Despite numerous futile attempts to identify an "alcoholic personality"—that is, someone likely to become alcoholic—clinicians recognize that while external circumstances and personality traits can increase vulnerability to alcoholism (e.g., loss of work, income, and significant others; difficulty in handling interpersonal conflict; rejection, and so forth), no one is immune from it. Alcoholism occurs among the upper, middle, and lower classes, women and men, young people and old. While the incidence of alcoholism among cross-sections of the population differs (e.g., rates are lower among Jews in comparison to non-Jews) no groups remain unaffected. Nor is alcoholism restricted to professional groups of one kind or another.

Whether or not the disease concept of alcoholism can be rationally or empirically proved or disproved is an academic debate that obscures the potential usefulness of that approach. If the notion of alcoholism as a disease were accepted, the public might be less likely to condemn the alcoholic and instead be more likely to initiate treatment referrals and encourage and maintain the human dignity of the troubled individuals. The disease concept suggests that there is a discontinuity between alcoholic imbibing and normal, nonalcoholic drinking. Alcoholism is not merely a bad habit (Szasz, 1972) nor is it evidence of lack of willpower (Bateson, 1971). The disease concept suggests that alcoholism will not disappear with enlarged doses of concentration or moralism or with a change in eating habits. It can be alleviated or cured only through a direct therapeutic approach.

Symptoms of Alcoholism

Problems of alcohol and drug addiction in health care organizations probably are more common than most people expect. Since the incidence of alcoholism, for example, is estimated at somewhere around 10 percent of the general population, the same percentage could be anticipated among those in the health care field. While alcoholism is increasingly recognized as one of the country's most significant health and social problems, many forces are at work attempting to conceal or at least minimize the situation, particularly in the work setting, as will be discussed.

From a clinical standpoint, end-stage alcoholism is fairly easy to detect from such symptoms as cirrhosis of the liver, jaundice, recurrent pancreatitis, seizures, and neurological impairment. The behavioral manifestations on the job also are readily apparent during this final stage. The individual has frequent, prolonged, and unpredictable absences; job performance is uneven and generally evidences periods of gross incompetence.

For the addicted physician, rounds may be made at unusual hours, with the doctor dressed in inappropriate clothes (e.g. tennis attire, athletic clothes) or rounds may not be made at all. Meeting schedules and individual patient appointments are likely to be missed. The physician's breath is heavy with the smell of alcohol, the gait is uneven. The general behavior is undependable and there is visible evidence of physical deterioration. The alcoholic complains of serious personal and/or family and financial problems that often are identified as the cause of the drinking, if that has been confronted and acknowledged.

At this point coworkers may continue covering up for the individual. However, the resulting extra work demands placed on them begin to take a toll. The alcoholic's job is on the line, with termination imminent. At this point, to revive the old vaudeville joke, work has interfered with drinking. Given that the probability of rehabilitation falls as the disease progresses, what earlier warning signs exist that may facilitate detection, treatment, and recovery at a stage when the likelihood of a successful outcome is greater?

Early stage difficulties are detected by specific symptoms as well as behavioral changes. Decreased efficiency, missed deadlines, increased error through inattention, poor judgment, lateness to appointments and meetings by individuals who typically had always been punctual are indicators suggesting further exploration of problems. An increase in cancelled appointments, leaving the job early, returning late from lunch, and absences also are signals. In this stage, the persons tend to overreact to real or imagined criticism, make excuses for the behavioral problems, and complain of not feeling well. It is likely that coworkers will complain about their behavior. It should be noted that these early stage symptoms, while associated with alcoholism (CompCare, 1976) also are indicators of work-related stress. What is critical is that problems be detected early without formal diagnosis (medical diagnosis can be made only by medical practitioners) and that steps be taken to remedy the difficulty.

Alcoholism should be considered when the symptoms point to multisystem involvement, particularly where certain patterns are apparent (Siegal & Faryna, 1980). A common set of physical symptoms involving the gastrointestinal system include early morning sickness and vomiting and intermittent abdominal pain. Meals are skipped frequently, with a high intake of caffeine and cigarettes, thus compounding and/or causing gastrointestinal difficulties. Psychological complaints including insomnia, nervousness, and generalized tension may be prevalent and may actually precipitate a request for medical help at this point (Siegal & Faryna, 1980).

Generally there is no awareness that alcohol is responsible for the symptomatology. Frequently there is a request for a psychotropic drug, such as Valium, to relieve symptoms. This may result in combined drug and alcohol addictions. Unlike those suffering from stress, alcohol-impaired individuals will deny personal or environmental stress, claiming instead that sleep will solve the difficulty. Neurological symptoms also are typical and point to the possibility of drug or alcohol problems. These generally include numbness and tingling sensations in the feet, frequent falls and injuries, particularly those for which no reasonable explanation exists, and sexual impotence (Siegal & Faryna, 1980).

Middle stage difficulties are characterized by increased difficulties in the factors noted earlier: attendance, performance, and general behavior. Attendance now is characterized by more frequent and longer time off for vague ailments or reasons that lack credibility. The persons may neglect to return from lunch, often not saying that they will not be back. Job performance shows general deterioration, further characterized by poor concentration, impaired judgment, and inattention. Statements are found to be unreliable, yet the individuals exaggerate work accomplishments, culminating in grandiose aggressive or belligerent behavior.

Money is likely to be borrowed from coworkers, with financial problems resulting in liens on property and/or salary garnishment. These persons tend to avoid discussion of their problems and begin avoiding contact with associates. Internally, some may experience guilt and are aware of their failure to control their behavior and drinking. They deny the problem to others and refuse to seek help on their own. Hospitalization is likely to increase, often the result of serious boating, fishing, hunting, or car accidents.

It is generally at this point that a crisis occurs in which the individuals come into conflict with the law, precipitating even more serious familial difficulties, with secondary effects on the job. The drinkers' jobs are in jeopardy, with punitive disciplinary action having been taken or recommended. The stage is set for the final phase of the illness.

While the distinction between the middle and final stages is considered arbitrary, the late stage is generally characterized by increased toxicity and damage to body organs and whole systems (Milam & Ketcham, 1981). The alcoholic's tolerance to alcohol lessens as a function of central nervous system damage; withdrawal symptoms increase in severity. At this point deterioration that began in the first two stages emerges rather dramatically. Both physical and mental health has deteriorated. Ironically, the drug that caused the disability also offers relief from what has now become constant emotional and mental agony and physical disability. Without treatment, death through continued drinking will result—typically from cirrhosis of the liver, heart failure, pancreatitis, respiratory problems, suicide, or accident. It should be noted that, as with other illnesses, treatment is available for alcoholics and their families. Critical to the successful outcome of therapy is early diagnosis, confrontation, and a program that requires the alcoholic to seek and participate in treatment. (The last point is of particular relevance to the work setting.) While Alcoholics Anonymous is often regarded as offering a treatment program for alcoholics, it is not. It has no professional counseling program, no 24-hour medical care or detoxification facilities and staff. Nor does it have any legal authority to ensure compliance with a treatment regimen. As a self-help group it does, however, offer tremendous support for recovering alcoholics and their families with its associated programs: Al-Anon and Al-Ateen.

DRUG ADDICTION: CAUSES AND SYMPTOMS

Recorded history is replete with stories of people who have used various means to escape what they believed was intolerable in life and/or to transcend into a "beyond." In its simplest form the use of drugs, like magic and ritual, reflects on the one hand an escape from, fight against, or defense against something (in this case, stress) and on the other hand a search for something new or better (Wurmser, 1975).

Discussions with drug abusers of various ages result in consistent explanations of their behavior: they report a desire to escape boredom, meaninglessness, lack of identity, and sense of not belonging. Deeper probing discloses such causes as a need to escape from painful feelings—anger, guilt, worthlessness, frustration, intense shame. Abusers seek the opposite: what they regard as excitement, fullness, belonging, pleasure, and a sense of meaning.

It is apparent, then, that the problem is not really drug abuse itself but the underlying set of serious difficulties that the users think the drugs will palliate. Of course, such a statement needs to be couched in a context— namely, that experimentation with drugs lies on one side of the continuum of abuse, with addiction or compulsive use on the other. Experimenters dabble in mind-altering drugs from peer pressure, curiosity, or as a symbol of independence and rebellion from authority. Chronic abusers who become addicts attempt to meet life problems through artificial means. Without the prop, other serious symptoms of conflicts and the inability to manage them appear: alcoholism, depression, violence, suicide attempts.

From a psychoanalytic perspective, these individuals are on a flight from loneliness, estrangement, and disillusionment, with the surcease provided through hallucinogens. Momentary escape from powerlessness, inadequacy, and boredom into mastery and control is gained through the use of amphetamines. Heroin yields a rush of peace, calm, and tranquillity, an escape from chronic grief, rage, and anxiety.

Three core conflicts have been suggested to highlight reasons for drug abuse (Vaillant, Brighton, & McArthur, 1970; Wurmser, 1975). The first entails an attempt to resolve a discrepancy between individuals' perceptions of themselves and their expectations. To the extent that they find an abyss between what they see and what they demand, they become disillusioned. They regard themselves as lacking in integrity, responsibility, and commitment. Without inner resources to adjust those self-imposed demands, change behavior, or develop more realistic appraisals, people are likely to turn to outside agents (drugs) to bridge the gap. The self-image now matches the idealized one with the help of those artificial means.

The second conflict reflects passivity and dependency in problem solving. As opposed to an approach oriented toward active environmental change, individuals turn inward, nurturing themselves with drugs that provide immediate, if only short-lived, relief.

The third conflict entails people's desire to be omnipotent and the realization that they are not. Drugs wipe out the real fact of human vulnerability, even if the effect is only illusion. As noted in Chapter 5, the particularly vulnerable individuals are those with histories of emotional deprivation themselves, those for whom the physician or nursing values of altruism, independence, emotional self-control, and self-assurance in judgment are carried to their logical extremes.

Symptoms common to drug abusers, regardless of the type of substance involved, typically include: changes in work or school attendance, performance, and discipline; general irritability; unusual flare-ups or outbreaks of temper; poor physical appearance (e.g., a well-dressed individual begins to look slovenly); furtive behavior; wearing of sunglasses at inappropriate times to hide dilated or constricted pupils; constant wearing of long shirt sleeves, regardless of the weather, to hide needle marks if drugs are being injected; borrowing money from associates for questionable purposes; being found in unusual places (e.g., storage rooms, closets, etc.); withdrawal from responsibility and associates; and general change in overall attitude (*Identification of Drug Abusers*, 1975). Manifestations of particular types of drug abuse differ, of course, and merit separate exploration.

Drugs Abused and Their Manifestations

Stimulants

Of particular importance in this category are the amphetamines—mood elevators that produce a stimulant effect on the central nervous system. Amphetamines potentiate the effects of norepinephrine, a neurohormone that activates parts of the sympathetic nervous system. They are used medically in certain types of Parkinson's disease, sometimes (very rarely) in manic-depressive or schizoid psychoses, and as an aid in dieting by depressing the appetite. They also are used to combat narcolepsy and are a frequent drug of choice self-prescribed by persons who need to remain awake over long periods of time. Ironically, while they do keep such individuals awake, they do not lead to good concentration and mental functioning.

Originally amphetamines were used as an antidepressant. This use has stopped because of their abuse potential, particularly their addictive properties. Some physicians still believe they have some value in counteracting mild, situational depression (e.g., bereavement) and in breaking an alcoholic cycle in which a person drinks because of being depressed over the last hangover. These latter uses are extremely controversial. In the case of bereavement, a psychodynamic perspective mandates the working through and expression of feelings of loss, a process that the drug blocks. In the case of alcoholism, it is questionable to prescribe drugs with a high addictive potential to a person who already is addicted, albeit to another substance.

Side effects of amphetamine abuse are rather noticeable, in particular anxiety, often with tremors. Dry mouth and nose associated with bad breath result in the abusers' licking their lips frequently and rubbing or scratching their noses. Users develop a tolerance to the pleasurable effects of the drug, leading to increased dosage to achieve the results of prior doses. The result is a tendency to increase the dose and to desire injections rather than pills because of their faster acting effects. Other side effects include loss of appetite, insomnia, marked restlessness, acute paranoia, delusions, irritability, argumentativeness, and combativeness (*The Medical Letter*, 1980).

One dose of 50 milligrams without a tolerance to amphetamines can precipitate a toxic psychosis with hallucinations and active paranoid delusions. Fatalities are rare but have occurred. An overdose typically is followed by chills, collapse, and loss of consciousness. Among the frequently used amphetamines are benzedrine, dexadrine, and methedrene ("speed"). (In nonabusive use, these drugs are taken under medical direction, particularly by people with high blood pressure and heart disease.)

Barbiturates

Because they have the opposite effect on the body from the amphetamines, barbiturates often are used in conjunction with them: the barbiturate is used to bring users "down" from an amphetamine "high." Generally known as sedatives, depressants, or hypnotics, barbiturates are associated with the highest incidence of addiction among the psychotropic drugs medicinally prescribed. Their side effects may be quite severe, including convulsions, coma, and death.

Barbiturates are associated with symptoms of alcohol intoxication but without the odor of alcohol on the breath: staggering or stumbling or falling asleep at meetings, home, or on the job. Abusers generally look drowsy and disoriented and manifest a general lack of interest in work or family activities. Other side effects include rashes, nausea, diarrhea, anxiety, and nervousness.

As a depressant on the central nervous system, barbiturates in small doses relieve tension and anxiety without causing excessive drowsiness. They are useful as an anticonvulsant (e.g., with epilepsy) or as an analgesic when minor pain prevents sleep. They also are a leading mode of suicide, often taken in combination with alcohol.

In part because of the tolerance nature of barbiturates, they are extremely dangerous. Tolerance will occur to get the desired effect but there is no parallel increase in the physically tolerated maximum dosage. Thus overdose, accidental or otherwise, is more likely to be fatal than with anything else, including heroin. Similarly, withdrawal reactions are very serious, again more so than in heroin withdrawal. Typical shock syndrome associated with a weak, rapid pulse; cold sweaty palms; and slow and shallow breathing is not uncommon.

Barbiturates come in several forms, depending on their short-term or long-term effect. Long-acting barbiturates include phenobarbital; intermediate short-acting drugs include Nembutal, sodium Amytal (also known as truth serum), and Seconal; very short-acting drugs include Pentothal.

Sleep Drugs

Another type of sedative includes the general category of sleep medications with effects similar to the barbiturates. Typical in this category are Doriden, which works over a six to eight-hour period, putting the individual into a sound sleep but is associated with a high incidence of addiction; chloral hydrate (Noctec); Placidyl, associated with a relatively low rate of addiction; and Dalmane.

Minor Tranquilizers

Minor tranquilizers are prescribed to relieve neurotic and situational anxiety and tension and are quite different in their effects and properties from the major tranquilizers (neuroleptics) used in the treatment of psychoses (*The Medical Letter*, 1980). Minor tranquilizers have no antipsychotic properties, do not influence cognitive processes, and do not have substantial influence on the psychomotor apparatus. For adolescent and geriatric populations they are most likely to have negative side effects. They have a high potentiating effect with liquor. Psychological dependence is possible with these drugs, and there are a few known cases of physiological addiction and problems of withdrawal, particularly with Valium (*The Medical Letter*, 1981a,b).

One of the most commonly prescribed minor tranquilizers is Valium, also known for its muscle relaxant properties. It interferes with judgment and concentration and can seriously impair driving. Since it alters the state of consciousness it can precipitate a psychotic reaction in borderline and psychotic persons in remission. Meprobamate, commonly referred to as Miltown and sold as Equanil, is associated with a fairly high rate of addiction among the minor tranquilizers. Dizziness is a prominent side effect. Librium, another common tranquilizer, has been shown to lower anxiety and raise aggression in people who are feeling both anxiety and aggression, thus increasing interpersonal difficulties. Vistaril, Tranxene, and Sinequan (which has an antidepressant and antianxiety agent) also are commonly prescribed.

Narcotics

Most typical narcotics abuse in medical settings seems to be associated with heroin and morphine. Inhaling heroin in powder form leaves traces of white powder around the nostrils, causing redness and rawness. Injecting heroin leaves scars on the inner surface of the arms and elbows, so users wear long-sleeved shirts all the time to cover the marks. Others may inject drugs in the body in places where needle marks will not be seen readily. Users may leave syringes, bent spoons, eyedroppers, cotton, and needles in lockers and rooms at work or home, unconsciously signalling the presence of an addiction. Abusers typically are lethargic and drowsy, and pupils of their eyes are constricted and fail to respond to light.

SIGNS OF EMOTIONAL DISTURBANCE

Those who have lived in or visited large urban centers frequently have come upon individuals referred to as "bag people." These people, predominantly women, check their wordly possessions into 24-hour lockers at bus or train stations, changing belongings from bag to bag, carrying some of these goods with them on their travels through the city during the day. They can be seen walking the streets, having conversations with the air, talking to individuals who are not there, arguing with others who walk by, shaking their heads or ignoring them. There is no question that these individuals manifest signs of emotional disturbance. But what about the emotional disturbance of others who walk the same streets, who are co-workers, whose signs are not as visible?

Unfortunately, for many types of emotional disturbance there may be no easily discernible red flag for the layman to identify early signs that colleagues may be in jeopardy. The key to emotional disturbance in many respects rests in what is "appropriate" behavior—and therein lies a very real danger in identifying someone as "emotionally disturbed." What is deemed "appropriate" often is a subjective assessment reflecting the observer's own values and behavioral preferences, not at all an indication of psychiatric disturbance in a clinical sense. Because of such subjectivity, observers' own perspectives can color what they label as emotional disturbance. Thus, if they do not like what other persons are doing, they may deduce that the others are out of their minds.

On the other hand, if individuals have had a history of behaving in questionable ways, especially with, for example, peers or other managers, such inappropriateness may be an indication that they have an emotional disturbance that is interfering with the job. One way of approaching the problem of emotional disturbance is to explore the dimension of mental health in relation to what constitutes mental illness.

Mental Illness vs. Mental Health

Mental illness has to be considered in a relative context—that is, relative to mental health. As Freud aptly noted, mental health is evidenced in emotional maturity, not the absence of conflict and stress in life but the ability to face those problems and still be able to love and work productively. A more contemporary view is reflected in the individuals' having adequate psychological reserves to deal with stress to maintain their adaptation (Dewald, 1971).

Psychopathology, or emotional disturbance, from a psychodynamic perspective, falls on a continuum ranging from nonneurotic, healthy functioning, to transient situational disturbances and simple stress reactions, on through neurotic disturbances (anxiety, dissociative, and conversion disorders; and others involving the obsessive-compulsive, posttraumatic stress, somatization, phobic, and depression or dysthymic disorders), moving to characteriological disturbances (e.g., substance use disorders, passive-aggressive or compulsive personality disorders, and borderline personality disturbances, etc.), through psychotic disturbances (e.g. major affective disorder— previously referred to as manic-depressive psychosis, schizophrenia, and psychotic or major depression).

(These clinical terms are reflective of the *Diagnostic and Statistical Manual III* (American Psychiatric Association, 1980), the accepted classification for psychiatric disturbances, while the continuum reflects this author's conceptualization of the range of disturbances reflecting nondiscrete clinical entities based on numerous years of clinical practice and teaching. The conceptualization has proved useful in gaining a perspective on the wide range and interrelationship of clinical problems.)

Underlying all emotional disturbance is an attempt to establish a dynamic equilibrium in the face of unconscious conflicts. Whereas all human behavior entails a compromise between inner drives and external reality, psychopathology, regardless of its severity, involves a compromise between an unacceptable wish that is buried from conscious awareness (i.e., repressed) and an unconscious fear (MacKinnon & Michels, 1971). Thus, neurotic behavior, in contrast to nonneurotic behavior, is a second-best solution to problems of living.

In addition to the compromise between inner drives and external reality, neurotic functioning provides an accommodation to the unconscious fear that leads to a restriction of functioning in the world. In essence there is a distortion of psychic functioning since factors outside of conscious awareness not related to rational thought processes (i.e., secondary process) are directing behavior. Regardless of how painful and restrictive psychological symptoms may be, it should be remembered that each one is an attempt to resolve a more disturbing, underlying conflict.

Boundaries Still Undefined

In this discussion of psychopathology or emotional illness it is important to remember that no satisfactory definition precisely articulates the boundaries of the concept "mental disorder." Some writers, Thomas Szasz and R.D. Laing in particular, have suggested that mental illnesses per se do not exist. In their views, what is socially defined as mental illness is best regarded as "problems in living" (Szasz, 1961) or as an attempt to deal with and respond to an essentially bizarre and crazy environment (Laing, 1972).

These are minority views in psychiatry and related clinical areas but they raise some important questions concerning the traditional medical model applied to emotional problems. However, let there be no misunderstanding that regardless of whether behaviors are defined as "illness" or "problems in living," they involve typically painful symptoms (distress) or impairment in one or more important areas of personal and/or social functioning (disability).

In the psychiatric classification schema (DSM-III), mental disorders are conceptualized as clinically significant behavioral or psychological syndromes that indicate behavioral, psychological, or biological dysfunction. Such dysfunction is considered to be more than a disturbance between an individual and society. Thus, conflict between an individual and society may represent "social deviance" and may or may not be desirable. However, such deviance is not considered a mental disorder. Homosexuality, for example, is not a mental disorder and is not listed in the classification.

There is no assumption in the classification system that individuals are being classified; rather it is the disorders that afflict people that are identified. Thus, it is possible to describe "a person with alcoholism" instead of an "alcoholic." Implicit in this reorientation is the attempt to remove stigmatizing labels from individuals as well as to provide the expectation that they no longer may have the disability at some point in the future. The disorder is seen as separate from the person's character.

This is not to suggest that nonneurotic, nonpathological functioning is devoid of conflict. Obviously, no life is free of conflict and no individuals ever are totally aware of all of their motivations in every situation. However, in nonneurotic functioning there is at least a partial conscious awareness of the underlying conflict. Secondary rational processes and logic are used to deal with it and resolve it in light of realistic environmental and personal constraints, with a minimum of regression and resort to unconscious defense mechanisms.

The Role of Defense Mechanisms

The use of psychological defense mechanisms is characteristic of all human behavior, regardless of whether people are healthy or emotionally disturbed. Part of what is considered ego functioning from a psychodynamic perspective involves the defense mechanisms that serve to protect individuals from a constant barrage of unconscious anxiety-arousing internal stimuli as well as external stimuli. According to psychoanalytic theories of personality, defense mechanisms become operative at various points in individuals' development.

What differentiates normal and disturbed functioning is the repertoire of defense mechanisms available to people in any given situation. Disturbed functioning is characterized by a narrow repertoire of more primitive defenses (i.e., those associated with earlier stages of psychological development) and/or an overutilization of particular mechanisms. Disturbed functioning tends to be less flexible and more prone to stereotyped, rigid responses with diminished ability to differentiate particulars of the situations in which individuals find themselves, leading to a tendency toward gross overgeneralization. The following list includes typically accepted defense mechanisms in their approximate relative emergence in development (they are discussed next):

- denial
- projection
- introjection
- identification
- magical undoing
- reaction formation
- isolation
- intellectualization
- regression
- repression
- suppression

- displacement
- conversion
- rationalization
- avoidance
- compensation
- substitution
- sublimation

Denial, one of the earliest defense mechanisms, corresponds to a negative hallucination. Something is believed not to exist (e.g., internal feeling, external event) when it, in fact, does. Projection, also a primitive defense mechanism, entails the denial of unacceptable or undesirable thoughts, traits, or actions and ascribing them to another. While all individuals at least periodically use these defenses in the face of anxiety-arousing issues they do not wish to confront, their frequent use becomes quite a problem, particularly since they entail a gross distortion of reality. They are the primary mechanisms at work in psychosis.

Introjection, the opposite of projection, involves the wholesale taking in of the good and bad qualities of another person with the individual's own loss of personal identity. Identification, a related process, occurs later in development involving the taking in of only selected aspects of another individual. Denial, projection, and introjection essentially are unconscious processes but do involve some conscious identification.

Magical undoing harks back to the magical thinking of the 2-year-old or 3-year-old. It is an attempt through symbolic behavior to abolish or control past experience or unacceptable thoughts, the consequences of which have been painful. The individuals often are unaware of what they are attempting to abolish, although the mechanism generally entails an act to eradicate an unconscious hostile wish. For instance, a person who has unacceptable hostile feelings toward a boss may act in "purely" positive ways toward the superior in attempting to undo any negative fallout anticipated from the hostile feelings. A related defense mechanism is reaction formation, which entails the development of convictions or traits exactly opposite to those that are perceived to be unacceptable by the unconscious. Thus, the woman who believes it unfeminine to be angry develops a kind, sweet view of herself in relation to the world, never allowing herself to express her anger.

Isolation involves the process of draining out the emotional components of events. Individuals who use isolation are seen as colorless and flat; they describe events without feeling. An example of isolation is the defense of intellectualization, a common style in which individuals' interactions are characterized by discussions of ideas that seem divorced from feeling.

Regression as a defense mechanism represents a retreat to earlier satisfactions, to earlier stages of psychic equilibrium. It typically occurs in neurosis where no satisfaction or insufficient satisfaction is available at the next stage of development. In healthy functioning "regression in service of the ego" is found as a temporary and needed escape through daydreaming, fantasy, sleep, and adult play.

Repression, a totally unconscious defense mechanism, involves the exclusion of unacceptable material from the conscious mind. While related to denial, it is less primitive and all-encompassing. Suppression, the most sophisticated of these three mechanisms (denial, repression, suppression), entails the conscious exclusion of unacceptable material from the mind.

Displacement involves shifting the emphasis of an individual's affect, or substituting feeling in response to unacceptable ideas or feelings. Unacceptability may stem from an internal perception based on earlier experiences with others who deemed certain things "unacceptable," as in the case of parents unable to tolerate their children's expressions of anger. Affect is shifted, for example, when an angry remark is said with a smile or made into a joke. The object of an affect also can be shifted, as in the case of someone with thoughts of killing a parent who instead becomes preoccupied with killing the president of the country. In its less extreme form, displacement occurs when individuals in positions of higher status are unable to tolerate direct expression of affect—in particular, anger. For instance, some physicians may not be confortable with a nurse's expression of anger or disagreement. The nurse, instead of becoming angry at the physician, turns on a peer, a "safe" target. This mechanism is commonly seen in organizations when anger toward a superior is displaced downward or across the hierarchy.

Conversion is a defense mechanism whereby unconscious "unacceptable" wishes or feelings are expressed through physical changes in the body. The classic case of this was hysterical paralysis, common in the days of Freud. Somatization entails a similar process in less extreme form.

Rationalization, a commonly used defense mechanism, involves an attempt to logically and rationally explain away behavior, thoughts, or feelings by finding acceptable excuses. In particular, rationalization may involve a conscious as well as unconscious component. Avoidance, another common mechanism, entails what its name suggests: the individual does not attend to a particular issue, feeling, or person that is the object of conflict. To skirt around or overlook certain sources of conflict may smooth an important relationship. The determination of whether or not the use of avoidance is healthy or constructive really depends on an analysis of several factors. Is the mechanism used selectively, based on a reasoned assessment of a specific situation? Or does the individual generally and consistently avoid confronting this person with, for example, disagreement? If so, is it a function of the recipient's actual inability to deal with disagreement constructively or does it reflect a generalized fear of confrontation on the part of this individual? To the extent that avoidance is selectively, consciously, and realistically based, its use can be considered reflective of healthy functioning. It is only when these qualities are consistently absent that possible emotional disturbance can be discussed.

Compensation, substitution, and sublimation were considered by Freud to be the most sophisticated and emotionally mature defense mechanisms. Compensation is related to a person's need for prestige. An individual who cannot accomplish in one area may repress a desire for accomplishment in that area and turn to another. For instance, someone who has difficulty writing may choose to excel in oral communications. Substitution operates by a similar principle: frustration, experienced in one area, is reduced by achieving gratification in another related area. A person who is rejected by medical school may go on to become a biologist. Finally, sublimation entails the diversion or redirection of the energy of an unacceptable wish into socially acceptable means and goals. Aggressive energies directed into competitive team sports is a classic example of sublimation at work.

Since everyone uses defenses, what guidelines might be helpful in identifying incipient signs of emotional disturbance? Most important for managers is attention to appropriate behavior on the job and consistent work performance. Lack of defensiveness and openness to constructive criticism are important indicators of emotional maturity and stability. Obviously, different people have different tolerances to criticism but apparent defensive attitudes and a lack of receptiveness to others' inputs are problems.

Regardless of how astute managers may be with regard to issues of a psychological nature, they are not psychotherapists or diagnosticians. As managers, their attention must be directed to effective coaching and counseling and to instituting disciplinary measures where mandated; they must not slip into the role of therapist. (Guidelines for coaching, counseling, and effective discipline among professional staff members are discussed in Chapter 9.)

CONFRONTING THE PROBLEMS OF STRESS

It is apparent from discussions with professional health managers across the country and from statements in the literature that there is a fairly pervasive tendency to avoid dealing with people experiencing excessive stress, whether they are exhibiting incipient symptoms or more serious evidences of (alcohol or drug) addiction or emotional disturbance. Typically avoidance is couched in such descriptions as fear of retaliation, concern for others' privacy, embarrassment, or a desire not to become involved. At a deeper level these comments seem to reflect managers' personal inadequacies in knowing what to do to be constructive, misguided attempts to protect the stricken individual, and fear of exposure of their own vulnerabilities and similar problems. In other cases avoidance reflects institutional norms that reward individuals for minding their own business and for not assuming responsibility. Given the costs of stress, addiction, and emotional disturbance for individuals and organizations, it is apparent that the ramifications of avoidance, for whatever reason, are profound.

Clark (1981) identifies four impediments to the diagnosis of alcoholism, in particular, that have relevance to the identification and handling of stress symptoms and emotional disturbance in general.

The first impediment involves a cognitive block in which people, including physicians, lack knowledge of the enormous variety and potential seriousness of the symptoms generated by stress, alcoholism, drug addiction, and emotional disturbance.

The second impediment pertains to deeply engrained social attitudes and values. To the extent that stress symptoms, problems of addiction, and emotional disturbance are perceived as character flaws, lack of "will," or—worse yet—willful self-destruction, the response to an individual in need will be to condemn and morally judge, not to help. Where these attitudes are coupled with feelings of helplessness, frustration, or general powerlessness in the face of such difficulties, condemnation may be used to justify individuals' (managers') own sense of impotence and subsequent avoidance.

The third impediment to appropriate handling involves communication problems. Since people with addictive disorders, stress symptoms, and emotional disturbances often are hostile, angry, anxious, moody, and misleading in their own communications (a tendency to deny difficulty is a pervasive theme) they typically provoke potential helpers into giving unhelpful, rejecting messages. An aggressive confrontation in the context of an emotionally tense and negatively charged atmosphere often makes it next to impossible for even well-trained clinicians to provide effective, compassionate communications.

Finally, Clark notes that "medicalization" of problems (i.e., a tendency to see only problems responding to medical technology as within the range of possible intervention) on the part of nurses and physicians, in particular, puts these difficulties outside the perceived range of jurisdiction of these professionals. Tied to a belief that such difficulties are the sufferer's "fault," avoidance is a typical response.

At another level there is an implicit expectation that providers of health care are somewhat immune from the negative effects of stress and vulnerability to emotional disturbance and addiction. Obviously, this is an erroneous and destructive belief but it does have profound implications. As noted in Chapter 5, the unspoken attitude toward the physician's ability to handle stress is reflected in the reactions of administrators, peers, and nurses. There are numerous instances in which administrators and health care professionals have attempted to ignore and/or deny the existence of seriously impaired physicians. How much this reflects a desire to maintain the myth that they are invulnerable is unknown.

However, physicians' professional ethos and the assumptions of the health care community in which they work require that they (1) not need a place to turn to, (2) not suffer from stress, addictions, and emotional disturbance, and (3) be able to make life-and-death decisions with absolute confidence. These demands rest on the assumption that there is a quantum difference between the limitations of physicians and of other mortals. It is time that the health care community undertook a critical reexamination of these attitudes.

Physicians are expected to be less vulnerable than nonphysicians. There is concern that if they show a flaw, such as in stress symptomatology, problems of addiction, or emotional illness, they will be prevented from ever practicing medicine again if that weakness is reported. Many are either "perfect" or not fit to be physicians. Most state medical boards recognize that revocation of a physician's license may not be the most useful response in the situation. In such cases the impaired physician may be removed from the practice of medicine while "recovering." The doctor then is sent back into the same system that tends to place its physicians on shaky pedestals of privilege, prestige, and status.

The irony of all this is reflected in the recommendation of one well-known doctor who suggests that alcoholic physicians should be treated with other alcoholics to give them an opportunity to recognize and to share their common humanity. The obvious question is, why should physicians wait until impairment to learn this important piece of living? The challenge facing the health care delivery system in this regard is how to restructure itself in order to better deal with the problems of stress, impairment, and vulnerability not only of physicians but of all professions in it. The need for early intervention cannot be underestimated, especially when the difficulty of treating these problems in their advanced stages is considered.

Chapter 9

The Organizational Response

There should be no question by now that organizations in many direct and indirect ways create potential stressors for their employees. In earlier days it could be argued safely that helping members of their staffs manage these stressors effectively should not be the organization's responsibility, and that institutions had little or no responsibility to minimize the existence of stressors known to have a harmful effect (e.g., poor communications, extreme ambiguity, too rapid change, extreme rigidity, and so forth). But it also has been shown that organizations pay a substantial price where employee stress and high levels of burnout exist. Therefore, from a survival and productivity standpoint, their own well-being dictates that organizations respond proactively to these problems, regardless of the organization's humanitarian concerns.

This chapter explores two major approaches to the management of job-related stress problems: (1) preventive and (2) monitoring and control. It should be noted that neither of these approaches is better than the other. Both in combination are likely to provide the most effective and comprehensive attempt at managing organizationally related stress. While many of the solutions will have particular intuitive appeal, it should be noted that rigorous empirically based research documenting general and comparative effectiveness of various alternatives is weak or lacking altogether.

For example, the University of Michigan Institute for Social Research has studied various dimensions of job stress for a quarter of a century. The work has focused on identifying stressors (i.e., cause of stress) and strains (effects of stress). But it has done little on stress management strategies. It is in the area of coping strategies in particular that the research is limited largely to anecdotal reports and testimonials documenting effectiveness. In large part this state of affairs reflects the complexity of the stress phenomenon itself.

As discussed earlier, for any given situation there will be a wide range of responses. Indeed, individual differences in relation to stress constitute probably the single most agreed-upon characteristic in the literature. Different individuals react differentially to the same stressor—what is a stressor for one person may not be for another. To complicate the picture further, these individual differences vary within the same person over time. People may react differently to the same stressor on different occasions.

The same differences across time and across individuals also occur in the area of coping strategies used to manage stress. Different individuals and even groups of individuals cope differently with the same stressor and a specific individual may handle a particular stressor differently on different occasions.

Similarly, what works for a particular organization with a particular history, culture, and climate may work less well for a different organization. It is incumbent on the organization to assess its needs systematically and develop or modify programs to meet them. In such an assessment it must be kept in mind that no organization is a monolithic whole. There are different environments within it and various programs may need to be designed to meet a variety of needs. Such an approach takes into account the complexity of stress and the fact that a single approach to its management and amelioration will be insufficient. Thus, what is presented here is a wide range of organizational interventions found to have some utility in reducing the negative effects of job-related and organizationally based stress.

Organizational diagnosis might reveal that some stressful jobs are characterized by low complexity or high routinization in the work, underutilization of skills and abilities, low participation in decision making, ambiguity with regard to job future, and organizationally induced insecurity. In short, some aspect of the organization—its policies, procedures, structures, programs, jobs, roles—may require modification. As is discussed later, specific interventions then could address these problems through job enlargement, increased participation and team building, job clarity, and improved organizational communications. The perspective adopted here places the organization in the role of "doer" in the task of improving the physical and mental health of employees. In designing programs the organization could focus on the causes or effects of stress (i.e., consequences for both individual and institution) or on some combination of them.

Prevention and treatment programs should be evaluated to determine their effect in reducing organizational stress and controlling and lowering negative stress outcomes among affected employees. However, as Newman and Beehr (1979) aptly note, the need for evaluative research or its lack should not imply that organizations should stop using "unproved" strategies to reduce stress. There also is no evidence that the strategies do not work. Given the economic, social psychological, and physical costs of stress, stopping such efforts would be grossly unwarranted.

PREVENTIVE MECHANISMS IN ALLEVIATING STRESS

Interventions at the Organizational Level

Numerous strategies aimed at modifying job stress through changes in organizational processes appear in the literature and the field. Among them are the following interventions:

- modification of organizational structure through such means as decentralization, increased integration, reduction in the levels of hierarchy, and communications channels necessary to accomplish work
- modification in the distribution of resources
- modification in the reward system and structure of priorities
- revision of selection, hiring, training, and development policies and procedures
- adaptation of the organizational socialization process
- modification of policies and opportunities for transfers and job rotation
- provision of integrated management development programs for all supervisory and managerial staff
- development of collaborative and noncompetitive work strategies (e.g., team building efforts), temporary work groups, and participative decision making
- reduction in role ambiguity and clarification of job responsibilities with the aim of improving person-environment fit
- establishment of audit management systems to systematically monitor the effects of organizational practices and policies.

The analysis begins with integrated management development since many other strategies aimed at reducing organizational stress can be understood from that perspective.

Integrated Management Development

In discussing management development in health care it is important to specify the context—in this case, the role of management in hospitals. Traditionally, management has been seen as the domain of business and industry and its role in health care institutions has been suspect. It was assumed that an individual who was loyal and competent in clinical and technical areas would make a good manager. While clinical or technical expertise and organizational loyalty are worthy qualities, they do not automatically add up to solid management competence.

In addition, as discussed in Chapters 5 and 6, managers in health care have tended to be promoted up from the ranks without specific training in management. This has resulted in a significant amount of stress for both the managers and the organization, in part because of the nature of that transition. Since the mid-1970s, in particular, there has been a strong and growing recognition that sound management practices are critically important to the well-being of health care institutions. In addition there has been a dramatic increase in the number of individuals trained with advanced degrees in health care management, for example masters in business administration (MBAs) and masters in health administration (MHAs).

However, because institutions on the whole have not recognized the need for an integrated approach to management, there are gaps between those with fairly sophisticated training and those without it. In some institutions this has resulted in frustration among managerially trained executives who are working with those who are less sophisticated in that skill. The price for these organizations has been high: rapid turnover of their best managers. One remedy for these problems calls for integrated management development systems.

There are three assumptions inherent in this.

First, organizations have a responsibility to teach managers the skills necessary to be effective.

Second, organizations have a responsibility to socialize managers to the institutions' values—that is, what it means to be a manager in this hospital. Part of that socialization involves building the personal networks across departments and up and down the hierarchy that are necessary to the successful operation of the institution. Such a process reduces the occurrence of "unit suboptimization," a phenomenon typical of many organizations in which departments, work units, or professional groups see their loyalty and concern merely in terms of these subunits, not in relation to the institution as a whole. Underlying unit suboptimization is an assumption of unit independence, in contrast to the more realistic and healthier notion of interdependence. Integrated development programs that provide a common managerial language, mutual understanding of executive tasks and roles, and an appreciation of functional interdependence have been extremely effective in minimizing the existence of unit suboptimization.

Third, there is an assumption in integrated management development that the nature of this approach itself is a continuing process. The skills required to be effective change over time, in part as a reflection of the growing complexity of the health care system. For example, not many years ago the topic of marketing was not regarded as worthy of discussion at a hospital meeting. This has changed greatly, as have the values involving marketing.

There are five components to integrated management development, as described in Figure 9-1. The climate analysis is a paper-and-pencil instrument used to assess the attitudes of the job force toward elements of the work environment that affect morale and productivity. Employee attitudes in such areas as clarity of responsibility, recognition, compensation, and

Figure 9-1 The Integrated Management Development System

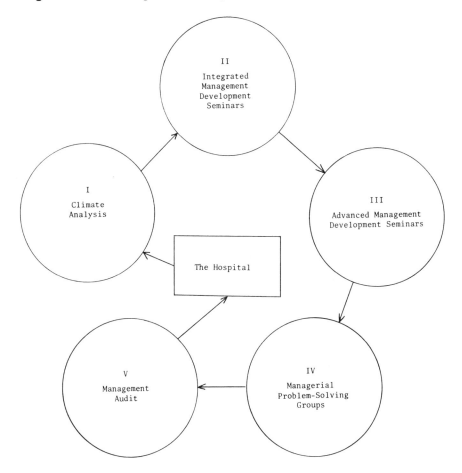

others are summarized statistically by department. Administered periodically, the climate survey is used to monitor the overall "health" of the
institution, to identify issues interfering with its performance, and to highlight aspects of its environment perceived as stress inducing. As a diagnostic tool it has been invaluable in the early detection of organizational
difficulties, thus paving the way for timely and appropriate intervention.

The second component consists of integrated in-house management
development seminars taught by experts in health care. These could include
a management development consultant or someone within the institution
in the position of internal consultant or management development specialist (e.g., human resource development specialist or trainer). Experience suggests that despite the plethora of "canned" seminars with high
participant satisfaction ratings, there are serious problems in the application and translation of these programs on the job. One reason for failure
is that seminars tend to be led by inexperienced trainees who are not able
to help participants adapt the general principles for their own use. Another
problem centers on organizational barriers that block implementation of
new concepts. Without adequate diagnosis of the specific knowledge needs
of managers and without a simultaneous assessment of organizational
variables impinging on implementation, these programs are likely to fail
abysmally.

While the specific content of the seminars presented here will differ
somewhat from institution to institution, several aspects remain constant.
Needs assessment identifies current areas of strength and weakness among
managers. The results of this process then are utilized in the seminars.
Regardless of specific content, such programs incorporate the following
broad objectives:

1. the development of a firm foundation of management principles,
   philosophy, and technique
2. the enhancement of management's identification with the institution
   and its objectives
3. the facilitation of interdepartmental communications.

When managers are provided with an overview of their roles and responsibilities, they gain a foundation and common framework for analyzing
various levels of management and how they fit in. Issues frequently reported
as stressful for managers in health care in particular also must be addressed;
they often are overlooked in traditional seminars (e.g., the influence of
professional socialization, administrative vs. clinical perspectives, the
problem of internal promotion, and the conflict of being liked vs. being
respected).

Considerable attention also must be focused on the communications process and on managing human relations. Managers need to be able to identify and respond effectively to dysfunctional communication, with the goal of establishing a productive work environment in which communications are open and directed and stress is kept at an optimal level (Numerof, 1982). The topic of motivation also must be explored in depth from the perspective of the individual, the work unit, and the organization. Similarly, personal style as a management tool must be addressed, particularly in relation to establishing effective teams.

The third component, the advanced management development seminar, then is established to provide more intensive, advanced training in limited areas of critical importance to effective management. Hiring and selection, advanced performance appraisal, budget and finance, and strategic planning are among the areas in which institutions might want to offer specialized work.

The fourth component, managerial problem-solving groups, entails structured small meetings attended by participants in the management development program and facilitated by the consultant responsible for the initial program. Discussion focuses on individual management problems within the theoretical and practical framework of the previous seminars.

The primary objective of this intervention is to provide managers with an opportunity to put into practice the skills they learned during the program. One inevitable result of training programs is that participants experience some anxiety and/or practical difficulty in implementing new ideas unless they have follow-up sessions in which they can get specific assistance with their situations. A second objective is to build a support and problem-solving network among managers so they can begin to use each other more effectively in the diagnosis and solution of problems.

The fifth component of this approach, management audit, has one primary objective: to assess the strengths and weaknesses of the management system at the departmental and organizational levels. The assessment, or systems analysis, is a broad process evaluation that examines organizational structures (e.g., communications networks, discipline systems, performance appraisal systems, compensation/benefits, grievance, planning processes, policy and procedures, tracking and controlling mechanisms, etc.) that are necessary for effective functioning. These structures provide the support that is crucial for managerial effectiveness. It is in the management audit that centralization or decentralization tendencies are identified and examined, reward structures are examined, and resource distribution is evaluated.

Managerial assessment, or individual performance analysis, uses different criteria for the various levels and functions. It examines the extent to which managers' objectives are reached and their relationship to overall organizational goals. Inherent in this assessment is the expectation that managers will be held accountable for implementing the practices laid out in the seminars.

Unfortunately, where management development efforts have been made but have not followed the guidelines presented here, they frequently fall into what has been called the "garbage pail" technique. This technique reflects a hit-or-miss approach in which topics for seminars are chosen at random, often with considerable political influence and without regard to an overall integrated management development system. In essence, they are programs looking for problems to address, with little or no attention to organizational diagnosis and assessment. Obviously, it would be difficult, if not impossible, to hold managers accountable for integrating and utilizing the contents of this type of program.

However, health care organizations have engaged in more strategic planning in recent years. This planning includes clinical programs, financial concerns, and building needs. It is ironic and rather telling that human resource development planning is not included—particularly in a service-intensive industry such as health care is.

Organizations face an interesting dilemma. If a hospital does institute integrated management development programs, how can it be determined whether they have any real effect? Are they worth the money spent on them? What should be done if evaluation indicates that cognitive knowledge was, indeed, imparted but the application assessment (i.e. the extent to which managers are using this knowledge to change their managerial behavior) shows abysmal results? What went wrong?

In this case the problem lies in the failure to provide managers with continued support in integrating the new knowledge and skills and in holding them accountable. Even where managers learn new ideas and skills, the daily stresses of managing can force them to shelve their good intentions to implement them until "the day when I have some time." Of course, that day just never seems to arrive. Since these managers are not expected to change (i.e., no one is holding them accountable for implementing these ideas), there is little incentive other than their own investment in change. What happens is that those who would change anyway, without the incentive, do so and those who really need to change do not, thus maintaining the pretraining status quo.

Unless, of course, something else happens. That something else is a philosophy inherent in management audit that says, "We will do more than pay lip service to good management practices and organizational development. We will hold you accountable, not only for productivity, however that is measured, but also for managing the climate of your department, unit, or staff. And, we will provide the structure and support necessary for you to do it.''

There are, of course, limitations to what parts of ''climate'' a manager is held accountable for. Some aspects, such as those that involve organizational structure, are beyond the control of individual managers. However, top administration can hold managers accountable for action plans in response to climate by assessing whether or not they carry out the agreed-upon plan. If the climate has not improved in the following year, it may be that something outside the managers' control was responsible, the plan was the wrong response to the problem, or the manager has been remiss in some way.

Job Design and Person-Environment Fit

Obviously no one can or would want to eliminate all of the stresses in organizational life. But stress levels do need to be held down to the needs and tolerance levels of individuals. One cause of job stress is a mismatch between the individual and the job. For instance, the job may exceed the person's capacities, causing high levels of debilitating anxiety, resulting in frustration and performance failure. Or the job may be too small, in which case the individual's abilities and training are not utilized fully, causing boredom, frustration, and, ironically, performance failure. Finally, the person's values may be at odds with the demands of the position, causing internal conflict and negatively affecting performance. This problem is seen most clearly in the case of the clinician who accepts a management position to satisfy needs for advancement when no avenues are available in clinical areas. As discussed earlier, the inherent value conflicts create role stress for the person.

A majority of job-fitting problems are the result of fairly rigidly defined work descriptions that attempt to fit people into predetermined slots as opposed to creatively matching their desires and talents to the needs and opportunities of the organization. How might an organization maximize the fit between its employees, the work needing to be accomplished, and the work environment?

It must be recognized that solutions to such problems require individual responses. It is not feasible to realign entire occupations (Caplan, 1976). General redesign programs that treat all employees the same will not reduce job stress for everyone. Organizations are best advised to identify high-level ''misfits'' who need individual attention. This is accomplished through job analysis, assessment of employee needs and abilities, and the degree of overlap between the two. The analysis should include the following job characteristics: clarity, complexity, workload, responsibility, variety, and autonomy, as well as resources available to sustain adequate role performance (Cascio, 1978; Hackman & Oldham, 1976; Kahn & Quinn, 1970; Numerof, 1982).

If the role is found to contain stress, it may be redefined; overload may be reduced by redistributing work; conflicting demands may be clarified; responsibility may be increased if the problem is one of underload or decreased if it is overload.

These responses are referred to as job redesign, attempts to alter the relation between the worker and the work. Where jobs are expanded, the process is known as job enrichment or job enlargement. The simplest way of doing this is to rotate tasks among employees, thus increasing variety. If the tasks are not simple and routine to begin with, boredom will be alleviated. However, merely adding variety among repetitive tasks results in only short-term solutions. Boredom, if it exists in one phase of the work, is likely to spread when an employee is assigned to another phase.

Vertical job loading, otherwise known as delegation of responsibility, is one way of overcoming boredom. In this strategy, selected managerial functions are transferred to subordinates, giving the employees greater autonomy and responsibility. Horizontal job loading is a form of work enrichment that expands the employee's number of responsibilities without rotating jobs or expanding that individual's degree of authority. Finally, autonomous work teams may be formed in which a group of employees, rather than an individual, is given an expanded, joint responsibility for an entire project.

Job redesign has significant implications for career development activities in health care. Because of the complexity and general controversy over such activities, it is explored separately.

Career Development

Career development has important implications for health care that have gone largely unrecognized. The concept generally is regarded as having little relevance to health care organizations because of their high prevalence of specialized professional groups whose practice is regulated by law. Such thinking leads some to the conclusion that career development is an issue of concern only to individuals whose behavior and advancement potential are dictated by forces outside the health care facility—namely, by the profession of which they are members. As a corollary to this reasoning, any application of career development would be limited to general management and the nonprofessional staff, omitting all professionals. However, career development has relevance to organizational effectiveness and long-range planning, particularly in relation to personnel planning.

Interdependence the Key Motif

At the root of career development is a perspective that emphasizes the interdependence of organizations and their employees. Organizations are dependent on the performance of their people, who in turn depend on organizations to provide jobs and career opportunities. Career development can become a mechanism to avert the negative effect of the primacy of professional identification and assumes that people do want to identify themselves as part of the organization, not merely the profession. This interdependence occurs not only at the point of entry but throughout the life of the person and the organization.

In this context, then, career development may include the following approaches, all of which can reduce organizational stress:

- planning and development of human resources at the organizational level
- planning individuals' careers (also geared to help people in difficult organizational situations cope better)
- improving the matching of all people within the organization at entry, midcareer, and late career points
- handling problems of obsolescence, demotivation, and leveling off
- maintaining the productivity/motivation of employees who are individual contributors and are not interested in the organizational ladder
- integrating changing work demands and family demands.

Implicit in this orientation is the recognition that people differ regarding their need to work and be career-involved and that these needs may change in a given individual over time. In addition there is the recognition that changes occur in key jobs and that new positions emerge, requiring training and retraining.

Job and Personnel Analysis

Essentially, career development, or career management, is best understood as a three-phase process entailing job analysis, personnel analysis, and matching people and jobs. Job analysis is conducted on current as well as anticipated positions. It includes a thorough assessment of the skills and interpersonal and cognitive abilities required to successfully perform a particular job. At the same time, existing personnel are analyzed. Through the use of structured interviews and survey instruments, the skills, deficiencies, and interests of incumbents are assessed. After those two analyses are completed, individual career development plans are mapped out in conjunction with each individual's manager and the personnel department.

To be successful, career development programs must provide the following:

- information about career opportunities within the organization
- thorough assessment and evaluation of employee capabilities and interests
- career counseling
- employee-centered career planning
- career growth and development opportunities
- job matching based on career interests and capabilities
- tracking systems to monitor program effectiveness.

Tracking systems are designed to answer the following questions: Were people whose promotions were successful matched to those jobs as a result of their performance in areas related to the requirements of the new position? Are employees counseled effectively by supervisors? Are supervisors held accountable for career development and counseling—that is, do they discuss career opportunities, counsel employees, and know where to refer them to explore development opportunities?

Presented in such a manner, career development offers unusual opportunities for organizations. In the short run it is an excellent method for overcoming tendencies toward unit suboptimization. Tracking systems that hold supervisors accountable for developing and promoting subordinates, can block their desire to hold onto particular employees because they are excellent performers. In organizations where the programs do not use monitoring, supervisors tend to want to keep star performers from leaving their departments, particularly if it means they may go to another department. Because these programs tie individual development needs to the organization, rather than to the department, they also tend to enhance employee commitment and morale, with secondary salutory effects on job satisfaction and performance. In that poor morale is a source of organizational stress, such an undesirable condition is alleviated.

Long-Range Planning Implications

Perhaps most importantly, career development has long-range planning implications for the organization. It answers such questions as: "Do we have the people to manage and run the organization we envision in the next one to five years? If not, how and where do we get them?'' If such questions cannot be answered directly, strategic decisions need to be rethought.

At another level, major organizational changes or departmental revampings require a career development approach. If the institution requires personnel changes, it must identify the employees whose behavior or skills are not commensurate with the new goals and explain to them why they no longer are needed. The organization's handling of these employees has an impact on the overall morale and motivation of those who remain. How the about-to-depart employees are treated sends clear signals to those remaining about their value to the institution and its attitude toward its key resource—its personnel. Where employees cannot be retained, they can be given guidance and help in locating another position. It is critical that employees understand that termination is not the result of ''poor'' skills but rather of the lack of fit between those skills and the employer's needs. Career development programs should minimize the likelihood that such terminations will occur.

High Visibility Essential

Assuming an organization decides to implement career development, certain factors must be present. The individual responsible for the success of the program must be high and visible in the hierarchy—for example, someone in the personnel department who sits on the administrative council. Administration must be clear about the program's goals, purpose, problems, methods of implementation, and analysis. It is important to provide sessions orienting members of the management staff to the new program. Their concerns must be considered in developing the goals, implementation, and analysis of the program. Following this initial phase, first-line supervisors and others responsible for career development and counseling are oriented as to what it is and how and why it is being implemented. Job and personnel analyses then are followed up and are reviewed yearly. Training in career counseling skills is designed and offered in a pilot program. Successes are identified and difficulties corrected before a full-scale organizationwide effort is mounted.

A frequent criticism of career development programs involves the limited number of management slots available as compared to the number of employees who are potentially interested in such positions. Critics contend that making career information available on an organizationwide basis will increase the competition for the few existing managerial positions and will lead to widespread demoralization since only a select few will ever reach them. Experience suggests that these fears are unfounded. Instead, employees feel more secure knowing what jobs exist, what they require, and what their strengths are relative to them. Where on-the-job training is not sufficient to justify a career change, as in the case of an activity therapy director wanting to become a clinical specialist in nursing, educational reimbursement programs underwritten by the hospital have proved very successful.

Implicit in the criticism is the belief that career development is equated with managerial opportunity. In actuality, many clinically and technically trained employees, particularly in nursing and laboratory technology, move into management positions because of limited advancement opportunities in their original areas. By introducing a dual career ladder (advancement tracks in both clinical/technical areas and management) with titles and remuneration commensurate with expertise, the organization and its employees gain.

Intradiscipline Job Enlargement

Another approach with a proven track record offers job enlargement within a professional discipline. For example, nurses with experience in obstetrics/gynecology who are interested in developing expertise in other specialty areas are afforded opportunities to do so. In addition to meeting their own needs for expansion and career development, they become more valuable to the organization.

One of the biggest drawbacks to the program is initial start-up cost of the analyses of jobs and of employee needs. A second problem is the fact that such open, systematic approaches to personnel planning and development can be incompatible with the "good ole boys" advancement network. In organizations where this network is entrenched and reinforced by administration, career development efforts will fail.

REDUCING ORGANIZATIONAL STRESS

Based on numerous research efforts on organizational stress and burnout discussed throughout the book, one common theme becomes apparent. Aside from specific stressors related to the work itself, the interpersonal environment of an organization, particularly from the standpoint of management–subordinate and interprofessional relations, plays a critical role in determining the level of stress there. How can organizations set an organizational climate to reduce stress? Perhaps most importantly, participation in decision making relevant to the work being performed, excellent communications, and interprofessional collaboration are necessary. For example, examination of the nurse-physician-administrator relationship shows how management efforts can reduce such stress-related consequences as turnover, low job satisfaction, low morale, etc.

According to the report of the National Commission on Nursing (1981), health administrators' support of collaborative practice models among nurses and physicians as well as of interdisciplinary teams is essential for the delivery of quality patient care as well as for improved job satisfaction and decreased job turnover among nurses. Despite their successes, inter-professional teams have faced numerous difficulties. One major point of resistance is the belief held by numerous physicians that the delivery of patient care in the hospital is not a team effort (Taxay, 1978). Where professional socialization in nursing, medical, and health administration training programs does not emphasize a team approach, it becomes the administrator's role to set the stage to bring about a collaborative team effort.

Even where team members are oriented to interprofessional collaboration, serious problems emerge. The members' vying for leadership often undermines the team's ability to accomplish its work. The roles of team members may be rigidly defined by professional training as opposed to individual expertise. Under such circumstances the team's ability to provide optimal care is diminished and the morale of its members suffers. Lack of agreed-upon policy and procedural guidelines further divert the teams' attention from the delivery of care. This frequently results in conflicts. Finally, without administrative support and specific skills in the effective resolution of conflict, team efforts often fail.

While the specifics of team building are beyond the scope of this book, it is useful to identify the characteristics of highly effective work groups: teams. The exploration begins with the cornerstones of team-building efforts: communication, participation, and collaboration.

Building Effective Teams

The effectiveness and level of stress of an organization are greatly influenced by the degree of cooperation within and between work groups. Integrating professionals into highly effective work groups has become increasingly important, particularly since organizations are being forced to do more with less. Such work groups, or teams, have identifiable characteristics and stages of development.

One of the most striking characteristics of the effective work group is its high degree of internal cohesion. This "stick-togetherness" results from forces that act on group members causing them to remain in the group. These forces involve the attractiveness of the group itself and the lesser attractiveness of alternatives. There are a number of determinants of group cohesion: the incentive properties of the group, the motive base of its members, the expectation of outcomes, and how the group compares to others (Cartwright & Zander, 1968). Each of these determinants is considered next separately.

Incentive properties include such variables as size and atmosphere, structure and leadership style, the nature of goals and tasks, the similarity of members, and their attractiveness. Where the group's atmosphere is characterized by high degrees of openness, mutual respect, and trust, it is more likely to be cohesive. For such trust to develop, members must have an opportunity to interact with each other directly. Large groups make face-to-face interaction and the establishment of trusting relationships increasingly difficult. A small group should have no more than six to eight members if there is to be adequate opportunity for that face-to-face interaction and the development of intimacy. Beyond this, size alone can change the quality of interactions so that relations are less intimate (Simmel, 1950).

Group structure and leadership style tend to be related. A democratic, participative structure in which all members have direct communications access with each other further reinforces the development of openness. An authoritarian, hierarchical structure in which communications are channeled through the leader impedes openness and trust and reduces individuals' involvement in group tasks. In contrast to the democratic group, interactions in the authoritarian group are characterized by one-way communications downward (from leader to group members), one-way accountability upward (from group members to leader), and unilateral decision making (the leader makes the decisions).

Research shows that such groups have low morale, with intermember scapegoating a frequent way of releasing the tensions that result from the structure (White & Lippit, 1960). Where the group's task is fairly unstructured and ambiguous, requiring the involvement of all members, work productivity and creativity tend to be impaired (Fiedler, 1967). Interestingly, in democratic groups where decision making, communications, and accountability are mutual, a highly structured, unambiguous task finds the group selecting a wheel-type communications network with the leader at the hub assigning tasks to members. With the completion of the specific task, the group reverts to an open all-channel type communications network. This flexible adaptive capacity, characteristic of teams, demonstrates the ability of such groups to respond appropriately to the demands of unique situations as they arise.

Goals, Activities, and Motivation

Group goals and activities, to the extent that they enhance the values and goals of individual members (that is, meet their needs), increase individuals' attraction to the group. The importance of the goals, their clarity, and the manner in which activities are structured also have a bearing on attraction. Members' similarity to each other on task-relevant characteristics further enhances attractiveness and group cohesion. On interprofessional teams, lack of similarity by profession also enhances team functioning where there is a shared (i.e., similar) belief in the value of interdisciplinary efforts to enhance patient care. Where that belief is not present, it is the leader's responsibility to instill it.

Intermember similarity in terms of motivation is important in facilitating group cohesion. Needs for affiliation, money, prestige, and security to some degree or another all can influence whether or not people join groups and the extent to which they then identify with them. In the case of health care delivery teams, similarity in terms of a common concern for quality care and commitment to the organization are important variables linking members together.

To the degree that members expect positive results from their group efforts, motivation to perform joint tasks will be strong. Such motivation is based on the belief that other group members will carry their responsibility for task completion and that the efforts of all of them are highly synchronized. Where the outcomes are seen as worthwhile, in and of themselves, motivation is enhanced.

Finally, how the group compares to others in terms of member attractiveness and the products or services produced will influence cohesion. Where member attractiveness and products are highly rated relative to other groups, cohesion will be affected positively.

If group cohesion is high, it is accompanied by the following desirable consequences:

- Team membership will be maintained over time, thus increasing opportunities for the development of interpersonal relations characterized by trust.
- Long-term maintenance of membership also produces short-term benefits, such as lowering absenteeism.
- The group will demonstrate high levels of loyalty and participation and will be able to exercise power and influence over its members.
- A degree of personal security will be experienced by each individual member, whose self-evaluation also will be high because of identification with the group.

The team, then, is an exceptional group that combines high loyalty, morale, energy, and commitment, resulting in effective task performance in something highly relevant to both the team and the organization, often in the face of what appear to be insurmountable obstacles.

The Difficult Developmental Process

The evolution of a group into a team is a developmental process. The fact that a number of people are engaged in a common enterprise does not ensure that a team will emerge. Groups get stuck at various points in their growth for a variety of reasons: poorly defined structures for decision making, lack of commitment and clarity regarding goals, inappropriate leadership, and unrecognized and unresolved conflict.

The relative scarcity of well-functioning teams points to the complexity of the developmental process. Good teams rarely happen by themselves. They must be created deliberately. This is the essence of team building: to create the conditions supporting, and to remove the blockages preventing, the development of highly effective groups. There are five stages in the development of teams.

Stage 1—Ambivalence: This involves the testing or approach-avoidance characteristic of any newly formed group. Despite eagerness for membership, there are doubts about the group's suitability, interpersonal compatibility, personal anxiety about belonging, and acceptance. People seek to learn about each other, gradually exchanging information concerning their values, attitudes, communications styles, and so forth. Issues are handled at a primarily superficial level but a degree of comfort is achieved when members are relatively satisfied when others evidence initial interest and commitment to the group. The group has not yet begun to work.

Stage 2—Power and Control: This entails the testing of individuals' influence and the limits of the group regarding its tolerance of disagreement and conflict. While the team leader has authority by virtue of that position, this authority is challenged overtly and covertly by team members. It is at this stage that the group is struggling with how it will go about its business. The norms are set with regard to issues of control (i.e., who controls the team and how that control is exercised) and deviance (how much and what kind is tolerated, how it is managed).

While there are no prescriptions for groups to follow in resolving these issues, certain typical problems set the stage for team blockage. For example, where the leader does not facilitate the open and constructive exploration of disagreement and conflict among all members, conflict is avoided but is expressed destructively through passive means (e.g., resistance to group discussion, sabotage of group effort, failure to contribute to group projects). Because personal views are not freely expressed and encouraged, the development of trust is impeded. The team is likely to become stalemated, characterized by low energy, low morale, and less than optimal performance. Control difficulties must be worked through in order to move on to Stage 3.

Stage 3—Affiliation and Work: This is characterized by positive inter-member relations, increased degrees of coordination, commitment, and energy toward the group's task and its completion. Individual differences are set aside as members improve their ability to listen receptively to one another. The team becomes concerned about efficiency and reviews performance, looking for alternative and better ways of accomplishing projects. A communications shorthand develops among members as the group strives to improve its methods of operation, becoming more flexible and creative in the process. This stage requires genuine understanding of various perspectives and that the members remain open to reevaluating team operating procedures, searching for improvement while keeping the goal in mind continuously. Without these latter elements, the group is likely to settle for performance adequacy as opposed to excellence.

Stage 4—Differentiation/Integration: This evolves from Stage 3. The emphasis is on the development of individual team members, supporting each to excel to fullest capacity. This development occurs in the context of cooperation among team members and the integration of different talents for the benefit of the group which, in turn, gives support for individual growth. While the formal leader is likely to remain in that position, members all have become skilled at leader and member roles. The result is a fluidity of leadership, depending on the requirements of a particular task or subtask and the abilities of particular members. Outside observers readily identify the tight-knit aspect of the team and its ability to accomplish work. However, the team is not an isolated unit within a system. Rather, it sees its role and function as intricately tied to the broader goals and objectives of the organization of which it is a part. At this stage, in particular, links to other teams and units in the organization are strengthened in the efforts to enhance interteam integration.

Stage 5—Dissolution: This entails the process of terminating the team. No group is forever. Many teams are formed to accomplish time-limited specific projects. Once the need is met and the team has no other mandate, it prepares for its ending. Because of the bonds that have developed and the immense satisfaction of working well with colleagues, resistance to the termination occurs at this stage. The effective team, however, will recognize the roots of such resistance and not create projects of small significance merely to keep itself alive. The team also experiences dissolution with the loss of one or more of its members, even if it continues as an entity. This occurs because the identity of the team cannot help but change with the loss of any member and/or the addition of a new one.

Despite the distinct advantages of such groups in improving organizational performance and reducing stress brought about by poor integration, lack of goal clarity, low levels of participation, trust, and the like, team building creates stress in the short run for members. If they are to be effective, teams require a degree of openness and self-disclosure that many individuals, regardless of their positions, find threatening. Because conflict is dealt with openly, those uncomfortable with its expression are likely to experience temporary stress and may try to block team development. These factors demand that the team leader be a strong, confident individual with the ability to facilitate discussion and development even when support seems minimal or lacking altogether. Often this requires specialized training. The end result, however, is more than worth the effort.

Team building has particular relevance in organizations in which the work is characterized by high levels of interdependence, frequent problem-solving efforts, and high demands for accuracy and/or timeliness. Given the nature of health care environments, the utility of teams and team building should not be underestimated, whether in the case of committees needing to work together, physician-nurse-administration collaboration, administration-board interaction, patient care teams, support service groups, and the like.

Quality Control Circles

Quality control circles, conceived originally in the United States during World War II, were introduced into Japanese companies after the war to improve productivity and quality control. Their start there stemmed largely from the concern of Japanese businesses over eliminating the reputation that their products were of poor quality. Indeed, it was not until the mid-1970s that these circles were introduced formally in the United States. Since then, interest in the concept has burgeoned, largely in the business and industrial sector, and has spread into the health care delivery sector as well.

One of the problems accompanying the widespread growth of quality control circles is that they often are implemented without a sufficient diagnosis of the organizational climate, without adequate preparation of management and members, and without adequate administrative support. Many of these problems occur as a result of an inadequately trained individual whose task it is to develop and facilitate them. Finally, circles have become somewhat of a fad, similar to management by objectives

(MBO) in its peak. They often are touted as a panacea to whatever currently ails an organization or might befall it in the future.

However, despite their misuse, circles can have substantial positive effects under the right conditions. A discussion of quality control circles in relation to the management style of an organization can provide a useful perspective for evaluating their potential effects.

Quality control circles probably are unnecessary in an organization which falls on the open end of a participative management continuum where team building already is in place. In institutions on the opposite end of the continuum (i.e., with closed management) quality control circles probably would increase organizational stress among employees. This would occur as a result of management's failure to respond to the circles' inputs. For institutions in the middle range, quality control circles are likely to be of some use in lowering organizational stress caused by low levels of worker participation, inadequate management-employee communications, low job clarity, and poor intragroup relations. The bottom line regarding an intervention such as quality control circles is that this technique should not be introduced if the organization is not willing to give a participative role to the work force.

What exactly are quality control circles?

Circles are small groups of people (four to ten members) doing similar work who meet regularly to identify, analyze, and solve productivity and quality problems related to their work. Meetings are held weekly, lasting one to two hours on work time in or near the job area itself. Membership is voluntary; leaders are work supervisors who have been trained in leadership techniques and in how to use the problem-solving tools necessary to perform the work of the circle. Typically a facilitator who has had fairly rigorous training in group dynamics and circle methodology trains the leaders and acts as a consultant once the circles are in place. Circle leaders generally are responsible for training their members in the skills required for effective problem solving.

Basically, leaders and members are trained in the techniques of brainstorming, e.g., establishing an open climate of discussion and dialogue without criticizing ideas until they all have been aired; looking for novel approaches to the identification of problems; using cause-effect diagrams to elucidate the nature of a problem; providing Pareto diagrams (i.e., special bar graphs that illustrate factors associated with a problem in descending, step-like order), histograms (i.e., bar graph), graphs, and checksheets to consolidate and compare information about problems to be examined; using graphs to illustrate trends; and including data collection, analysis procedures, and simple statistics. Leaders and members also are trained in techniques that are particularly helpful in making presentations to management concerning the problems identified and the solutions suggested to remedy them. Presentations are utilized to inform management about the circle's progress and to gain its recognition and support of the suggestions made.

Setting a Climate for Evaluation

Subordinate/superior relations are characterized by unequal power. As a result, continuing lack of trust characterizes most such relationships. Both parties, but particularly the subordinate, are watching their "p's and q's"—never completely open because they never are really sure when a constructive criticism or disagreement will boomerang and come back at them in a poor performance appraisal. Under the best of circumstances performance appraisal itself, the culmination of the continuous year-long evaluation, frequently is characterized by a high degree of anxiety and thus loses much of its effectiveness. But because they are always watching themselves, subordinates' performance suffers. Their creativity is stifled. Upward communication is distorted as people increasingly are concerned, not about the organization and the work, but about covering themselves.

This may sound unethical and something everyone would like to say does not exist in health care organizations. Unfortunately, in studies of organizations across the country in 1981 and 1982, the author has found that health care managers and nonmanagerial employees are no different from other mortals. When they feel abused by the system through what is described as "creeping expectations" (i.e., what is expected increases constantly and surreptitiously) or unfair use of power, especially in performance appraisal situations, their typical response is to do only what is needed to get by. How this affects the clinical and technical care delivered in institutions is not really clear since the author lacks data on that question. However, to the extent that the data show decreased morale, organizational sabotage (e.g., through organizational noncompliance), and reduced sensitivity to patient concerns, it is likely that care is, indeed, affected negatively.

The challenge is to create a climate in which evaluation is perceived as a positive and integral part of the job, essentially part of professional development. To accomplish this it is necessary to reverse the process of low trust and tendencies toward power abuse. This can be done only when evaluation is seen as a mutual accountability process between superior and subordinate. It will happen only when the system and the superior regard the professional subordinate as someone with special competencies whose contributions are critical to the supervisor's survival and the organization's overall well-being. The underlying premise here is that human resources in a professional organization are its most valuable capital. If that premise is not operative, this approach will not work.

From a mechanical standpoint the implementation of this approach is fairly straightforward. First, the entire process of evaluation is mutual. The subordinate is expected to give feedback to the superior regarding: (1) what has been helpful in enhancing the subordinate's ability to do the job, (2) what has not been helpful in that regard, and (3) what behaviors might be helpful that are not now in evidence. The premise is that a manager who is not facilitating the development of the subordinate and the person's ability to get the job done should not be there.

Second, managers must themselves be held accountable for climate. Data on which to base such accountability stem from the results of yearly climate studies that all employees fill out anonymously. There are, of course, limitations as to which parts of climate managers are held accountable for. For instance, they are held responsible for management practices and for action plans designed as a response to climate.

There are, of course, some real obstacles to this approach. Among them are low levels of trust, built-in resistance to change, and personal feelings of threat experienced by all parties. Employees often are not willing to take risks or to expose themselves in areas they perceive to be outside their domain. Unconsciously or consciously, managers may sabotage the program.

Ironically, people want to trust—they are merely reluctant to do so. Most individuals have had experiences in which people in whom they have put that trust have violated it. Trust is earned. Once it has been seriously violated, it is extremely difficult to regain.

Organizational Structures and Communications

While the subject of how best to structure organizations is beyond the scope of this book, several points concerning structure need to be addressed because of their relevance to organizational stress. Two dimensions of organizational design, the centralization-decentralization continuum and the relationship between authority and knowledge, are explored.

Centralization of authority and responsibility occurs when most decisions are made at the top of the organizational hierarchy. Theoretically, the most centralized institution would be one in which the administrator at the top knew all aspects of the work and made all important decisions. In all but the smallest organization, the demands upon such an executive would be impossible to meet.

Decentralization entails moving decision-making authority lower in the chain of command. The notion of continuum is important here, for no organizations are entirely centralized or decentralized; rather, they tend to be more or less decentralized. There is no theoretical advantage of one over another, assuming that decisions concerning degree of centralization are made on the basis of the tasks to be performed and in regard to the needs of the people performing them. Organizational performance might be identical in both (1) a decentralized institution in which managers at lower levels have the knowledge and expertise to make appropriate decisions and in (2) a centralized structure in which the central administrator is most expert and knowledgeable.

Centralized authority offers more control to top-level management. As a result, in times of crisis (financial or otherwise), organizations have a tendency toward centralization of authority. The central authority, whether this be the chief executive officer or the chiefs of key professional areas such as medicine and nursing, can oversee all organizational needs, make all the necessary but unpopular decisions, and maintain a higher level of confidentiality on important matters. Centralization ensures that the person or people at the top will have access to the information necessary to make decisions. It is likely to develop when competition increases or when financial or other problems arise.

However, in noncrisis situations, decentralized authority, particularly in professional organizations, offers some advantages. In such complex organizations, top management cannot maintain central control. It may not possess the clinical or technical knowledge necessary to make decisions. In such cases authority should be vested in the managers and staff members most knowledgeable about their work. In this manner, small, more manageable units are created that afford more people in the organization an opportunity to participate meaningfully in decision making, thus increasing job autonomy. Such decentralization means that managers must delegate responsibility and authority to subordinates.

One distinct disadvantage to such decentralization is that departments tend to perceive themselves and their needs as most essential (unit suboptimization). It is senior level administration's responsibility to make sure that the functional departments maintain an integrated perspective with regard to the needs of the entire organization. Each department is critically important; no one is more important than the others. Coordination and integration remain the challenge for administration.

The tendency toward uniting authority and knowledge in the person or team that possesses the most pertinent knowledge necessary for making a particular decision has important implications for organizational communications. Herbert Simon (1976) emphasizes that the flow of information should become an important, conscious aspect of organizational design, as important as job descriptions and the authority system itself. Structures should be determined by such considerations as the type of information needed for specific decisions, the identification of persons who have access to or possess that information, the identification of other individuals with whom the information possessors should communicate, and an assessment of how these people can best communicate with each other. A case study highlights the serious obstacles that occur when these principles are not followed. The case demonstrates communications structured on the basis of organizational hierarchy without regard to professional competencies, efficiency, and effectiveness. While the example describes communications within the personnel function of a corporate structure, similar difficulties occur in clinical and technical areas as well. (Even the first names in this case have been changed.)

Mitchell N., corporate director of organization development and evaluation, has an office across the hall from John T., vice president of nursing home services. John T. was interested in a series of climate studies to be conducted in the nursing homes. He had discussed this with Carol B., human resource manager for the homes, whose office was in a separate facility eight miles from corporate headquarters. She endorsed the idea. To facilitate the process John T. (who enjoyed a friendly professional relationship with Mitchell N.), contacted Pat B., corporate vice president for human resources and training who was Mitchell N.'s superior. John T. telephoned the request for climate analysis to Pat B., who called Mitchell N., requesting that he contact Carol B. to pursue the matter. This accomplished, Mitchell N. sent a memo to Pat B., informing her officially where the matter stood. Carol B. memoed her superior, John T., notifying him.

This is a classic example of bureaucratic communications controls that impede efficiency and undermine employee morale.

RETHINKING SOCIALIZATION

One of the important tasks of an organization is to find suitable means through which individuals can and will internalize and identify with its goals. The process of affiliation and the employees' subsequent personal identification with the organization take place in part through such experiences as initial training and orientation. In this process, those who approve the organization's goals to some degree by accepting employment then put aside personal aims and adopt organizational objectives. The individuals are being socialized to the culture of the organization.

Culture as a Potential Stressor

Culture is best understood as a concept embodying the mores, values, attitudes, institutions, behavioral norms, and expectations of a group in a given period of time. Culture, while it does change over time, is resistive to change and in that sense exerts a long-lasting, fairly pervasive influence over people within it. Such influence may be direct or indirect. Organizations can be said to have unique cultures that are a product of their individual histories in interaction with their internal and external environments. Organizational cultures determine protocol and norms of deference regarding professional and hierarchical status. Norms regarding how individuals dress, how much deviance is tolerated, and what behaviors are prohibited altogether are important aspects of organizational culture.

Climate is a function of culture. It is the translation of culture into more current and specific perceptions of what it feels like to work in the organization. Climates differ within an organization. While there may be subcultures in an institution, it is reasonable to view culture as a more pervasive, overarching aspect whose influence endures over time.

Culture shock, which afflicts those ill equipped to the adaptations required by rapid, continuing technological change, has been popularized through the work of Alvin Toffler (1970). Hospital cultures also are responding to technological and professional change, as noted in previous chapters. However, they need to respond to yet another drastic shift, perhaps in part because of changes in the broader financial environment affecting them. This entails the creation of large, multi-institutional arrangements. Whether it is the for-profit chain, the not-for-profit chain, the smaller mergers, or the corporate acquisition of a for-profit operation, each expansion changes the organization's culture that has given structure and meaning to employees' lives. As with any change, a stress condition occurs. Depending on how it is managed and how employees are integrated and socialized into the new situation or culture or environment, negative consequences for both the organization and the individuals are likely.

Where employees lack information regarding the reasons for, and the impact and specific consequences of, the change, particularly for them, anxiety will be high and performance will suffer. To the extent that job security is an issue, the organization is vulnerable to unionization attempts. Whether or not unions actually can win security or gains is a moot point. What is important is that where employees perceive that the organization is unconcerned about them, they are more willing to turn to outside parties to protect their interests.

Such lack of concern may be evidenced in the absence of (or inadequate and unclear) communications, insufficient opportunity for the expression of employee concern about the tangible (e.g., position security, reporting relationships, job shifts, salary and benefit changes) and less tangible (e.g., climate modification, change in identifications, loyalties, and support systems) consequences associated with the broad-scale change. The remedy for these problems is straightforward: Administrators need to devote as much time and attention to the resocialization, orientation, and integration of employees as they do to fiscal and program concerns.

Internal Support Systems

The use of various types of support groups to alleviate or prevent the harmful effects of job-related stress events is reported frequently in the literature. Social support is believed to reduce the physiological consequences of stress (anxiety, tension, worry, low self-esteem) but it may have little effect in reducing the psychological effects (Pinneau, 1976). Given that social support groups generally do not engage in direct action to modify the sources of stress, it also is questionable whether this approach can have lasting effects in terms of being able to buffer people against job-related stressors.

At the base of the social support interventions is the assumption that by talking to a colleague who has experienced similar feelings, a person is relieved of the burden of carrying inner tensions alone. Feelings of comradeship develop; the individual has a "fellow traveler" with whom to share the troubles, thus bolstering the person's energy to perform the work. To the extent that social support pairs or groups digress into "bitch" sessions, the coping strategy actually may become a source of stress as members reinforce each other's perceptions of how awful things are.

It seems likely, however, that time-limited and/or problem-focused support groups may have very positive short-term effects on preventing or alleviating members' negative stress outcomes. Several studies of social support groups for new employees as they face identity stress during their early months at work have shown positive benefits as a result of the experience (Graen, 1976; Mansfield, 1972; Wanous, 1977). Professional support groups begun in numerous medical schools and residency programs across the country have reported positive results, although most of them have not been studied empirically. Support groups for professionals in intensive care units of various types and oncology units have been described as helpful in increasing participants' abilities to handle death and dying and to provide more humanistic care to patients and their families. Experience suggests that support groups also seem to increase staff members' collegiality and willingness to help each other out. These groups almost always are voluntary and generally are facilitated by consultants from outside the department. Frequently, supervisory and managerial staff persons do not attend these meetings, viewing their presence as a deterrent to openness.

Managerial effectiveness groups, with which this author has had extensive experience, have been extremely effective in establishing problem-solving networks among executive staff members, decreasing their feelings of isolation, and improving their professional abilities. While these small, time-limited groups (six to eight members) have been facilitated by an outside consultant, they have been structured in such a way that they develop the tools to continue on their own.

Anecdotal reports of managers in health care facilities in different parts of the country suggest that social support, if it is to be effective in the sense of providing general emotional backing for work-related stress, cannot be mandated institutionally. People in organizations generally have problems regarding who they can trust. Because of the personal nature of what is discussed, many believe that individuals must be given the freedom to select such support on their own as it is needed. Furthermore, there are some who, because of professional socialization and/or personal expectations, tend not to use support even when it is available and could be helpful. The most obvious examples of this are physicians in general and administrative level personnel, particularly men. However, it is possible to begin to approach even the problems of physician stress. For the administrator who recognizes the need for general intervention, several actions are recommended.

First, the administrator needs to take the initiative in developing, in cooperation with the chief of the medical staff, a support system that is acceptable to all concerned. The administrator might begin by identifying the problem of stress and its importance, delineating its systemic roots, and exploring ways in which the health care organization can offer preventive programs. Depending upon what form the needs of the group(s) might take, this could include workshops in stress management, provisions for administrative leave, modification of residents' inflexible and unrealistic time demands, problem-oriented workshops for physicians in communications, and staff training to recognize signs of stress and strategies for coping.

In addition, there needs to be a reexamination of the double standard with regard to differential behavior tolerance among health care providers. A large range of physicians' behavior that is tolerated by nonphysicians would not be acceptable if exhibited by the latter. Included in this would be irritability, unusual working hours, failure to complete charting, failure to chart, etc. It could be argued that the "tolerated behaviors" really are manifestations of stress that would be handled as such if they were exhibited by someone else. However, the complexity of identifying early warning signals and handling people under stress sensitively cannot be overstated. For example, it might be difficult to differentiate between the physician who generally is irritable and the one on the verge of an emotional breakdown. (It also would be useful to know why this general irritability exists. Is it, too, a manifestation of stress?) A reluctance to confront individuals under stress may stem from a lack of knowledge concerning its symptoms and a lack of skill in handling such persons. It seems clear that the health care community no longer can afford to ignore such situations. It can begin to meet these problems by educating staff members about the manifestations of stress and their consequences.

Regardless of the lack of substantive empirical evidence in favor of social support groups within the organization, self-reports indicate that this modality does help members cope in the short run. To the extent that burnout is typified by a sense of social isolation and the lack of someone to talk to about the problems encountered at work, reversing this phenomenon makes intuitive and rational sense.

This leaves the task of defining more specifically what types of social support are useful in ameliorating what types of stressors for which people. How do the effects of these support groups differ? Essentially it is necessary to know whether social support is equally relevant to all types of stress and/or stress outcomes. It also is important to know by what processes social support may mitigate the effects of stress on health. It is apparent that health care professionals still are grossly ignorant concerning the concept.

MONITORING AND CONTROL MECHANISMS

When high pressure becomes chronic in an institution, as frequently is the case in health care, a pattern of stress-reducing behavior develops that helps members cope but is dysfunctional for organizational performance (Harrison, 1981). Activity level remains high but problem solving decreases. Time perspective decreases as people look for short-term solutions. Perception narrows and there is a decrease in the number of solutions considered for problems. Resistance to new data springs up and people fail to consider related problems and their ramifications. Cooperation and helping decrease, while blaming and avoidance of responsibility increase. Stress symptoms increase, leading to withdrawal.

Obviously, this scenario calls for measures beyond prevention. The negative stress effects that have occurred already must be remedied. Monitoring and quality control mechanisms need to be in place to handle such occurrences. Performance appraisal and discipline systems are the monitoring and control mechanisms used most widely in organizations. Coaching, counseling, and quality control circles are newer approaches. None of these measures is geared specifically toward the alleviation of stress. All focus on measures of performance and on behaviors relevant to the job. However, because excessive stress may manifest itself in poor performance—either in terms of quality or quantity, or both—and in behavioral changes, these measures afford the organization a means for intervening through employees' immediate superiors.

Performance Appraisal: Role and Guidelines

Performance appraisal is a means by which people are held accountable for achieving specific results. It aims to improve performance and results. If properly designed, appraisals identify the strengths and weaknesses of peoples' performance, indicate where the individuals stand in relation to department expectations, encourage self-development, give them recognition for their accomplishments, and suggest areas for improvement. The evaluation, based on assessments over a designated period, helps in promotion and transfer decisions, salary recommendations, and remedial action in the case of substandard performance.

To be effective, performance appraisals should be cooperative ventures (Numerof, 1982). That means a supervisor cannot be out to "get" a subordinate and the subordinate should not be left feeling defensive. Most people sincerely want to know how they are doing and how they can improve. Despite this natural desire, they frequently respond with less openness to even the most constructive criticism when they feel that their abilities are being judged. In anticipation of subordinates' sensitivity, supervisors may couch their remarks in such a manner that the truth is shaded, leaving the subordinates with an unrealistic evaluation of their performance or with a great deal of anxiety regarding how it really has been perceived.

If the relationship between supervisors and subordinates is open and direct, the performance appraisal should be less eventful than when communication is not direct. The matters discussed should come as no surprise to either party. The performance appraisal is not a substitute for regular, continuing supervision.

If the supervisors perceive themselves as guides or facilitators to improve performance, the evaluation is likely to be less traumatic for all concerned and far more beneficial than if they regard their role as that of inspectors or taskmasters driving subordinates on to higher achievements.

Appraisals can be conducted with regard to either of two factors, or some combination of them both: performance results and subordinate traits. The former method uses a management-by-objectives approach. The latter appraises certain characteristics that are believed to lead to good results. The advantages of performance appraisal by results achieved are numerous. When implemented properly, both supervisors and subordinates understand exactly what is being evaluated, minimizing the potential for misunderstanding and misapprehension. Because the subordinates are involved in setting the goals in terms of how or on what they will be evaluated, they have a vested interest in seeing that the objectives are achieved. When feedback is given regarding performance at the time goals should have been reached, it will mean more to the subordinates than if it is offered six months or a year later.

There are, however, significant limitations to this approach, which is why a combination of the traits and results appraisals is useful. Merely looking at the accomplishments says nothing about what type of person the subordinates are, an especially important consideration if appraisals are to be used for promotion and transfer. Do the subordinates show initiative, creativity, and courage? Do they demonstrate cooperation and facilitating capacities? How do they react to change? A subordinate with high initiative and creativity whose performance record is high but who reacts poorly to a frequently changing work environment would not be an especially appropriate person to manage the emergency room. However, that same person might be an excellent candidate for a more stable environment such as the housekeeping department.

Trait assessment might include such qualities as dependability, cooperativeness, enthusiasm, judgment, initiative, and quantity and quality of work produced. Traits range from the abstract and highly personal to the more concrete and impersonal (such as quantity of work). It is preferable, whenever possible, to make traits as specific as possible. One means of achieving such specificity is through behavioral anchoring. Such a procedure provides a scale on which each trait can be defined and measured (Exhibit 9-1).

Although no predetermined number of traits is more beneficial than another to use on an evaluation, six to ten provides a manageable number—neither too few nor too many. Traits that are job specific probably are the most useful in appraisal. Thus it is advisable for individual supervisors to use discretion in choosing which ones they will select for performance appraisal. In addition, it is an excellent idea to solicit employee feedback regarding which traits they think might reflect appropriate dimensions for evaluation. Unfortunately, subordinate input into the design of

Exhibit 9-1 Sample Trait Performance Appraisal Form: Initiative

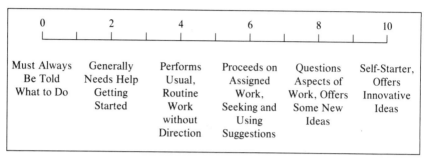

0	2	4	6	8	10
Must Always Be Told What to Do	Generally Needs Help Getting Started	Performs Usual, Routine Work without Direction	Proceeds on Assigned Work, Seeking and Using Suggestions	Questions Aspects of Work, Offers Some New Ideas	Self-Starter, Offers Innovative Ideas

evaluation instruments and selection of their dimensions does not occur as frequently as it might.

Despite the fact that many supervisors would prefer having someone else do performance evaluation, there is no avoiding the fact that this appraisal is their responsibility. No one else is in a position to judge a particular person's performance. Given that they work closely together on a regular basis, the supervisor has access to the particulars of the subordinate's work. The supervisor is judged on what the department accomplishes and that, in turn, depends on how well each department member performs. The supervisor thus has a vested interest in the performance appraisal process.

In the evaluation, the supervisor should focus on the time period for which the subordinate is being evaluated. It does little good to evaluate earlier work or just the most recent period. The most effective appraisal should offer an overview of all work over the entire period, not focusing on isolated incidents.

Appraisal that occurs on a daily basis integrated into a regular work cycle is recommended. With such a format, it is not an isolated, once-a-year experience but a continuous process that helps to ensure that the appraisal does aim to improve performance. To be sure that the subordinate is engaged in the process to the fullest extent possible, the supervisor should encourage the subordinate to ask questions and seek assistance and clarification. To check the tendency to concentrate on the most recent occurrences or to think in terms of one brief period, the supervisor should keep notes on a regular basis regarding performance over time, and not trust to memory. These notes can be filed and used later to document the evaluation.

The supervisor is cautioned to guard against the tendency to rate a subordinate on all traits in a similar manner. This tendency not to discriminate in ratings on different items is called a halo effect. When this is operative, the supervisor allows the judgment of one item to influence the appraisal of others.

Last, the supervisor should look at trends in appraisals of each subordinate and of the group as a whole over time. Is the individual advancing, backsliding, or standing still? Is progress being made in areas that were identified previously as needing improvement? If not, why not? If the appraisal is used as a means for defining where help and assistance are needed, it tends to keep the process on more positive ground than if it emphasizes what the person or the group lacks.

The Discipline System

Managers and supervisors have various demands made of them. Among these is the expectation that they reach the objectives of their departments and work groups through the efficient use of the people under their direction. If supervisors and managers have established solid work relationships with their staff by communicating clearly what is expected of them and by showing appreciation of their cooperation and performances aimed at meeting department objectives, they generally will not encounter personnel problems.

However, there are times when a particular person's work or personal behavior fails to meet the organization's standards. The first-line supervisor is responsible for correcting the problem. In part a result of today's emphasis on employee rights and the existence of grievance procedures and arbitration, it is necessary to correct these problems by using acceptable methods that spell out the appropriate action to be taken and the general principles that are being followed. Each of these is considered next separately.

Progressive Steps in Discipline

Disciplinary action should (in unionized situations, must) follow progressive steps that are outlined in the employee handbook that also gives consequences associated with each step. The sequence is useful in that it allows time for the person to correct unacceptable behavior. It also gives people adequate warning as to the seriousness of the problem and the possible consequences. Generally, the progressive steps are: (1) a verbal warning, (2) a first written warning, (2) a second written warning, and, if necessary, (3) suspension or termination. While physicians, for example, are not generally employees in the strict sense of the word, they are accountable to the institution; these approaches can be modified to meet their particular situation.

Verbal Warning: For most problems, including attendance and work habits, the supervisor calls in the subordinate to discuss the situation. If the organization is unionized, the employee working under a collective bargaining agreement usually has the option of having a union representative present. During the meeting, the unacceptable behavior and the necessary corrective action are discussed in a friendly manner and in such a way that the employee knows what the problem is. Counseling and attempts to help the employee remedy the problem should be made and documented. The person should not be embarrassed by having coworkers other than the union delegate overhear the warning. A memorandum is written and placed in the person's file to document the oral warning. The verbal warning should describe the nature of the offense and possible consequences. It is general practice for the person, union, and personnel department not to receive copies of the memorandum.

Written Warnings: The person who does not heed the verbal warning and continues with the same problem is spoken to in a more formal way and is informed that a written notice will be forthcoming on the problem and what was said in the interview. The interview and the subsequent written notice should mention the rule violated, specific details, prior verbal or written warnings, the seriousness of the problem, the difficulty it imposes on the department, what is expected of the person to correct the situation, and the consequences of not correcting it. Copies of the written warning are sent to the person, the union (where appropriate), and the personnel department, with one retained by the supervisor in the individual's file.

Suspension: If the person does not heed the oral and written warnings within a reasonable time (or immediately, in the case of very serious offenses), the department head may approve suspension of the worker. In some cases, especially those involving absenteeism, if an employee improves temporarily after a written warning, then falls back into unacceptable behavior, another written warning without suspension may be issued.

It is advisable for supervisors to refer recommendations for suspension to department heads, who may consult with the personnel department regarding the merits or duration of such action in a particular case. Suspension is a serious disciplinary measure that imposes an economic penalty on the staff person. It usually is considered the final warning: future incidents involving the same offense within a specified period will result in automatic termination. Where it is the final warning, the supervisor should state clearly that termination will be the next step unless there is sustained improvement. Suspension is valuable in that it forcefully notifies the subordinate of the seriousness of the problem. Suspensions usually should be limited to one or two days.

As with the written warning, an interview is held before the suspension, with the details documented and made part of the subordinate's permanent record. (In a unionized institution, the union representative should be present.) The documentation should include the same facts as in the written warnings: the rule violated, the specific details, prior verbal and written warnings, the seriousness of the problem, the difficulty it imposes on the department, what is expected of the subordinate to correct it, and the consequences of not correcting it. The supervisor or department head generally must notify the director of personnel and the employee relations manager (where one exists) that the person has been suspended. The director of personnel usually takes responsibility for notifying union representatives.

Discharge: Especially in a tight job market, discharge is close to the economic death of the employee, with its corresponding psychological and social ramifications. Regardless of that, however, discharge is necessary when an employee cannot or will not meet the organization's standards after appropriate disciplinary steps have been taken. Termination may take place after consultation with the personnel department. In any case, when an employee is terminated, the union representative (where there is a union) usually is present as the documentation on the previous steps is reviewed. The final (termination) notice is presented to the employee detailing the offense, the rule violated, prior warnings, the seriousness of the problem, and steps taken to remedy it. Copies of the notice are kept in the employee's file in the department, in personnel, and in the union file.

General Principles in Discipline

The purpose of disciplinary action is not punishment but correction and rehabilitation. Therefore, the tone and climate of the interview should be hopeful while remaining firm and strict. Essentially, the supervisor is conveying a hope that the subordinate will correct the problem, recognizing that if this is not done, the person will suffer the consequences. Verbal warnings generally should be less strict and formal than written warnings. The cause of the problem should be sought and the employee counseled. Efforts at helping the worker should be documented.

In taking disciplinary action, the supervisor may learn that the poor performance is, in part, the result of poorly defined rules and procedures. Department rules must be reasonable, must be clear, and must be circulated to all members (and the union). People cannot be held responsible for rules that are vague or known only to a few. When procedures and rules exist, they should be posted in the department; otherwise, each employee should receive a copy of them and sign for it.

When employees are disciplined it is important to follow the progressive procedures for less serious problems so as to give them adequate warning that they are not meeting standards. This gives them ample time to take corrective action.

Regardless of the type of action taken, it is important that supervisors gather all the facts and details about the situation. Often, they suffer embarrassment when their warning notices, suspensions, and terminations are retracted because procedures were not followed or because they were issued before all the facts were known. It is important for employees to be given a hearing on their side of the situation before a judgment is made. Written notices never should be prepared before the supervisor has given the employee a chance to speak. Extenuating circumstances should be considered in deciding on discipline. Here again the supervisor's own conduct will affect the measure taken. Supervisors who are argumentative and shout at employees probably will see offenses as far more serious than if they were in control of their own behavior.

Disciplinary action must fit the offense. It is unreasonable to fire an employee for the first absence or the first poor work performance. Issues of seniority, the person's previous work record, and the amount of time between offenses should be considered. More serious violations require more serious discipline. Promptness in taking action is of critical importance. It makes little sense to issue a warning three weeks after an infraction. To be legally acceptable, as well, warnings should be issued on the heels of the offense. If a behavior is important enough to merit a warning, it is important enough to issue the notice promptly.

Objectivity in the application of rules is another important element. Rules are established to facilitate the work of the organization. An employee's failure to comply reflects the person's inability to meet reasonable standards that coworkers do without difficulty. It is important that all employees understand that the supervisor is not out to get any one of them. If employees abide by the rules, discipline will not be necessary. The need for impartiality in the application of such rules is a mandatory principle. The supervisor must apply the rules to all subordinates across the board, not only to those less favored subordinates.

In addition, the supervisor must be consistent. If rules are to have validity, they must always be enforced. If they are not, the supervisor is giving tacit approval for their violation, leading to inconsistent standards and confused expectations. Similarly, the supervisor's failure to follow through once corrective action has been initiated gives tacit approval of whatever behavior the employee exhibits subsequently. It is advisable to mark a calendar at a reasonable time in the future to review the employee's recent record.

Finally, the supervisor should consider the time elapsing between offenses in imposing discipline. An employee with lateness and absence problems may have shown significant temporary improvement after discipline. The improvement may be followed by a return of the undesirable behavior. Because of the temporary improvement, the disciplinary process should not advance from the written warning to suspension but should consist of an additional warning of the same degree as used previously. In discipline, supervisors should:

- get all the facts and details
- hear the subordinate's perspective
- consider extenuating circumstances
- have the penalty fit the offense
- be prompt in taking action
- be objective
- be impartial
- be consistent
- do follow-up
- consider the time elapsed between offenses.

Failure to Exercise Discipline

Supervisors have the authority to discipline subordinates for cause but often fail to exercise it. They may not accept their authority because management has not delegated it clearly. They may be unaware of proper procedures to follow. They may be afraid of exercising the authority for fear they may be disliked. They may be afraid of employee retaliation, either from the individual disciplined or from coworkers. In the case of individual retaliation, the supervisor may fear legal action in the form of a discrimination suit or unfair labor practice case. In the case of group retaliation, the supervisor may anticipate work slowdowns or increased absenteeism. Finally, supervisors may fear that upper-level management will not back their decisions once disciplinary measures are taken.

Whether or not any or all of these fears are based on reality is immaterial. If supervisors believe that any of these responses are potential consequences of disciplinary action, the probability that such action will be taken, even when warranted, will diminish.

From the reasons cited for failure to exercise disciplinary authority, several generalizations can be made. Some of the difficulty lies with upper-level management and some with the supervisor. It is management's responsibility to ensure that disciplinary procedures are specified clearly, that supervisors are trained in their proper use, and that management supports disciplinary action when taken appropriately. Supervisors must exercise their authority in disciplining when necessary. It is their delegated responsibility to do so. Supervisors who attempt to win a popularity contest while acting as a boss are likely to fail in both roles.

Chapter 10

The Personal Response

Many centuries ago the philosopher Epictetus is believed to have said, "People are disturbed not by things, but by the views which they take of them." More recently Hans Selye produced a more elaborate version of essentially the same theme, with a series of maxims for reducing the negative effects of stress:

> [d]on't waste your time trying to befriend a mad dog; don't strive for perfection (it doesn't exist), rather strive for the best in the category; genuine simplicity in life style earns much good will and love; keep your mind on the pleasant aspects of life and on actions which can improve your situation; forget ugly events; when frustrated, take stock of your past successes and rebuild your confidence; when faced with a very painful task yet very important, don't procrastinate—ease the pain instead of prolonging it by gently rubbing the surface; love your neighbor and work hard to earn your neighbor's love. (1974, pp. 134–135)

As any therapist can attest, such prescriptions to depressed, anxious, and highly stressed clients/patients inevitably fall on deaf ears. However, as coping strategies that individuals freely adopt, many of these and similar maxims appear to work well for certain persons under particular circumstances. Changing perspective, for example, was a frequently used helpful strategy used by participants in the research reported in Chapter 4.

INDIVIDUAL STRESS REDUCTION TECHNIQUES

Personal strategies for reducing stress effects are numerous, ranging from behavioral change through physical and psychological change. In an excellent review of the literature, Newman and Beehr (1979) suggest that personal coping strategies be aimed at modifying some aspect of the person (i.e., psychological condition, physical condition, behavior, or performance in the work environment). However, the literature lacks empirical research documenting actual effectiveness of coping strategies in reducing work-related stress for particular people under certain stressful conditions. Despite this deficit, an exploration of the approaches seems warranted. Given the costs of negative stress consequences, even anecdotal reports of positive effects may spark others to try approaches they believe may be helpful to them personally. Since evidence pro or con is lacking, such efforts could have considerable merit.

Psychological and Physiological Approaches

McLean (1974), for example, offers a psychoanalytic approach to occupational stress in which personal strategies involve the recognition and management of individuals' own character defenses in the face of tasks that are specific to their life stage and age, as well as complementary to the usual way in which they maintain their equilibrium. In this context, being able to adapt implies an ability to manage intrapsychic drives, cope with the gap between the ego ideal and self-image (large discrepancies can be a source of stress), and maintain a perspective on one's central conflicts in the face of institutional requirements that may magnify or intensify them.

For instance, individuals who, because of childhood experiences of not being trusted, are sensitive about situations in which they perceive their judgment is being questioned, may respond defensively to a superior who asks about a rationale for a particular decision. That request for clarification may not involve a question of judgment but such individuals respond as though it were. If they maintained a perspective on the central conflict, they would be able to evaluate the request on its face and recognize that it implied no questioning of their judgment so they should not experience stress. On the other hand, their judgment may indeed be questioned but, separating historically based issues (i.e., from childhood experiences) from present ones, they would be able to respond to the demands of the immediate situation without confusing their reactions with previous experiences. This also would reduce stress.

Other personal strategies geared toward changing individuals' psychological characteristics or conditions include meditation, progressive relaxation, relaxation response, autogenic training, self-hypnosis, yoga, and biofeedback. These strategies are performed primarily away from the workplace. While transcendental meditation and biofeedback have been shown to modify general stress, there is no evidence to date regarding their effectiveness or lack thereof on work related stress. Since the popular literature describes each of these approaches in considerable detail, only an overview is offered here.

Meditation

Also referred to as transcendental meditation (TM), meditation is a process of gaining mastery over one's mental attention (Le Shan, 1974) that requires regular exercise. The goal is to still the conscious mind so that cognitive processes are suspended during the meditation. Meditation also involves a physiological process in which the relaxation response (see below) is triggered and the rate of various body processes are slowed (e.g. heart, breathing). Numerous anecdotal reports speak to the effectiveness of meditation but do not document that meditation increases job effectiveness.

Progressive Relaxation

Progressive muscle relaxation, also known as the Jacobson relaxation technique, is based on the belief that emotions and muscular tension are directly related to each other. The process involves tensing muscle groups, holding them tensed, then relaxing them. For example, the individual might begin with tensing the toes and feet, working up the body to the face, then relaxing each part in reverse order. The result is a relaxed body. The objective of the exercise is to learn what it feels like to be tense and then to be relaxed.

Relaxation Response

The relaxation response (Bensen, 1974), like meditation, involves deeper physiological changes in the body. Specifically, it reverses the stress cycle in the body and is the normal reaction following the fight-flight reaction. In it the heart rate, pulse, and blood pressure all go down and oxygen consumption decreases. Bensen argues that the relaxation response could be induced and is a useful antidote to stress.

The response is built on the following four components: (1) a quiet, calm environment with few distractions; (2) being seated in a comfortable position; (3) development of a passive attitude; and (4) focus on a mental device while paying attention to breathing. Such a device might include counting one through four on each breath inhalation and continuing for five to ten minutes. It is important that this exercise not be done within two hours after meals since digestion interferes with it.

Autogenic Training

Autogenic (self-generated) training combines specific exercises and autohypnosis to bring about deep mental and physical states of relaxation. The result is a general feeling of warmth throughout the body and of heaviness in the torso. The warmth is from dilation of the arteries that occurs with relaxation and the heaviness from the actual relaxation of the muscles. While there are many variations in the exercise, one method is to repeat the following phrases slowly four or five times while breathing in and out deeply and slowly:

I am . . .	relaxed.
My arm . . .	is heavy.
My leg . . .	is heavy.
My arm . . .	is warm.
My leg . . .	is warm.
My heartbeat . . .	is calm and regular.
My breathing . . .	is free and easy.
My abdomen . . .	is warm.
My forehead . . .	is cool.
My mind . . .	is quiet and still.

Some recommend a cancellation message after each statement series to relax each body part separately. Autogenic visualization occurs after the individual has successfully mastered the physical aspect of the exercise. The person then focuses on a calm, serene setting in the mind while in the physically relaxed state or clearly visualizes having reached a self-determined goal.

Self-Hypnosis

Self-hypnosis, another personal relaxation technique, frequently is confused with daydreaming or sleep yet it is very different from either of those states. Under self-hypnosis the individuals do not loosen control of self but do relax the feeling of conscious control. Under hypnosis they allow themselves to respond to someone else's suggestions while allowing free reign to their own imaginations. In self-hypnosis they respond to their own suggestions.

Self-hypnosis can be brought about through a number of procedures, including the eye-fixation method. In this situation individuals sit in a comfortable position and focus on a stationary object, concentrating and silently telling themselves that their eyelids are getting heavier and heavier, that the eyelids will close, and soon they will be very relaxed yet also aware. This statement is repeated every minute until the eyelids close. The subjects then take a deep breath, hold it for 10 to 15 seconds, exhale, and say the word "relax." To go deeper, they imagine themselves on an escalator, going into deeper states of relaxation. They then visualize self-change suggestions such as telling themselves: "I will be more relaxed when I face deadlines in the future."

Yoga

Yoga, a complex series of physical positions (exercises), diet, and mental attitude is believed to be one of the most successful methods of decreasing stress through a mixture of mental and physical approaches (Pelletier, 1977). Yoga means union or fusing and aims to bring about inner tranquillity and harmony by gaining better control over body and mind.

Many Yoga practitioners focus their energy on attempts to alter "involuntary" physiological processes, such as heart rate, breathing, and digestion through various meditations (Ornstein, 1972). Meditation in Yoga typically involves a mantra—words that may or may not be of significance but serve as a focal point for conscious awareness. In this type of meditation (of which Transcendental Meditation is one example) the person repeats the words over and over, either silently or aloud. Mantras are flowing, pleasurable sounding words that are easily repeated. Other types of Yoga use visual meditation with continuous concentration on a single object replacing the repetition of the mantra. Finally, Yoga may involve more or less complex physical postures and repetitive movements of various limbs. In the latter, awareness is directed toward the process of making the movements that serve the same functions as the visual meditation and mantra.

Biofeedback

Finally, biofeedback provides a means for learning to control automatic functions—pulse rate, muscle tension, and sweating—through electronic monitoring. For example, muscle tension can be measured through an electromyograph, electrical conductivity of the skin through a galvanic skin response (GSR) monitor. While hooked up to the monitors, the respondent receives feedback through a light, tone, or meter and in this way begins to learn responses that have the effect of reducing pulse rate, etc., monitoring success by the feedback mechanisms.

Wellness, employee health, and stress management programs have sprung up around the country in recent years in business and industry and are growing at a fairly rapid rate. These programs offer many of the techniques just described, with the underlying assumption being that the institution and its employees share the responsibility for worker fitness. A number of authors (Gavin, 1971; McLean, 1974; Oates, 1971) describe anecdotal success in handling personal stress through many of these techniques but no research examining their utility in reducing or managing job stress is reported.

In a similar vein, proper diet and regular exercise have always been considered important determinants of individuals' health and productivity. Yet the role of diet and exercise in helping people cope with or ameliorate job stress has not been researched. An important question to consider is how these factors (relaxation, diet, exercise) affect employee resistance to job-related sources of stress. The implication in many of these approaches to stress management is that people may (and do) learn to exercise control over their own psychological and physiological responses to stressful events. Having learned such control, they can easily practice many of these approaches at work, making them attractive personal strategies for handling job stress (Newman & Beehr, 1979). The validity of the implication remains to be tested.

COGNITIVE AND BEHAVIORAL APPROACHES

The maxim "plan ahead" seems to be used often by health care managers in the national study reported in Chapter 4 as an effective strategy for coping with job-related stress. This is expressed in a variety of ways such as: "I prepare myself with as many facts as possible" and "I make a plan for getting things done." It seems likely that people who think about events in advance, identifying potential stressors that might arise from them, would be in a better position to deal with them than those who merely move from one event to another.

It is interesting to note that the ten most helpful and frequently used coping strategies by the health managers in the national study (Table 4-7, supra) did not refer to any of the psychological and physiological mechanisms discussed previously. The strategies they identified as most helpful and frequently used can be divided into five groups:

1. perspective taking (e.g., I realize that some conflict is inevitable, I put things in perspective, I look at the stresses as part of the job)
2. planning ahead (I make a plan for getting things done, I think about alternative ways of dealing with the situation, I prepare myself with as many facts as possible)
3. interpersonal (I am sensitive to staff needs and feelings, I let others air their grievances, I try to keep communications channels open in the entire organization)

4. acceptance of limits (I recognize that others have ideas that may be different from mine that also are useful, I recognize and accept my limits to bring about changes alone)
5. managerial action (I delegate responsibility downward, I get the staff to participate as a team, I have open discussions with staff, I use the organization's chain of command to solve problems)

The only strategy appearing in the ten most frequently used and helpful list for all positions was keeping communications channels open throughout the organization.

While it would be valuable to have definitive evidence linking perceived job-related stress, coping strategies, and stress symptoms, the national study of health managers can provide only speculative answers to several important questions. In particular, does the use of certain coping strategies ameliorate negative stress symptoms regardless of the perceived level of job-related stress? Examination of the data on personal stress symptoms shows medical directors and nurses reporting few symptoms, as compared to other managerial groups. In addition, nurses report far greater stress than do medical directors. Could it be that the type of coping strategies used by nurses, in particular, reduces the likelihood that they will experience negative stress symptoms?

Table 4-8 (supra) indicates that nurses are not likely to "think about something else during meetings" as other managers might, nor are they as likely to "fulfill others' expectations of them." However, they are more likely than some other managerial groups to get the staff to participate as a team, prepare themselves with as many facts as possible, focus on the positive aspects of an issue, tell staff members their expectations, talk over issues with people who are directly involved, and look at mistakes as learning experiences.

In a Gallup poll commissioned by *The Wall Street Journal* to investigate sources of stress among top corporate executives in industry, respondents identified interpersonal stresses (e.g., staff conflicts) as the most serious sources of stress they experienced at work (Ricklefs, 1982). This finding parallels the results of the study of national health managers. Once again, these point to potential problems in stress management techniques that aim at symptom reduction (e.g., alleviation of tension and anxiety) resulting from stress rather than focusing on and alleviating the causes of stress (e.g., poor interpersonal communications, maladaptive organizational structures, jobs that subvert autonomy as well as employee participation in decision making, and irrational thinking on the part of individuals).

Behavior modification techniques, for example, have been employed for Type A individuals who are concerned with actual or potential cardiac stress. In one study participants were helped to change their life styles, lower their drive intensity, and modify rigid, unrealistic self-imposed deadlines (Suinn, 1976). By learning to ease up using relaxation exercises and through emotional desensitization (i.e., retraining emotional reactions to stressful situations), they were able to exercise active control over their environments. They responded to stress in a relaxed, controlled manner, while generally slowing down their life paces. More specifically they were better able to say no, to allocate time more realistically, and to meet others' demands. Cholesterol and blood pressure dropped to normal levels after training, as well. To the extent that Type A managers such as these participants are likely to cause stress for subordinates and colleagues, a change in their behavioral styles has significant consequences for themselves and for the organization.

As noted in Chapter 3, stress in the interpersonal environment of the organization often is the result of individuals' faulty perceptions that cause a distortion in the interaction; it also stems from poor interpersonal communications. Since the latter also are influenced by perceptual difficulties, it is useful to explore a technique that helps clarify self-perceptions and expectations, thus improving interpersonal effectiveness.

Cognitive Reframing

Many people believe that other individuals and the events in their own lives cause them to feel the way they do. As a result, they blame external factors that usually are beyond their control for their upsets. Seeing the solution to these as beyond their control, they become even more upset and stressed. The problem lies in their own definition of the situation and in their own thinking, which can lead to stress.

Behavioral therapists in particular have focused on cognitive structuring—how individuals connect their thoughts and their relationships to feelings and behavior—as an important component in stress. For example, a supervisor has criticized an employee for failing to complete a project on time. The person becomes mildly depressed, upset, and nervous about work performance. In this case, the activating event is the criticism that the employee thinks has resulted in these feelings and behavior. In actuality, the person's thoughts about the event ("I forgot all about it, I ought to be fired") have been the real causes of the feelings of anxiety. This is diagramed in Exhibit 10-1 and contrasted with a more rational, functional thought process, the outcome of which is a feeling of disappointment—considerably less stressful than depression and anxiety.

The key in this approach is to recognize that each event can be perceived in a variety of emotional responses. It is not the stress event per se that

Exhibit 10-1 Irrational and Rational Processes

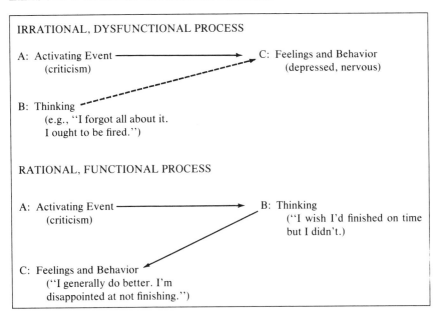

creates tension but how the person thinks about it (i.e., the meaning attached to it). If individuals believe that poor performance is unfortunate, inconvenient, awful, catastrophic, and likely to lead to failure, then they are going to experience depression, anxiety, and tension. As a result, their performance will be diminished.

In an interpersonal situation, if someone acts in a way individuals do not like, and they begin thinking "that person absolutely should not act this way," they are likely to experience anger and hostility. This thinking suggests that people believe they have control over others' behavior when in fact they do not, thereby setting themselves up for stress and negative outcomes. In short, their thoughts about what they want can result in their feelings. Therefore, they have the ability to change unwanted or irrational thoughts voluntarily to produce different (and better) emotional feelings and reduce stress. The process is referred to here as cognitive reframing.

At the base of cognitive reframing is the need to differentiate between rational and irrational beliefs and unrealistic performance expectations or role myths. The following list of irrational beliefs provides examples of stress-inducing attitudes:

- If I don't receive love and approval from the people I care about, I'm worthless.

- If I show my anger, that tells others I'm losing control.
- If I don't live up to my potentials, I'm a failure as a person.
- If I disagree with my boss and people in authority, I'll lose my job.
- If others don't appreciate my assistance, that shows it was worthless (or they are ungrateful).
- If I make a mistake, that shows I'm inadequate.
- If I admit my weaknesses, then no one will respect me.
- If I rely on my past, it will determine what I do in the present.
- If my way is the only right way of doing things, then others' ways are irrelevant.
- If I share my doubts with someone, they will take advantage of me.

Obviously, each of these beliefs guides behavior vis-à-vis others'. Thus, the beliefs are sources of unrecognized stress to the individuals and to those with whom they relate.

Role myths, another source of stress, refer to images or expectations about the peoples' roles that are unrealistic and are guaranteed to lead to stress. (It will be recalled that one of the most frequently mentioned sources of stress in the health managers study in Chapter 4 pertains to their unrealistic expectations and performance standards.) These myths refer to self-imposed demands: the need to appear perfect to selves or others. For instance, the perfect doctor or nurse always responds to patients' needs, always is sensitive, always has the answer to questions that arise and doesn't need to reference things (i.e., "Let me look that up and get back to you"). Role myths may hold that supervisors should have all the answers to problems that may come up, should always be responsive to the staff's professional requests, should never or rarely admit they are wrong, and should keep themselves aloof from their subordinates.

Individuals can use these ideas as a stress management technique by listing their major roles, then the major role myths associated with each, and finally how the myths can be made rational. Guidelines for differentiating between rational and irrational beliefs that individuals might find useful in such an endeavor include questions similar to the following:

- Are the beliefs based on objective reality?
- Are the beliefs helpful? (Self-destructive beliefs invariably are irrational.)
- Are the beliefs helpful in reducing conflict with others? (Irrational beliefs generally lead to interpersonal strife, setting up "we-they" situations.)

- Do the beliefs reduce emotional conflict? (Do they help create a miserable feeling—a sign of an irrational belief—or do they help generate a better feeling?)
- Do the beliefs help in reaching short-term and long-term goals or do they get in the way of their accomplishment? (The latter indicates an irrational belief.)

Recognizing that the way people think determines the way they feel is a key to reducing the stress they bring on themselves. However, that does not mean a devaluation of personal standards for themselves and others. It is important to maintain a high personal standard, one that stretches capacities but that is within reach. However, not always meeting high standards does not imply failure.

Directed Communications

Unfortunately, the author of the following wonderful story about communications assumptions is unknown:

> This is a story about four normal people—Everybody, Somebody, Anybody, and Nobody. There was an important job to be done and Everybody was asked to do it. Everybody was sure that Somebody would do it. Anybody could have done it but Nobody did it. Somebody got angry about that because it was Everybody's job. Everybody thought that Anybody could do it and Nobody realized that Everybody wouldn't do it. It ended up that Everybody blamed Somebody when actually Nobody blamed Anybody.

Communications assumptions run rampant in most organizations, leading to the kinds of problems outlined in Chapter 3. The task here is to identify communications techniques that minimize distortion and increase the probability that a given individual's needs will be met without resulting in loss for others. Key assumptions in directed communications rest on the combination of individuals' active listening skills and focusing on their own needs and feelings directly, assuming responsibility for their open and clear expression. Specifically, these assumptions include:

- Individuals have a right to their own feelings, thoughts, and opinions.
- Individuals have the right and freedom to express these as long as they do not impinge on others' right to their own feelings, thoughts, and opinions.

- Individuals thus acquire responsibility for their own feelings and respect for those of others.

Thus, directed communications place the expression of personal feelings and opinions in a social context. People must assume responsibility for their feelings and display sensitivity for the possible effect they may have on receivers. Freedom for self-expression is not akin to license to say anything with impunity.

Individuals who utilize directed communications find that they feel better about themselves. They demonstrate an ability to:

- express positive and negative emotions (e.g., I like . . . , I appreciate . . . , I don't like . . . , I'm angry that . . .)
- get their needs met (e.g., I need . . . , I would like . . .)
- say no to what they believe are unreasonable requests (e.g., No, I would prefer that you do not borrow my car. No, I cannot get the report in by 9 a.m. tomorrow. How would the day after be?)
- begin and end conversations (e.g., I have a meeting beginning soon, can we pick this up later? I'd like to talk with you about . . .).

The essence of this approach is to take responsibility in communications by using "I messages" without hinting around, using sarcasm, or intentionally hurting or embarrassing the receiver.

One model the author has utilized in organizations across the country has demonstrated excellent results in minimizing communication distortions, particularly in situations involving conflict. The model is called DESC (description, expression, specification, and consequences) and is based on a four-step communication sequence:

Step 1 involves the behavioral description (D) of an event that is to be discussed. The key here is in describing the event objectively so the receiver fully understands the subject. Beginning with a behavioral description increases the likelihood that a positive resolution of the situation will occur, for two reasons. First, behavioral descriptions require the sender to put aside personal emotions for the moment. Since people in conflict situations tend to begin with a burst of anger that usually puts receivers on the defensive, avoiding this error keeps communication lines more open and less defensive. Second, the receiver is given a road map, so to speak, of what is to follow. This minimizes the likelihood of crossed communications resulting from the parties' responding in terms of two different situations.

Step 2 entails the expression (E) of the sender's feelings about the situation described in Step 1 in terms of an I-message that reflects personal responsibility for these feelings without blaming another.

Step 3 involves specifying (S) what the sender would like the receiver to do differently in the situation.

Step 4 points out the positive consequences (C) in store if the receiver complies with the request.

The use of such a framework minimizes the chances of a battle for control or interpersonal putdowns resulting in situations involving actual or potential conflict. While the model leaves both communicators with their dignity intact, it does not guarantee that the sender will, in fact, gain what was desired. In the area of interpersonal processes, it is possible to predict with certainty what receivers will do; the sender cannot control their behavior.

Active listening skills comprise the other component in directed communications. Active listening, particularly in the face of heated conversation, can be an extremely effective stress reducer in that an initial response that acknowledges the intensity of the sender's feelings (e.g., "You sound angry about that") serves to diffuse the emotion because the message has been received. Such a response also gives the receiver an opportunity to clarify the direction of the emotion (i.e., "Is he angry at me or someone else?") without becoming defensive and escalating the intensity of the interaction. Finally, the initial listening response gives the sender time to decide how best to then respond.

EMPLOYEE ASSISTANCE PROGRAMS

During the 1940s two of this country's major industrial corporations, Eastman Kodak Company and E.I. du Pont de Nemours & Co., established the first alcoholism assistance programs in the United States. These programs grew out of the realization that alcoholism was having adverse effects on their employees' lives and on the companies themselves—particularly in the areas of absenteeism, medical benefit costs, safety, motivation, discipline, and the like. As a result of the success of these initial efforts, other corporations introduced similar programs.

Within the next 25 years companies with alcoholism assistance programs began to realize that other problems affected job performance—financial concerns, interpersonal conflicts, intrapersonal issues, and marital or family difficulties. With the recognition and acceptance of the fact that the existence of these problems did not necessarily involve alcohol abuse came the concept of broad spectrum employee assistance programs (EAPs). Generally, EAPs offer help to any employee with problems in the areas mentioned.

The benefits for both employees and companies have been substantial, according to corporations that have installed EAPs. The companies report considerable cost savings, particularly in reduced absenteeism, and the retention of valuable employees who might otherwise have been terminated. In addition, EAPs serve a role in fulfilling the companies' aims of social responsibility. They also are described as helpful in reducing employee grievances, accidents on the job, work disruptions caused by personal and familial problems adversely affecting job performance, and excessive medical and compensation claims for illness. In that they increase employee retention they reduce the amount of time, energy, and money companies otherwise would have to channel into the hiring and training of new employees.

Since the mid-1970s, the spread of EAPs has been rapid, with the focus expanding beyond alcohol and drugs. All across the country EAPs now incorporate a wider range of employee difficulties (personal and marital problems) but the emphasis still is on drugs and alcohol.

Employees covered by most EAPs are able to talk with an organizationally based counselor on a self-referral or by referral from a supervisor. The counselor generally refers the employee to an appropriate agency or professional in the community for the actual counseling primarily because of confidentiality. Despite the fact that the content of the counseling interview is confidential and does not appear in the employee's personnel file, a supervisor's referral and acknowledgement of the worker's follow-through are noted in cases that are not self-referred. Self-referred individuals frequently express concern that seeing an organizationally based employee counselor will "somehow get out." Of course, from a practical standpoint, organization counselors could not be expected to provide the wide range of services likely to be required by employees of even medium-sized institutions.

EAP: Basic Services

EAP programs differ widely from organization to organization in both their components and their level of sophistication. Typically, however, they offer some if not all of the following services:

Assessment

The assessment interview is the employee's first contact with the EAP regardless of whether or not the person is self-referred. A trained professional (clinical social worker or counselor) determines the problem in conjunction with the employee, identifies a course of treatment, and refers the individual to the appropriate services.

Continuing Counseling

Some EAPs offer short-term counseling (e.g., three sessions) of a problem-solving nature and refer those needing and wanting more long-term help to selected community agencies and private practitioners. Depending on the nature of the initial referral (i.e., supervisor or self), an EAP counselor may monitor the employee's follow-through and progress in treatment. For example, where job performance mandates a referral for personal/family issues, an employee's participation in the prescribed treatment is monitored, as is job performance.

Supervisory Training

EAP counselors also provide training for supervisors in job performance monitoring. The training includes an emphasis on the constructive handling of employees whose poor performance based on personal issues must be confronted and who need to be referred for EAP help. It is not expected that supervisors have or should be given the training to assess an employee's personal problems. Referrals are made when unsatisfactory job performance continues and the usual channels (e.g., appraisal and discipline) do not yield improvement.

Employee Education

General orientation about the EAP typically is provided to all employees through promotional materials including initial orientation sessions, newsletters, brochures, movies, and so forth.

Program Evaluation

Periodic reports (quarterly or semiannually) are provided by the EAP staff to the organization, identifying the types of referrals to the program, the number and type of employees involved, and the type of service provided. The more sophisticated programs also offer cost analyses and follow-up evaluations assessing degree of success.

Regardless of the type of program instituted, in no case does a properly installed EAP in any way impinge upon or alter existing collective bargaining agreements, disciplinary policies, grievance procedures, or expectations regarding job performance, should work problems persist.

IN RETROSPECT

The journey through various aspects of the stress phenomenon is complete. It has examined the complex interrelationship of physiological and socioemotional components of stress and its far-reaching effects. The focus has been on the job-related stress of health care professionals—in particular, physicians, nurses, and administrators. More specifically, it has looked at the relationship between aspects of the individual—professional and personal socialization, individual needs, age, sex, and so forth—and aspects of the organization.

It has emphasized repeatedly that work-related stress management is the responsibility of both the individual and the organization. Unlike other approaches that place the burden of stress management solely on the shoulders of the individual, the thrust here suggests that organizations are responsible for monitoring and correcting stress, including management practices and organizational structures and policies.

Individual stress management techniques can be very effective in ameliorating the negative effects of some job-related problems. However, to the extent that these are reactions to situations over which the individual may have little or no control, the person will be exposed constantly to stress-inducing events with no real way to escape them. Under these circumstances only an approach that modifies the source of stress itself is likely to have any long-range benefit for the individual and for the organization.

While some might argue that organizational responses to alleviate unhealthy amounts of stress are merely humanitarian acts, that view is quite simplistic. Ironically, it is in the organization's self-interest to respond proactively in setting up healthy environments. Armed with effective coping strategies at the level of both individual and organization, society is likely to see increased productivity, effectiveness, and health for all participants in the health services system.

Questionnaire Used in Health Administrators Stress Study

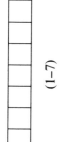

(1–7)

This questionnaire is being filled out by a national sample of administrators, directors/chiefs of medical staffs. Your responses will be kept strictly confidential. Data will be reported by group response only. This questionnaire has been assigned a code number (upper right-hand corner) to analyze the data by regional groups (East Coast, Midwest, West Coast).

We would appreciate it if you would return the completed questionnaire in the enclosed envelope within 48 hours of receiving it. The average time to complete the questionnaire is 50 minutes. We would also welcome your comments. Thank you again for your cooperation.

Please choose the appropriate answer to each question and put the number of your answer in the *box* next to each question.

(8)

Sex: (1) Male   (2) Female

(9–10)

Age:

(11)

Marital Status:

(1) Single
(2) Married
(3) Divorced
(4) Separated
(5) Widowed
(6) Other (specify): _____

(12–13)

Number of children

(14) ☐   Professional Degree

(1) M.D.
(2) R.N.
(3) B.S.N.
(4) M.S.N.

(5) B.A.
(6) M.A.
(7) Ph.D.
(8) Other (specify): _____

(15–16) ☐☐   Number of years in Administration:

(17–18) ☐☐   Number of years in present position:

(19–20) ☐☐   Number of years with this facility:

(21) ☐   Position:

(1) Chief Executive Officer
(2) Associate Administrator
(3) Director of Nursing
(4) President, Medical Staff
(5) Medical Director
(6) Other (specify): _____

(22) ☐   Type of Hospital:

(1) University
(2) Voluntary, Religious Affiliated
(3) Voluntary, Community, Nonreligious
(4) Proprietary
(5) Government
(6) Other (specify): _____

(23–26) ☐☐☐☐   Number of Beds:

(27) ☐   On a scale of 1 to 5, with 1 = almost no stress at all and 5 = high stress: How would you rate the degree of stress you generally experience?

(28–29) ☐☐   How many hours do you work on a typical day?

(30–31) ☐☐   How many days have you spent on vacation this year?

Source: Reprinted with permission of Numerof and Associates, Inc., Copyright © 1981 by R.E. Numerof, K. Cramer, and S. Shachar Hendin.

Appendix A continued

The following list of situations has been identified as stressors by others in positions similar to yours. (By stressors is meant any situation that places demands on you that require you to respond or take action. Stressors can be positive or negative.)

Please *circle* how often you deal with each situation *and* the degree of stress you experience as a result of it. We have found that the first response that comes to mind is likely to be the most characteristic of your experience. Therefore, we recommend that you give your first response without deliberating.

Situation	Does Not Apply	Never	Yearly	Quarterly	Monthly	Weekly	Daily	No Stress	Little Stress	Moderate Stress	Much Stress	Very Much Stress
				Frequency of Occurrence						Degree of Stress		
1. Meeting your own expectations for excellence.	NA	0	1	2	3	4	5	0	1	2	3	4
2. Having a lot of responsibility for projects and little authority to accomplish them.	NA	0	1	2	3	4	5	0	1	2	3	4
3. Working with administrative people who are not clear about the direction in which we need to go.	NA	0	1	2	3	4	5	0	1	2	3	4
4. Seeing problems within the organization and not having the resources to correct them.	NA	0	1	2	3	4	5	0	1	2	3	4
5. Attending meetings I don't want to attend.	NA	0	1	2	3	4	5	0	1	2	3	4

Item			
6. Having an active and outspoken staff which states its demands and wants action right away.	NA 0 1 2 3 4 5	0 1 2 3 4
7. Learning that patients/families have received less than the best care/understanding from hospital staff.	NA 0 1 2 3 4 5	0 1 2 3 4
8. Dealing with board members.	NA 0 1 2 3 4 5	0 1 2 3 4
9. Being chewed out by those upon which I depend for support.	NA 0 1 2 3 4 5	0 1 2 3 4
10. Being given responsibility to accomplish a project and then being undercut.	NA 0 1 2 3 4 5	0 1 2 3 4
11. Dealing with community groups who do not feel fairly treated.	NA 0 1 2 3 4 5	0 1 2 3 4
12. Being confronted by professions/professionals fighting over turf.	NA 0 1 2 3 4 5	0 1 2 3 4
13. Having to respond to demands which I cannot fulfill because of personal inadequacies (i.e., limited knowledge, attitudes, etc.)	NA 0 1 2 3 4 5	0 1 2 3 4
14. Dealing with conflicts of needs or interests between people in the organization.	NA 0 1 2 3 4 5	0 1 2 3 4
15. Dealing with the strong personalities of staff.	NA 0 1 2 3 4 5	0 1 2 3 4
16. Making an error in judgment with respect to a major decision for the organization.	NA 0 1 2 3 4 5	0 1 2 3 4
17. Making decisions with long-term, major implications for institution.	NA 0 1 2 3 4 5	0 1 2 3 4
18. Making presentations to boards or committees.	NA 0 1 2 3 4 5	0 1 2 3 4
19. Handling patients' or families' complaints about care.	NA 0 1 2 3 4 5	0 1 2 3 4
20. Responding to government agencies/regulations.	NA 0 1 2 3 4 5	0 1 2 3 4
21. Attempts by staff to unionize.	NA 0 1 2 3 4 5	0 1 2 3 4
22. Balancing time between work and family.	NA 0 1 2 3 4 5	0 1 2 3 4
23. Disagreement between board and management about the role of each.	NA 0 1 2 3 4 5	0 1 2 3 4
24. Financial cutbacks.	NA 0 1 2 3 4 5	0 1 2 3 4
25. Staff resistance to innovations in clinical areas.	NA 0 1 2 3 4 5	0 1 2 3 4

Appendix A continued

Situation	Degree of Stress					Frequency of Occurrence						
	No Stress	Little Stress	Moderate Stress	Much Stress	Very Much Stress	Does Not Apply	Never	Yearly	Quarterly	Monthly	Weekly	Daily
26. Conflict between line and executive staff.	0	1	2	3	4	NA	0	1	2	3	4	5
27. Trying to demonstrate community need for program to obtain HSA approval, in face of consumer activist groups which are antiprovider.	0	1	2	3	4	NA	0	1	2	3	4	5
28. Trying to get others to be committed to achieve objectives/outcomes which I feel are important.	0	1	2	3	4	NA	0	1	2	3	4	5
29. Being embarrassed or publicly criticized for the operation of the institution.	0	1	2	3	4	NA	0	1	2	3	4	5
30. Staff's lack of response to the quality assurance program.	0	1	2	3	4	NA	0	1	2	3	4	5
31. Public expectations for more services than institution can or wants to provide.	0	1	2	3	4	NA	0	1	2	3	4	5
32. Dealing with people who do not think quickly and flexibly.	0	1	2	3	4	NA	0	1	2	3	4	5
33. Trying to be a role model for others in the institution.	0	1	2	3	4	NA	0	1	2	3	4	5
34. Doing things others consider a high priority but I don't.	0	1	2	3	4	NA	0	1	2	3	4	5
35. Nursing staff seeking equal status with physicians and increased pay.	0	1	2	3	4	NA	0	1	2	3	4	5
36. Lack of understanding from administrative staff.	0	1	2	3	4	NA	0	1	2	3	4	5
37. Dealing with the stress of those who report to me.	0	1	2	3	4	NA	0	1	2	3	4	5

Item	Scale 1	Scale 2
38. Personal experience of discrimination (e.g., minority or gender status).	NA 0 1 2 3 4 5	NA 0 1 2 3 4
39. Being responsible for, but not having direct control over, the quality of patient care.	NA 0 1 2 3 4 5	NA 0 1 2 3 4
40. Making decisions about priority expenses in times of economic constraint.	NA 0 1 2 3 4 5	NA 0 1 2 3 4
41. Dealing with staff reactions to the hiring of new personnel who bring new expertise or new services to the organization.	NA 0 1 2 3 4 5	NA 0 1 2 3 4
42. Creating a well-functioning staff team.	NA 0 1 2 3 4 5	NA 0 1 2 3 4
43. Competing demands and needs of consumers in community.	NA 0 1 2 3 4 5	NA 0 1 2 3 4
44. Getting others to carry out their job responsibilities.	NA 0 1 2 3 4 5	NA 0 1 2 3 4
45. Dealing with public media.	NA 0 1 2 3 4 5	NA 0 1 2 3 4
46. Dealing with union problems.	NA 0 1 2 3 4 5	NA 0 1 2 3 4
47. Miscommunication with staff.	NA 0 1 2 3 4 5	NA 0 1 2 3 4
48. Moderating committees (being prepared, keeping meetings orderly while allowing all to speak).	NA 0 1 2 3 4 5	NA 0 1 2 3 4
49. Serving as resource person from hospital to the community.	NA 0 1 2 3 4 5	NA 0 1 2 3 4
50. Dealing with patients for whom medical care has not been effective (e.g., chronic or traumatic problems for which medicine has no cure).	NA 0 1 2 3 4 5	NA 0 1 2 3 4
51. Dealing with staff incompetence.	NA 0 1 2 3 4 5	NA 0 1 2 3 4
52. Administration done by an elected rather than appointed official.	NA 0 1 2 3 4 5	NA 0 1 2 3 4
53. Representing clinical staff positions to administration.	NA 0 1 2 3 4 5	NA 0 1 2 3 4
54. Being a buffer between the staff and administration (management).	NA 0 1 2 3 4 5	NA 0 1 2 3 4
55. Staff who have unreasonable expectations.	NA 0 1 2 3 4 5	NA 0 1 2 3 4
56. Having to say no to people even though what they want is worthwhile.	NA 0 1 2 3 4 5	NA 0 1 2 3 4

Appendix A continued

Situation	Degree of Stress						Frequency of Occurrence							
	No Stress	Little Stress	Moderate Stress	Much Stress	Very Much Stress		Daily	Weekly	Monthly	Quarterly	Yearly	Never	Does Not Apply
57. Giving direction and clarification to the role my profession should play in the hospital.	0	1	2	3	4		5	4	3	2	1	0	NA
58. Having to work through a decision-making process with others rather than being able to make decisions on my own.	0	1	2	3	4		5	4	3	2	1	0	NA
59. Not having the support of my immediate superior or board.	0	1	2	3	4		5	4	3	2	1	0	NA
60. Having inadequate opportunity to influence important, hospitalwide policies.	0	1	2	3	4		5	4	3	2	1	0	NA
61. Having too many time demands.	0	1	2	3	4		5	4	3	2	1	0	NA
62. Seeing ineffective treatment/procedures being used with patients.	0	1	2	3	4		5	4	3	2	1	0	NA
63. Not having things done as quickly as I would like (waiting for others to participate).	0	1	2	3	4		5	4	3	2	1	0	NA
64. Dealing with staff complaints.	0	1	2	3	4		5	4	3	2	1	0	NA
65. Responding to multiple demands and not having time to see how those responses affect the department or hospital overall.	0	1	2	3	4		5	4	3	2	1	0	NA
66. Keeping staff informed.	0	1	2	3	4		5	4	3	2	1	0	NA

	Scale 1	Scale 2
67. Getting staff's participation in policy/program development.	NA 0 1 2 3 4	5 0 1 2 3 4
68. Having no one to talk to about the job.	NA 0 1 2 3 4	5 0 1 2 3 4
69. Deciding what's important to get done.	NA 0 1 2 3 4	5 0 1 2 3 4
70. Getting board to approve policies.	NA 0 1 2 3 4	5 0 1 2 3 4
71. Inability of staff to understand overall picture.	NA 0 1 2 3 4	5 0 1 2 3 4
72. Getting staff to accept new policies/procedures.	NA 0 1 2 3 4	5 0 1 2 3 4
73. Dealing with community groups wanting staff privileges.	NA 0 1 2 3 4	5 0 1 2 3 4
74. Dealing with power problems or infighting among staff.	NA 0 1 2 3 4	5 0 1 2 3 4
75. Having to resolve interdepartmental conflicts and jealousies.	NA 0 1 2 3 4	5 0 1 2 3 4
76. Having to develop a power base to accomplish change.	NA 0 1 2 3 4	5 0 1 2 3 4
77. Having colleagues question my judgment in an area outside their expertise.	NA 0 1 2 3 4	5 0 1 2 3 4
78. Having to sacrifice/compromise professional ideals.	NA 0 1 2 3 4	5 0 1 2 3 4
79. Not having responsibility nor authority to take needed action.	NA 0 1 2 3 4	5 0 1 2 3 4
80. Having to work with administrators who are insensitive to clinical issues.	NA 0 1 2 3 4	5 0 1 2 3 4
81. Having my words twisted around.	NA 0 1 2 3 4	5 0 1 2 3 4
82. Having to meet deadlines.	NA 0 1 2 3 4	5 0 1 2 3 4
83. Dealing with organizational disorganization (re policies and procedures).	NA 0 1 2 3 4	5 0 1 2 3 4
84. Covering staff shortages.	NA 0 1 2 3 4	5 0 1 2 3 4
85. Delegating work.	NA 0 1 2 3 4	5 0 1 2 3 4
86. Attracting qualified staff.	NA 0 1 2 3 4	5 0 1 2 3 4
87. Retaining qualified staff.	NA 0 1 2 3 4	5 0 1 2 3 4
88. Organizing staff to operate efficiently and effectively.	NA 0 1 2 3 4	5 0 1 2 3 4
89. Not having the support of my subordinates.	NA 0 1 2 3 4	5 0 1 2 3 4
90. Other (specify):	NA 0 1 2 3 4	5 0 1 2 3 4

Personal Stress System Assessment

To give us a better understanding of how stress affects people, we would appreciate your identifying those symptoms you experience by circling the frequency with which each occurs.

	Almost Never	Rarely	Sometimes	Often	Almost Always
1. Headaches	1	2	3	4	5
2. Stomachaches	1	2	3	4	5
3. Backaches	1	2	3	4	5
4. Stiffness in neck/shoulders	1	2	3	4	5
5. Elevated blood pressure	1	2	3	4	5
6. Fatigue	1	2	3	4	5
7. Crying	1	2	3	4	5
8. Forgetfulness	1	2	3	4	5
9. Blaming self	1	2	3	4	5
10. Blaming others	1	2	3	4	5
11. Yelling	1	2	3	4	5
12. Bossiness	1	2	3	4	5
13. Irritability	1	2	3	4	5
14. Loss of or excessive appetite	1	2	3	4	5
15. Compulsive smoking	1	2	3	4	5
16. Worrying	1	2	3	4	5
17. Depression	1	2	3	4	5
18. Agitation	1	2	3	4	5
19. Impatience	1	2	3	4	5

20. Anger (strong)	1	2	3	4	5
21. Frustration	1	2	3	4	5
22. Loneliness	1	2	3	4	5
23. Inflexibility	1	2	3	4	5
24. Teeth grinding	1	2	3	4	5
25. Nail biting	1	2	3	4	5
26. General tension	1	2	3	4	5
27. Drinking	1	2	3	4	5
28. Use of stimulants or tranquilizing drugs	1	2	3	4	5
29. Pounding of the heart	1	2	3	4	5
30. Dryness of the throat and mouth	1	2	3	4	5
31. Impulsive behavior	1	2	3	4	5
32. Trouble concentrating	1	2	3	4	5
33. Anxiety or nervousness	1	2	3	4	5
34. Trembling	1	2	3	4	5
35. Nervous tics	1	2	3	4	5
36. Tend to be easily startled	1	2	3	4	5
37. Stuttering	1	2	3	4	5
38. Insomnia	1	2	3	4	5
39. Sweating	1	2	3	4	5
40. Frequent need to urinate	1	2	3	4	5
41. Diarrhea	1	2	3	4	5
42. Indigestion	1	2	3	4	5
43. Queasy stomach	1	2	3	4	5
44. Vomiting	1	2	3	4	5
45. Premenstrual tension/painful menstruation	1	2	3	4	5
46. Nightmares	1	2	3	4	5
47. Accident proneness	1	2	3	4	5
48. Not feeling good about self	1	2	3	4	5
49. Minor physical ailments (colds, flu, etc.)	1	2	3	4	5
50. Major physical disorders	1	2	3	4	5
51. Constipation	1	2	3	4	5

Appendix B continued

	Almost Never	Rarely	Sometimes	Often	Almost Always
52. Weight loss or gain	1	2	3	4	5
53. Inability to relax	1	2	3	4	5
54. Other (specify): _____	1	2	3	4	5

Source: Reprinted with permission of Numerof and Associates, Inc., Copyright © 1981 by R.E. Numerof and S.A. Shachar Hendin.

Coping Strategies

The following list of coping strategies has been identified by others in positions similar to yours for dealing with stress. Please circle how often you use each strategy and how helpful or harmful it has been for you in reducing stress.

Coping Strategy	Frequency of Use					Degree of Helpfulness				
	Almost Never	Rarely	Sometimes	Often	Almost Always	Harmful	Somewhat Harmful	Neutral	Somewhat Helpful	Helpful
1. I reduce my involvement in one or more roles.	1	2	3	4	5	1	2	3	4	5
2. I engage in regular physical activity.	1	2	3	4	5	1	2	3	4	5
3. I negotiate to change deadlines.	1	2	3	4	5	1	2	3	4	5
4. I realize that some conflict is inevitable.	1	2	3	4	5	1	2	3	4	5
5. I realize that some of the demands I feel now are only temporary.	1	2	3	4	5	1	2	3	4	5
6. I think about alternative ways of dealing with the situation.	1	2	3	4	5	1	2	3	4	5
7. I think about something else during meetings.	1	2	3	4	5	1	2	3	4	5
8. I postpone dealing with the situation.	1	2	3	4	5	1	2	3	4	5
9. I change my standards.	1	2	3	4	5	1	2	3	4	5
10. I get the staff to participate as a team.	1	2	3	4	5	1	2	3	4	5
11. I meet demands.	1	2	3	4	5	1	2	3	4	5
12. I am sensitive to staff's needs and feelings.	1	2	3	4	5	1	2	3	4	5

#	Item											
13.	I get psychological support from others by sharing my pressures.	1	2	3	4	5	1	2	3	4	5
14.	I call in outside consultants.	1	2	3	4	5	1	2	3	4	5
15.	I keep my roles separate (e.g., I don't bring work home with me).	1	2	3	4	5	1	2	3	4	5
16.	I meditate.	1	2	3	4	5	1	2	3	4	5
17.	I ask others involved to have different expectations of me.	1	2	3	4	5	1	2	3	4	5
18.	I get people to focus on the positive aspects of an issue.	1	2	3	4	5	1	2	3	4	5
19.	I remind myself that I am experiencing conflict because I am engaged in demanding but fulfilling activities.	1	2	3	4	5	1	2	3	4	5
20.	I rationalize why things are not being solved.	1	2	3	4	5	1	2	3	4	5
21.	I prepare myself with as many facts as possible.	1	2	3	4	5	1	2	3	4	5
22.	I think about what I should have done differently.	1	2	3	4	5	1	2	3	4	5
23.	I do something to take my mind off the problem.	1	2	3	4	5	1	2	3	4	5
24.	I express my feelings about things.	1	2	3	4	5	1	2	3	4	5
25.	I specify corrective action for staff to take.	1	2	3	4	5	1	2	3	4	5
26.	I agonize.	1	2	3	4	5	1	2	3	4	5
27.	I get frustrated.	1	2	3	4	5	1	2	3	4	5
28.	I spend time with family.	1	2	3	4	5	1	2	3	4	5
29.	I try to keep communications channels open in the entire organization (across/up and down the formal hierarchy).	1	2	3	4	5	1	2	3	4	5
30.	I politic with those who can influence others.	1	2	3	4	5	1	2	3	4	5
31.	I decide time will solve the problem.	1	2	3	4	5	1	2	3	4	5
32.	I focus on the positive aspects of the issue.	1	2	3	4	5	1	2	3	4	5
33.	I find myself blocking things out of my mind.	1	2	3	4	5	1	2	3	4	5
34.	I lose my temper.	1	2	3	4	5	1	2	3	4	5
35.	I tell staff my expectations.	1	2	3	4	5	1	2	3	4	5
36.	I drink.	1	2	3	4	5	1	2	3	4	5
37.	I become indifferent.	1	2	3	4	5	1	2	3	4	5
38.	I let others air their grievances.	1	2	3	4	5	1	2	3	4	5
39.	I rely on my religious faith.	1	2	3	4	5	1	2	3	4	5
40.	I establish relationships with key people outside the	1	2	3	4	5	1	2	3	4	5

Appendix C continued

Coping Strategy	Frequency of Use					Degree of Helpfulness				
	Almost Never	Rarely	Sometimes	Often	Almost Always	Harmful	Somewhat Harmful	Neutral	Somewhat Helpful	Helpful
41. I try to cajole or calm people down.	1	2	3	4	5	1	2	3	4	5
42. I try to stay unemotional in conflict situations.	1	2	3	4	5	1	2	3	4	5
43. I recognize that others have ideas which may be different from mine that are also useful.	1	2	3	4	5	1	2	3	4	5
44. I make a plan for getting things done.	1	2	3	4	5	1	2	3	4	5
45. I compartmentalize the difficult problems.	1	2	3	4	5	1	2	3	4	5
46. I decide to prepare myself better next time.	1	2	3	4	5	1	2	3	4	5
47. I talk about it with someone who is not directly involved.	1	2	3	4	5	1	2	3	4	5
48. I have open discussions with staff.	1	2	3	4	5	1	2	3	4	5
49. I worry.	1	2	3	4	5	1	2	3	4	5
50. I put things in perspective.	1	2	3	4	5	1	2	3	4	5
51. I adopt the attitude "not everything can be accomplished."	1	2	3	4	5	1	2	3	4	5
52. I anticipate the demands/expectations/actions of others.	1	2	3	4	5	1	2	3	4	5
53. I develop patience (e.g., in regard to the process of organizational decision making).	1	2	3	4	5	1	2	3	4	5
54. I tend to keep my personal opinions and feelings to myself.	1	2	3	4	5	1	2	3	4	5

55. I make lists of things I need to do.	1	2	3	4	5	1	2	3	4	5
56. I think about how I handled similar things in the past.	1	2	3	4	5	1	2	3	4	5
57. I say no.	1	2	3	4	5	1	2	3	4	5
58. I terminate personnel.	1	2	3	4	5	1	2	3	4	5
59. I develop physical symptoms (e.g., headaches, stomach problems).	1	2	3	4	5	1	2	3	4	5
60. I handle only the most urgent demands now.	1	2	3	4	5	1	2	3	4	5
61. I try to organize my schedule better.	1	2	3	4	5	1	2	3	4	5
62. I institute penalties for noncompliance to policy/procedure.	1	2	3	4	5	1	2	3	4	5
63. I work harder than usual.	1	2	3	4	5	1	2	3	4	5
64. I hire extra personnel to cover shortages.	1	2	3	4	5	1	2	3	4	5
65. I decide certain role obligations can wait.	1	2	3	4	5	1	2	3	4	5
66. I travel to get away from it all.	1	2	3	4	5	1	2	3	4	5
67. I ask superiors to clarify priorities.	1	2	3	4	5	1	2	3	4	5
68. I've learned to take risks and assume responsibilities.	1	2	3	4	5	1	2	3	4	5
69. After a situation is over, I forget and let go of it.	1	2	3	4	5	1	2	3	4	5
70. I prioritize.	1	2	3	4	5	1	2	3	4	5
71. I give myself positive reinforcement for jobs and efforts well done.	1	2	3	4	5	1	2	3	4	5
72. I recognize and accept my limits to bring about changes alone.	1	2	3	4	5	1	2	3	4	5
73. I decide not to meet others' demands.	1	2	3	4	5	1	2	3	4	5
74. I take matters into my own hands even when they are not my responsibility.	1	2	3	4	5	1	2	3	4	5
75. I eat.	1	2	3	4	5	1	2	3	4	5
76. I develop a sense of humor.	1	2	3	4	5	1	2	3	4	5
77. I spend whatever time is necessary to meet deadlines.	1	2	3	4	5	1	2	3	4	5
78. I clarify others' expectations.	1	2	3	4	5	1	2	3	4	5
79. I fulfill others' expectations of me.	1	2	3	4	5	1	2	3	4	5
80. I decrease my social life.	1	2	3	4	5	1	2	3	4	5
81. I extend the work day.	1	2	3	4	5	1	2	3	4	5

Appendix C continued

Coping Strategy	Frequency of Use					Degree of Helpfulness				
	Almost Never	Rarely	Sometimes	Often	Almost Always	Harmful	Somewhat Harmful	Neutral	Somewhat Helpful	Helpful
82. I use the organization's chain of command to solve problems.	1	2	3	4	5	1	2	3	4	5
83. I learn to lower my commitment—doing an adequate job in the time available.	1	2	3	4	5	1	2	3	4	5
84. I engage in leisure activities.	1	2	3	4	5	1	2	3	4	5
85. If other people are involved, I talk the situation over with them.	1	2	3	4	5	1	2	3	4	5
86. I do something physical to blow off steam (e.g., hit tennis balls, clean, etc.)	1	2	3	4	5	1	2	3	4	5
87. I realize that my problems are less serious than those of many others.	1	2	3	4	5	1	2	3	4	5
88. I ask other people to do more.	1	2	3	4	5	1	2	3	4	5
89. I recognize that I don't have total responsibility for a situation.	1	2	3	4	5	1	2	3	4	5
90. I look at the stresses as "part of the job."	1	2	3	4	5	1	2	3	4	5
91. I ignore the problem.	1	2	3	4	5	1	2	3	4	5
92. I get conflicting parties together and try to moderate to achieve a compromise.	1	2	3	4	5	1	2	3	4	5

93. I remember that I have handled similar problems successfully in the past.	1	2	3	4	5		1	2	3	4	5
94. I try not to personalize all problems and disagreements.	1	2	3	4	5		1	2	3	4	5
95. I talk it over with people who are directly involved.	1	2	3	4	5		1	2	3	4	5
96. I look at my mistakes as learning experiences.	1	2	3	4	5		1	2	3	4	5
97. I lessen the demands on myself by changing what I expect of myself.	1	2	3	4	5		1	2	3	4	5
98. I mandate staff policies.	1	2	3	4	5		1	2	3	4	5
99. I become depressed.	1	2	3	4	5		1	2	3	4	5
100. I sleep.	1	2	3	4	5		1	2	3	4	5
101. I inform staff in writing about an issue.	1	2	3	4	5		1	2	3	4	5
102. I try to be sympathetic.	1	2	3	4	5		1	2	3	4	5
103. I get support from my superior(s).	1	2	3	4	5		1	2	3	4	5
104. I delegate responsibility downward.	1	2	3	4	5		1	2	3	4	5
105. Other (specify): _____	1	2	3	4	5		1	2	3	4	5

Appendix C continued

For those of you with time left, we would appreciate your comments on the following question.

If your time is particularly short, please go on to the next page. For your *most* important source of stress please *describe* the situation and give specific examples to illustrate it. Please identify *what* happened, *who* was involved (e.g., immediate superior, administrator, physician, nurse, allied health professional, government agency, patient, family of patient, laboratory, housekeeping, etc.), your *action* and the *outcome*.

Situation:

Who Was Involved:

Action:

Outcome:

From the stress situation list choose the *three most important* sources of stress for you and write the item number and phrase in the spaces provided below under the heading "stress situation." Next to each situation identify the ways in which you handle the stress and the degree to which that strategy is helpful. Finally, please identify how you feel the organization might respond to help alleviate this stress.

Stress Situation	Coping Strategy	Degree of Helpfulness					Organizational Response
		Helpful	Somewhat Helpful	Neutral	Somewhat Harmful	Harmful	
Most Important Source of Stress Item Number: ___							
Second Most Important Source of Stress Item Number: ___							
Third Most Important Source of Stress Item Number: ___							

Individual Profile of Stressors

Purpose:

This questionnaire is designed for the purpose of identifying and describing the sources of stress (stressors) that are present for you at this point in your life. Your answers to these questions will provide information about stress that you experience:

- Personally
- Psychosocially
- Physically

The results of this questionnaire will be processed and given back to you in the form of a printed profile. A Stress Center staff member will discuss the results with you.

The questionnaire *does not* assess physical, mental, or emotional illness and, therefore, is not appropriate for use as such. The questionnaire was designed for normal, healthy individuals who wish to either maintain or further improve their state of well-being.

Use of the Questionnaire

Information from this questionnaire will be used to help you assess your current sources of stress. Otherwise, for purposes of protecting your confidentiality, all information is coded anonymously. In this way this information can be compiled without identifying you personally with your answers.

Name: _____ Date: _____

Age: _____ Sex: _____ Highest grade attained in school: _____

Occupation: _____

Instructions

Please work on this questionnaire when you can spend a period of uninterrupted time to complete an entire section.

Please respond to each statement or question using the scale to the right. Follow the instructions preceding each set of items. There are no right or wrong answers and some may be hard to respond to, but please make a sincere effort. If none of the available responses fits perfectly, pick one that seems closest to your answer. Since your completion of this questionnaire is voluntary, it is not necessary to respond to an item if you find it objectionable; however, the results will be more useful if you will complete every item.

Appendix D continued

Circle the numbers that represent how these statements describe your general style of life: *AN* is Almost Never, *R* is Rarely, *S* is Sometimes, *O* is Often and *AA* is Almost Always.

	AN	R	S	O	AA
1. I feel motivated to do things.	1	2	3	4	5
2. I am patient.	1	2	3	4	5
3. I fit in well with the people around me.	1	2	3	4	5
4. I know what others expect of me.	1	2	3	4	5
5. Day-to-day living is monotonous for me.	1	2	3	4	5
6. I watch television more than two hours each day.	1	2	3	4	5
7. My present job is routine and dull.	1	2	3	4	5
8. When I feel good about some one, I tell them.	1	2	3	4	5
9. I have difficulty concentrating.	1	2	3	4	5
10. I have aches or pains.	1	2	3	4	5
11. I have a clear conscience.	1	2	3	4	5
12. Things that happen to me are unfair.	1	2	3	4	5
13. I feel no strong commitment to major goal or set of goals.	1	2	3	4	5
14. Drinking beer or alcohol makes problems for me.	1	2	3	4	5
15. I feel physically strong and capable.	1	2	3	4	5
16. When I have problems, I work on finding a solution right away.	1	2	3	4	5
17. My memories of the past are unpleasant.	1	2	3	4	5
18. I accomplish things that are important to me.	1	2	3	4	5
19. My present job is a big source of satisfaction for me.	1	2	3	4	5
20. I take care of the most important things first.	1	2	3	4	5
21. I find it hard to be by myself.	1	2	3	4	5
22. When there is a job to be done, I don't let my feelings interfere.	1	2	3	4	5
23. I get what I want.	1	2	3	4	5
24. I have what I need to carry out my responsibilities.	1	2	3	4	5
25. My work is stressful.	1	2	3	4	5
26. I think I am living fully.	1	2	3	4	5
27. My life is dull and uninteresting.	1	2	3	4	5
28. I feel anxious when I am by myself.	1	2	3	4	5
29. There seems to be a big difference between how I am and how I should be.	1	2	3	4	5
30. I look forward to my future years.	1	2	3	4	5
31. I have trouble saying "No" to people.	1	2	3	4	5
32. I feel loved by someone important to me.	1	2	3	4	5
33. When I have problems with someone, it's hard for me to let them know.	1	2	3	4	5
34. I have the standard of living I deserve.	1	2	3	4	5
35. I worry about my weight.	1	2	3	4	5
36. In competition, I feel angry if I don't win.	1	2	3	4	5
37. I get daily physical exercise.	1	2	3	4	5
38. My stomach bothers me.	1	2	3	4	5

Appendix D continued

	AN	R	S	O	AA
39. Finding words for how I feel is easy.	1	2	3	4	5
40. I take pills or drink to relax.	1	2	3	4	5
41. Being alone leads to recharging and clear thinking for me.	1	2	3	4	5
42. I have the stamina and endurance I need.	1	2	3	4	5
43. At this point in my life I am making important decisions.	1	2	3	4	5
44. I feel in control of my appetite.	1	2	3	4	5
45. When I'm tense or upset, I eat something.	1	2	3	4	5
46. I have a sense of direction in my life.	1	2	3	4	5
47. I can remember important things.	1	2	3	4	5
48. I feel well organized and clearheaded.	1	2	3	4	5
49. I am happy and contented.	1	2	3	4	5
50. I feel relaxed.	1	2	3	4	5
51. Other people expect me to do things that are not my responsibility.	1	2	3	4	5
52. I feel sad or down in the dumps.	1	2	3	4	5
53. I feel guilty about eating.	1	2	3	4	5
54. I am proud to do my line of work.	1	2	3	4	5
55. I enjoy unscheduled time alone.	1	2	3	4	5
56. I have pleasant feelings.	1	2	3	4	5
57. I worry about how things will turn out.	1	2	3	4	5
58. I enjoy being with the people around me.	1	2	3	4	5
59. I eat nutritious meals.	1	2	3	4	5
60. I feel resentment about things that have happened to me in the past.	1	2	3	4	5
61. It's hard for me to get close to people.	1	2	3	4	5
62. I react to problems in an easygoing manner.	1	2	3	4	5
63. I feel nervous or upset.	1	2	3	4	5
64. Interesting things happen to me.	1	2	3	4	5
65. I keep my feelings to myself.	1	2	3	4	5
66. I feel I belong where I am.	1	2	3	4	5
67. I have trouble knowing my priorities.	1	2	3	4	5
68. I smoke cigarettes.	1	2	3	4	5
69. I take on more than a person could realistically handle.	1	2	3	4	5
70. I accomplish things that are important to me.	1	2	3	4	5
71. I am lethargic and lack energy.	1	2	3	4	5
72. I am lonely.	1	2	3	4	5
73. I would like to start all over.	1	2	3	4	5
74. I feel good about my eating habits.	1	2	3	4	5
75. My sleep is disturbed.	1	2	3	4	5
76. There are situations in which I cannot be myself.	1	2	3	4	5
77. This stage of life is rewarding.	1	2	3	4	5
78. I cannot keep up with all the demands made on me.	1	2	3	4	5
79. I feel excluded by people.	1	2	3	4	5
80. I feel like I am part of a family.	1	2	3	4	5

Source: Reprinted with permission of Department of Health Promotion, St. Louis University Medical Center, © 1981.

References

Abdel-Halim, A.A. Employee affective responses to organizational stress: Moderating effects of job characteristics. *Personnel Psychology*, 1978, *31*(4) 561–579.

Abdel-Halim, A.A. Individual and interpersonal moderators of employee reactions to job characteristics: A reexamination. *Personnel Psychology*, 1979, *32*(1) 121–137.

Abdel-Halim, A.A. Effects of role stress: Job design-technology interaction on employee work satisfaction. *Academy of Management Journal*, June 1981, *24*(2), 260–273.

Abrams, M.N., & Numerof, R.E. Collective bargaining among nurses in health care: Current issues and future prospects. Health Care Management Review, accepted for publication, 1983.

Achterberg, J., & Lawlis, G.F. *Imagery of cancer: An evaluation tool for the process of disease*. Champaign, Ill.: Institute for Personality and Ability Testing, 1978.

Achterberg, J., & Lawlis, G.F. *Bridges of the bodymind*. Champaign, Ill.: Institute for Personality and Ability Testing, 1980.

Achterberg, J.; Lawlis, G.F.; Simonton, O.C.; & Simonton, C. Psychological factors and blood chemistries as disease outcome predictors for cancer patients. *Multivariate Clinical Experimental Research*, December 1977.

Adams, E.F.; Laker, D.R.; & Hulin, L. An investigation of the influence of job level and functional specialty on job attitudes and perceptions. *Journal of Applied Psychology*, 1977, *62*, 335–343.

Adams, J.S. The structure and dynamics of behavior in organizational boundary roles. In M.D. Dunnette (Ed.), *Handbook of Industrial and Organizational Psychology*. Chicago: Rand-McNally Publishing Company, 1976, 1175–1199.

Aiken, L.H.; Blendon, R.J.; & Rogers, D.E. The shortage of hospital nurses: A new perspective. *Annals of Internal Medicine*, 1981, *95*, 365–372.

Albrecht, K. *Stress and the manager: Making it work for you*. Englewood Cliffs, N.J.: Prentice-Hall, Inc., 1979.

Aldrich, H., & Herker, D. Boundary-spanning roles and organization structure. *Academy of Management Review*, June 1977, *2*(2) 217–230.

Allen, M.; Jackson, D.; & Youngner, S. Closing the communication gap between physicians and nurses in the intensive care unit setting. *Heart and Lung*, 1980, *9*, 836–840.

Alutto, J.A., & Belasco, J.A. Determinants of attitudinal militancy among nurses and teachers. *Industrial Labor Relations Review*, January 1974, *27*(2), 216–227.

317

American Medical Association. Fifth conference on the impaired physician. Portland: Fall, 1982.

American Medical Association. Fourth conference on the impaired physician. Baltimore: Fall, 1980.

Amkraut, A., & Solomon, G.F. From the symbolic stimulus to the pathophysiologic response: Immune mechanisms. *International Journal of Psychiatry in Medicine*, 1975, *5*(4), 541–563.

Anslinger, H.J. An interview with H.J. Anslinger. *Modern Medicine*, 1957, *25*, 170–191.

Appelbaum, S.H. *Stress management for health care professionals.* Rockville, Md.: Aspen Systems Corporation, 1981.

Appley, M.H.E., & Trumbell, R. *Psychological stress.* New York: Appleton-Century-Crofts, Inc., 1967.

Ausubel, D.P. *Theory and problems of adolescent development.* New York: Grune and Stratton, 1954, 46–48.

Ayres, P.R. *Do you know a sick doctor?* Paper presented at the ALC 80: International Conference on Alcoholism, Batte, England, September 1980.

Bach, G.R., & Goldberg, H. *Creative aggression: The art of assertive living.* New York: Doubleday and Company, Inc., 1974.

Bardi, C.A. Job-sharing alternative draws nurses back to the hospital. *Hospitals,* June 16, 1981, *55*(12), 71–72.

Bardwick, J.M., & Donovan, E.M. Ambivalence: The socialization of women. In Judith M. Bardwick (Ed.), *Readings on the psychology of women.* New York: Harper & Row Publishers, Inc., 1972.

Barnard, J. *Women and the public interest.* New York: Aldine Publishing Co., Inc., 1971.

Bates, E.M., & Moore, B.N. Stress in hospital personnel. *The Medical Journal of Australia,* 1975, *2,* 20, 765–767.

Bateson, G. The cybernetics of self: A theory of alcoholism. *Psychiatry,* 1971, *34,* 1–18.

Battling employee alcoholism. Dunn's *Business Month.* June, 1982.

Becker, H.S.; Geer, B.; Hughes, E.C.; & Strauss, A.L. *Boys in white: Student culture in medical school.* Chicago: University of Chicago Press, 1961.

Beckhard, R. *Organization development: Strategies and models.* Reading, Mass.: Addison-Wesley Publishing Co., Inc., 1969.

Beehr, T.A. Perceived situational moderators of the relationship between subjective role ambiguity and role strain. *Journal of Applied Psychology,* 1976, *61,* 35–40.

Beehr, T.A., & Newman, J. Job stress and employee and organizational effectiveness: A facet analysis, model and literature review. *Personal Psychology,* 1978, *31*(4), 665–700.

Beehr, T.A.; Walsh, J.T.; & Taber, T.D. Relationship of stress to individually and organizationally valued states: Higher order needs as a moderator. *Journal of Applied Psychology,* 1976, *61,* 41–47.

Bem, S.L., & Bem, D.J. Training the woman to know her place: The power of a nonconscious ideology. In S.L. Bem & D.J. Bem (Eds.), *Women's Role in Contemporary Society.* New York: Avon Books, 1972.

Benson, H. Your innate asset for combating stress. *Harvard Business Review,* July/August 1974, *52,* 49–60.

Benson, H., & Allen, R.L. How much stress is too much? *Harvard Business Review,* September/October 1980, *58,* 86–92.

Bergan, T., & Hirsch, G. *Analysis and planning for improved distribution of nursing personnel and services: A national model of supply, demand, and distribution.* Washington, D.C.: U.S. Department of Commerce, 1976.

Block, A. Combat neurosis in inner-city schools. *American Journal of Psychiatry,* October 1978, *135,* 10, 1189–1193.

Bloom, J.R.; O'Reilly, C.A.; & Parlette, G.N. Changing images of professionalism: The case of public health nurses. *American Journal of Public Health,* January 1979, *69*(1), 43–46.

Bloom, J.R.; Parlette, G.N.; & O'Reilly, C.A. Collective bargaining by nurses: A comparative analysis of management and employee perceptions. *Health Care Management Review,* 1980, *5*(1), 25–33.

Borsay, M.A., & Leff, A.M. Physician drug addiction: A challenge to medical educators. *Ohio State Medical Journal,* November 1977, 740–742.

Brayfield, A.H., & Crockett, W.H. Employee attitudes and employee performance. *Psychological Bulletin,* September 1955, *52,* 396–424.

Brief, A.P., & Aldag, R.J. Correlates of role indices. *Journal of Applied Psychology,* 1976, *61,* 404–409.

Buck, V.E. *Working under pressure.* London: Staples Press, 1972.

Bullough, B. Barriers to the nurse practitioners movement: Problems of women in a women's field. *International Journal of Health Services,* 1975, *5*(2), 225–233.

Burchfield, S.R. The stress response: A new perspective. *Psychosomatic Medicine,* 1979, *41*(8), 661–672.

Burke, R.J., & Weir, T. The type A experience: Occupational and life demands, satisfaction and well-being. *Journal of Human Stress,* December 1980, 28–38.

Caldwell, T., & Weiner, M.F. Stresses and coping in ICU nursing. *General Hospital Psychiatry,* 1981, *3,* 119–134.

Calhoun, G.L. Hospitals are high stress employers. *Hospitals,* June 16, 1980, *54*(12), 171–176.

Cannon, W.B. *Bodily changes in pain, hunger, fear and rage* (2nd ed.). Boston, Mass.: Charles T. Bradford Co., 1953.

Caplan, R.D., & Jones, K.W. Effects of work load, role ambiguity, and type A personality on anxiety, depression, and heart rate. *Journal of Applied Psychology,* 1975, *60,* 713–719.

Cartwright, D., & Zander, A. *Group dynamics: Theory and research* (3rd ed.). New York: Harper & Row Publishers, Inc., 1968.

Cascio, W.F. *Applied psychology in personnel management.* Reston, Va.: Reston Publishing Co., Inc., 1978.

Cassem, N.H., & Hackett, T.P. Sources of tension for the CCU nurse. *American Journal of Nursing,* 1972, *72,* 1426–1430.

Chafetz, J.S. Women in social work. *Social Work,* September 1972, *17,* 12–19.

Charlesworth, E.A.; Murphy, S.; & Beutler, L. Stress management skill for nursing students. *Journal of Clinical Psychology,* April 1981, *37,* 284–290.

Charns, M., & Beattie, H. *Organizational correlates of house staff burnout.* Paper presented at the 42nd annual meeting of the Academy of Management. New York, August 1982.

Charns, M.; Stoelwinder, J.; Millen, R.; & Schaefer, M. *Coordination and patient-unit effectiveness: A study of organizational factors affecting patient care.* Paper presented at the 41st annual meeting of the Academy of Management. San Diego, August 1981.

Cherniss, G. *Professional burnout in human service organizations.* New York: Praeger Publishers, 1980.

Clark, W.D. Alcoholism: Blocks to diagnosis and treatment. *The American Journal of Medicine,* August 1981, *71,* 275–286.

Cobb, S. Role responsibility: The differentiation of a concept. In A.A. McLean (Ed.), *Occupational Stress.* Springfield, Ill.: Charles C Thomas, Publisher, 1974, 62–69.

Cobb, S. Social support as a moderator of life stress. *Psychosomatic Medicine,* 1976, *38*(5), 300–314.

Cofer, C.W., & Appley, M.H. *Motivation: Theory and research.* New York: John Wiley & Sons, Inc., 1964.

CompCare. *How an alcoholic employee behaves.* Minneapolis: CompCare Publications, 1976.

Conference of the East-West Association of the Healing Arts. Washington, D.C.: 1977.

Conference report: The role of stress in hypertension. *Journal of Human Stress,* June 1979, *5*(2), 7–27.

Connelly, S.V., & Connelly, P.A. Physicians' patient referrals to a nurse: Practitioner in a primary care medical clinic. *American Journal of Public Health,* January 1979, *69*(1), 73–75.

Controlling managerial stress: A manager's manual. Waterford, Conn.: Bureau of Business Practice, 1980.

Cooley, E.J., & Keesey, J.C. Moderator variables in life stress and illness relationship. *Journal of Human Stress,* September 1981, *7*(3), 35–40.

Coombs, R.H. *Mastering medicine: Professional socialization in medical school.* New York: The Free Press, 1978.

Cooper, B., & Sylph, J. Life events and the onset of neurotic illness: An investigation in general practice. *Psychological Medicine,* 1973, *3,* 421–435.

Cooper, C.L., & Marshall, J. *Understanding executive stress.* Petrocelli Books, Inc., 1977.

Cramer, K.D. *Individual profile of stressors.* St. Louis: St. Louis University, School of Medicine, Stress Management Center, Department of Health Promotion, 1981.

Crooks, E. Nurses' associations and collective bargaining. *RN,* April 1979, *42,* 83–84, 88.

Cunningham, R.M. Get all the working parts together. *Hospitals,* November 16, 1980, *54*(22), 70–74.

Dana, B. Value dilemmas in the delivery of social health services: Caring, coping, and curing. In H. Rehr (Ed.), *Ethical dilemmas in health care: A professional search for solutions.* New York: Prodist, Neale Watson Academic Publications, Inc., 1978.

DeVries, R.A. CEOs don educator's cap. *Hospitals,* January 16, 1980, *54*(2), 108–111.

Dewald, P. *Psychotherapy: A dynamic approach* (2nd ed.). New York: Basic Books, Inc., 1971.

Dohrenwend, B.P. Life events as stressors: A methodological inquiry. *Journal of Health and Social Behavior,* 1973, *14,* 167–175.

Dohrenwend, B.P., & Dohrenwend, B.S. The conceptualization and measurement of stressful life events: An overview of the issues. In J.S. Strauss, H.M. Babigian, & M. Roff (Eds.), *Proceedings of the Conference on Methods of Longitudinal Research in Psychotherapy.* New York: Plenum Press, 1977.

Donnelly, J.C. *The internship experience: Coping and ego development in young physicians.* (Doctoral dissertation, Harvard University, 1979).

Dossett, S.M. Stress: Nursing staff in high dependency areas. *Nursing Times,* 1978, *78*(21), 888–889.

Dossett, S.M. Stress: The patient in the intensive therapy unit. *Nursing Times,* 1978, *78*(21), 890–891.

Drucker, P. *Management: Tasks, responsibilities, and practices.* New York: Harper & Row, Publishers, Inc., 1973.

Eaton, W.W. Life events, social supports, and psychiatric symptoms: A reanalysis of the New Haven data. *Journal of Health and Social Behavior,* 1978, *19*(2), 230–234.

Edelwich, J., with Brodsky, A. *Burnout: Stages of disillusionment in the helping professions.* New York: Human Sciences Press, Inc., 1980.

Elling, R.H. The shifting power structure in health. *Milbank Memorial Fund Quarterly,* January 1968, *46,* 119–143.

Elliott, C.L. Hospitals must face heavy unionization drives in '80s—Part II. *Hospitals,* July 16, 1981, *55*(14), 99–102.

Ellis, B. Winds of change sweep nursing profession. *Hospitals,* January 1, 1980, *54*(1), 95–98.

Epstein, C.F. *Woman's place.* Berkeley, Calif.: University of California Press, 1970.

Etzioni, A. *The Semiprofessions and their organization.* New York: The Free Press, 1969.

Fahlberg, W.J., Jr. *A comparative study of the perception of work-related stress between the registered nurses in medical intensive care and the general medical unit.* (Unpublished Master's thesis, Washington University, Health Administration and Planning Program, May 1972.)

Fairbank, D.T., & Hough, R.L. Life event classifications and the event-illness relationship. *Journal of Human Stress,* September 1979, *5*(3), 41–47.

Felch, W.C. Physician-nurse relationships. *The Hospital Medical Staff,* July 1976, *6,* 6–8.

Fiedler, F.E. *A theory of leadership effectiveness.* New York: McGraw-Hill Book Company, 1967.

Filipowicz, C.A. The troubled employee: Whose responsibility? *The Personnel Administrator,* June 1979, *24*(6), 17–22.

Fottler, M.D. Physician attitudes toward physician extenders: A comparison of nurse practitioners and physician assistants. *Medical Care,* May 1979, *17*(5), 536–549.

Fraiberg, S.H. *The magic years.* New York: Charles Scribner's Sons, 1959.

Francis, D., & Young, D. *Improving work groups.* San Diego: University Associates, Inc., 1979.

Frederick, C.J. (cited by M.M. Manber). Being a doctor may be hazardous to your health. *Medical World News,* August 20, 1979, 68–78.

Freidson, E. *Professional dominance: The social structure of medical care.* New York: Aldine Publishing Company, Inc., 1970.

French, J.D. The reticular formation. *Scientific American, 196*(5), May 1957, 54–60.

French, J.R.P. and Caplan, R.D. Organizational stress and individual strain. In A.J. Marrow (Ed.), *The failure of success.* New York: AMACOM, American Management Associations, 1973.

French, W.L., & Bell, C.H. *Organization development.* Englewood Cliffs, N.J.: Prentice-Hall, Inc., 1978.

Friedman, M., & Rosenman, R.H. *Type A behavior and your heart.* New York: Alfred A. Knopf, Inc., 1974.

Friedman, R.C.; Bigger, J.; & Kornfeld, D.S. The intern and sleep loss. *The New England Journal of Medicine,* July 22, 1971, *285,* 201–203.

Friedman, R.C.; Kornfeld, D.S.; & Bigger, R.J. Psychological problems associated with sleep deprivation in interns. *Journal of Medical Education,* May, 1973, *285*(4) 436–441.

Fuchs, V. *Who shall live? Health, economics, and social change.* New York: Basic Books, Inc., 1974.

Fuller, S.S.; Endress, M.P.; & Johnson, J.E. The effects of cognitive and behavioral control on coping with an aversive health examination. *Journal of Human Stress,* 1978, *4*(1), 18–25.

Gardner, E.R. *Fundamentals of neurology.* Philadelphia: W.B. Saunders Co., 1968.

Gardner, E.R., & Hall, R.C.W. The professional stress syndrome. *Psychosomatics,* August 1981, *22*(8), 672–680.

Gardner, E.R., & Hall, R.C.W. Protracted stress syndrome in health care providers. *Texas Medicine,* 1980, *73,* 63–65.

Garmezy, N. Children under stress: Perspectives on antecedents and correlates of vulnerability and resistance to psychopathology. In A.I. Robin, J. Aronoff, A.M. Barcley, & R.A. Zucker (Eds.), *Further Explorations in Personality.* New York: John Wiley and Sons, 1981.

Garvey, M., & Tuason, V. Physician marriages. *Journal of Clinical Psychiatry,* March 1979, *40*(3), 129–131.

Gavin, J.F. Occupational mental health—Forces and trends. *Personnel Journal* (1977): *56*(4), 198–201.

Georgopoulos, B.R. (Ed.). *Organization research on health institutions.* Ann Arbor, Mich.: University of Michigan, Institute for Social Research, 1972.

Gibb, J.R. Defensive communication. *The Journal of Communication,* September 1961, *9*(3), 141–148.

Gillanders, W., & Heiman, M. Time study comparisons of three intern programs. *Journal of Medical Education,* 1971, *46,* 142–149.

Gillespie, D.F. *Protective service worker study.* Lansing, Mich.: State of Michigan Department of Social Services, Protective Services Division, 1979.

Gillespie, D.F. Correlates for active and passive types of burnout. *Journal of Social Service Research,* Winter 1980/81, *4*(2), 1–16.

Goffman, E. *The presentation of self in everyday life.* New York: Doubleday and Company, Inc., 1959.

Gray-Toft, P., & Anderson, J.G. The nursing stress scale: Development of an instrument. *Journal of Behavioral Assessment,* 1981, *3*(1), 11–23.

Green, D. Hospital opts for "greenhouse" atmosphere in staff dining area. *Hospitals,* February 16, 1981, *55*(4), 137–138.

Guytin, A.C. *Textbook of medical physiology* (4th ed.). Philadelphia: W.B. Saunders Company, 1971.

Hackett, T.P.; Cassem, N.H.; & Wishnie, H. Detection and treatment of anxiety in the coronary care unit. *American Heart Journal,* 1969, *78,* 727–730.

Hackman, J.R., & Lawler, E.E. Employee reactions to job characteristics. *Journal of Applied Psychology,* 1971, Monograph No. 3, 259–286.

Hackman, J.R., & Oldham, G.R. Development of the job diagnostic survey. *Journal of Applied Psychology,* 1975, *60,* 159–170.

Hackman, J.R., & Oldham, G.R. Motivation through the design of work: Test of a theory. *Organizational Behavior and Human Performance*, 1976, *16*(2) 250–279.

Hackman, J.R., & Oldham, G.R. *Work redesign*. Reading, Mass.: Addison-Wesley Publishing Company, Inc., 1980.

Hall, D.T., & Lawler, E.E. Job characteristics and pressures and the organizational integration of professionals. *Administrative Science Quarterly*, 1970, *15*, 271–281.

Hall, R.C.W.; Gardner, E.R.; & Perl, M. The professional burnout syndrome. *Psychiatric Opinion*, 1979, *16*, 12–17.

Hampton, D.R.; Summer, C.E.; & Webber, R.A. *Organizational behavior and the practice of management* (3rd ed.). Glenview, Ill.: Scott, Foresman & Company, 1978.

Handbook of labor statistics. Washington, D.C.: U.S. Department of Labor, Bureau of Labor Statistics, Bulletin 1905, 1976, 327.

Harrison, R. Startup: The care and feeding of infant systems. *Organizational Dynamics*, Summer 1981, *10*(1). 4–29.

Harrison, R.F., O'Moore, A.M., O'Moore, R.R., & McSweeney, J.J. Stress profiles in normal infertile couples: Pharmacological and psychological approaches to therapy. In V. Insler & G. Bettendorf (Eds.), *Advances in Diagnosis and Treatment of Infertility*. New York: Elsevier/North-Holland, 1981, 143–157.

Hay, D., & Oken, D. The psychological stresses in intensive care unit nursing. *Psychosomatic Medicine*, 1972, *34*(2), 109–118.

Herman, J.B.; Dunham, R.B.; & Hulin, C.L. Organizational structure, demographic characteristics, and employee responses. *Organizational Behavior and Human Performance*, 1975, *13*(2), 206–232.

Holmes, G.L., & Mills, E. Contribution of a nurse clinician to office practice productivity: Comparisons of two solo primary care practices. *Health Services Research*, Spring 1976, *11*(1), 21–33.

Holmes, T.H., & Masuda, M. Life change and illness susceptibility. In B.P. Dohrenwend & B.S. Dohrenwend (Eds.), *Stressful life events*. New York: John Wiley & Sons, Inc., 1974.

Holmes, T.H., & Rahe, R.H. The social readjustment rating scale. *Journal of Psychosomatic Research*, 1967, *11*, 213–218.

Hooyman, N.R., & Kaplan, J.S. New roles for professional women—Skills for change. *Public Administration Review*, 1976, *36*, 374–378.

Horowitz, M. Phase-oriented treatment of stress response syndromes. *American Journal of Psychotherapy*, 1973, *27*, 506–515.

House, J.S. Occupational stress and coronary heart disease: A review and theoretical integration. *Journal of Health and Social Behavior*, 1974, *15*(1) 12–27.

House, R.J., & Rizzo, J.R. Role conflict and ambiguity as critical variables in a model of organizational behavior. *Organizational Behavior and Human Performance*, 1972, *7*, 467–505.

Hunter, R.C.; Lohrenz, J.G.; & Schwartzman, A.E. Nosophobia and hypochondriasis in medical students. *Journal of Nervous and Mental Disorders*, 1964, *139*, 147–152.

Huse, E. *Organization development and change* (2nd ed.). St. Paul, Minn.: West Publishing Company, 1980.

Identification of drug abusers. Harrisburg, Pa.: Pennsylvania Department of Health, Division of Drug Control, 1975.

Imparato, N. Relationship between Porter's need satisfaction questionnaire and the job descriptive index. *Journal of Applied Psychology*, 1972, *57*, 397–405.

Ivancevich, J.M., & Matteson, M.T. Nurses and stress: Time to examine the potential problems. *Journal of Nursing Leadership Management,* 1980, *11,* 17–22.

Ivancevich, J.M., & Matteson, M.T. Optimizing human resources: A case for preventive health and stress management. *Organizational Dynamics,* Autumn 1981, *9,* 5–25.

Jacobs, S.C.; Prusoff, B.A.; & Paykel, E.S. Recent life events in schizophrenia and depression. *Psychological Medicine,* 1974, *4,* 444–453.

Jacobson, S.P. Stressful situations for neonatal intensive care nurses. *The American Journal of Maternal Child Nursing,* May/June 1978, 144–151.

Jellinek, E.M. *Disease concept of alcoholism.* New Haven, Conn.: Hill House Press, Publishers, 1960.

Jenkins, C.D. Psychosocial modifiers of response to stress. *Journal of Human Stress,* December 1979, *5*(4), 3–15.

Johnson, R.L. How much process is due? *Trustee,* October 1979, *32*(10), 12–20.

Johnson, R.L. Boards are remodeled as hospitals merge. *Hospitals,* May 1, 1980, *54*(9), 101–105.

Johnson, T.W., & Stinson, J.E. Role ambiguity, role conflict, and satisfaction: Moderating effects of individual differences. *Journal of Applied Psychology,* 1975, *60,* 329–333.

Joint Commission on Accreditation of Hospitals. *Accreditation manual for hospitals.* Chicago: JCAH, 1980.

Jones, L.F. How 92% beat the dope habit. *Bulletin of Los Angeles County Medical Association,* 1958, *88*(19), 37–40.

Jourard, S.M. *The transparent self.* New York: Van Nostrand Reinhold Company, 1971.

Juris, H.A. Collective bargaining in hospitals. *Labor Law Journal,* August 1977, *28,* 504–511.

Kahn, R.L. Conflict, ambiguity and overload: Three elements in job stress. In A.A. McLean (Ed.), *Occupational stress.* Springfield, Ill.: Charles C. Thomas, Publisher, 1974, 47–61.

Kahn, R.L., & Quinn, R.P. Role stress: A framework for analysis. In A.A. McLean (Ed.), *Occupational mental health.* New York: Rand-McNally Publishing Company, 1970.

Kahn, R.L.; Wolfe, D.M.; Quinn, R.P.; Snoek, J.R.; & Rosenthal, R.A. *Organizational stress: Studies in role conflict and ambiguity.* New York: John Wiley & Sons, Inc., 1964.

Kalisch, B.J., & Kalisch, P.A. An analysis of the sources of physician-nurse conflict. *Journal of Nursing Administration,* January 1977, *7,* 51–7.

Kane, R.L.; Hammer, D.; & Byrnes, N. Getting care to nursing home patients: A problem and a proposal. *Medicare Care,* January 1977, *15*(1), 174–180.

Kanter, R.M. *Men and women of the corporation.* New York: Basic Books, Inc., 1977.

Kantner, T.R., & Vastyan, E.A. Coping with stress in family practice residency training. *The Journal of Family Practice,* September, 1978, *7,* 599–600.

Katz, D., & Kahn, R.L. *The social psychology of organizations.* New York: John Wiley & Sons, Inc., 1966.

Keller, R.T.; Szilagyi, A.D.; & Holland, W.E. Boundary-spanning activities and employee relations: An empirical study. *Human Relations,* 1976, *29,* 699–710.

Kelly, J.A.; Bradlyn, A.S.; Dubbert, P.M.; & St. Lawrence, J.S. Stress management training in medical school. *Journal of Medical Education,* February 1982, *57,* 91–99.

Kim, J., & Kohout, F.J. Multiple regression analysis: Subprogram regression. In N.H. Nie, C.H. Hull, J.G. Jenkins, K. Steinbrenner, & D.H. Bent (Eds.), *Statistical package for the social sciences* (2nd ed.). New York: McGraw-Hill Book Company, 1975, 320–367.

Kissen, D.M. Psychosocial factors, personality, and lung cancer in men aged 55–64. *British Journal of Medical Psychology*, 1967, *40*, 29 ff.

Kohn, M. *Class and conformity*. Homewood, Ill.: The Dorsey Press, 1969.

Korman, A.K.; Wittig-Berman, M.; & Lang, D. Career success and personal failure: Alienation in professionals and managers. *Academy of Management Journal*, June 1981, *24*, 342–360.

Kornhauser, A. *Mental health of the industrial worker*. New York: John Wiley & Sons, Inc., 1965.

Kovner, A.R., & Norville, J.L. *CEO-board relationships*. Paper presented at the annual meeting, Association of University Programs in Health Administration, May 1979.

Krakowski, A.J. Stress and the practice of medicine—the myth and the reality. *Journal of Psychosomatic Research*, 1982, *26*(1) 91–8.

Laing, R.D. *The politics of the family and other essays*. New York: Vintage Books, 1972.

Langs, R. *The technique of psychoanalytic psychotherapy* (Vols. 1 and 2). New York: Jason Aronson, Inc., 1974.

Latack, J.C. Person/role conflict: Holland's model extended to role-stress research, stress management and career development. *Academy of Management Review*, January 1981, *6*(1), 89–104.

Lawler, E.E., & Porter, L.W. The effect of performance on job satisfaction. *Industrial Relations*, 1967, *7*(1), 20–29.

Lawrence, P.R., & Lorsch, J.W. *Organization and environment: Managing differentiation and integration*. Cambridge, Mass.: Harvard University Press, 1967.

Lazarus, A. *I can if I want to*. New York: William Morrow & Company, Inc., 1975.

Lazarus, R.S. A strategy for research on psychological and social factors in hypertension. *Journal of Human Stress*, 1978, *4*(1) 35–40.

Lee, A.A. Still the handmaiden. *RN*, July 1979, *42*, 21–30.

LeShan, L. *How to meditate: A guide to self-discovery*. New York: Bantam Books, Inc., 1974.

LeShan, L., & Worthington, R.E. Some recurrent life-history patterns observed in patients with malignant disease. *Journal of Nervous and Mental Disease*, 1956, *124*, 460–465.

Levine, J.I. The nurse practitioner role: Physician utilization, patient acceptance. *Nursing Research*, July-August 1978, *27*(4), 245–254.

Levinson, H. The changing role of the hospital administrator. *Health Care Management Review*, Winter 1976, *1*(1) 79–89.

Levinson, H. The abrasive personality. *Harvard Business Review*, May-June 1978, *56*(4), 86–94.

Levinson, H. Power, leadership, and the management of stress. *Professional Psychology*, 1980, *11*(3), 497–508.

Levinson, H. When executives burn out. *Harvard Business Review*, May/June 1981, *59*(3), 72–81.

Lewis, F.M. The nurse as lackey: A sociological perspective. *Supervisor Nurse*, April 1976, *7*, 24–27.

Lief, H.I. Personality characteristics of medical students. In R.H. Coombs & C.E. Vincent (Eds.), *Psychosocial aspects of medical training*. Springfield, Ill.: Charles C Thomas, Publisher, 1971.

Litwin, G.H., & Stringer, R.A. *Motivation and organizational climate.* Cambridge, Mass.: Harvard University Press, 1968.

Lochoff, R.V.; Cane, R.D.; Buchanan, N.; & Cox, H.J.E. Nursing staff stress in an intensive care unit. *South African Medical Journal,* 1977, *52*(24), 961–963.

Lynn, N.B.; Vadem, A.G.; & Vadem, R.E. The challenges of men in a women's world. *Public Personnel Management,* January 1975, *4*(1), 4–17.

MacKinnon, R., & Michels, R. *The psychiatric interview in clinical practice.* Philadelphia: W.B. Saunders Company, 1971.

Mahler, M.; Pine, F.; & Bergman, A. *The psychological birth of the human infant.* New York: Basic Books, Inc., 1975.

Mahoney, T.A., & Frost, P.J. The role of technology in models of organizational effectiveness. *Organizational Behavior and Human Performance,* 1974, *11,* 122–138.

Marshall, R.E., & Kasman, C. Burnout in the neonatal intensive care unit. *Pediatrics,* June 1980, *65*(6), 1161–1165.

Maslach, C. Burned-out. *Human Behavior,* September 1976, *5,* 16–22.

Maslach, C. Job burnout: How people cope. *Public Welfare,* Spring 1978, *36,* 56–58.

Maslach, C., & Pines, A. The burnout syndrome in day care settings. *Child Care Quarterly,* Summer 1977, *6*(2) 100–113.

Maslach, C., & Pines, A. Burnout of professionals in mental health settings. *Hospital and Community Psychiatry,* April 1978, *29,* 233–237.

Mason, J.L. *Guide to stress reduction.* Culver City, Calif.: Peace Press, Inc., 1980.

Mattern, C.L. Make your credentialing procedures work for you. *Trustee,* August 1979, *32*(8), 8–15.

Matteson, M.T., & Ivancevich, J.M. Organizational stressors and heart disease: A research model. *Academy of Management Review,* July 1979, *4*(3), 347–358.

Mawardi, B.H. Satisfactions, dissatisfactions, and causes of stress in medical practice. *Journal of the American Medical Association,* 1979, *241,* 1483–1486.

McClelland, D.C., & Jemmott, J.B. Power motivation, stress and physical illness. *Journal of Human Stress,* December 1980, *6*(4) 6–15.

McCue, J.D. The effects of stress on physicians and their medical practice. *The New England Journal of Medicine,* February 25, 1982, *306*(8), 458–463.

McGrath, J. (Ed.). *Social and psychological factors in stress.* New York: Holt, Rinehart & Winston, Inc., 1970.

McGrath, J.E. Stress and behavior in organizations. In M.C. Dunnette (Ed.), *Handbook of industrial and organizational psychology.* Chicago: Rand McNally Publishing Company, 1976, 1351–1390.

McKenna, J.F.; Oritt, P.L.; & Wolff, H.K. Occupational stress as a predictor in the turnover decision. *Journal of Human Stress,* December 1981, *7,* 4, 12–17.

McLean, A.A. (Ed.) *Occupational stress.* Springfield, Ill.: Charles C Thomas, Publisher, 1974.

McLean, A.A. (Ed.) *Reducing occupational stress. Proceedings of occupational stress conference,* May 1977. Washington, D.C.: U.S. Department of Health, Education, and Welfare, National Institute for Occupational Safety and Health, Publication No. [NIOSH] 78-140, 1978.

McLean, A.A. *Work stress.* Reading, Mass.: Addison-Wesley Publishing Company, Inc., 1979.

Mechanic, D. The management of psychosocial problems in primary medical care: A potential role for social work. *Journal of Human Stress,* December 1980, *6*(4) 16–21.

Mechanic, D. Stress, illness, and illness behavior. *Journal of Human Stress,* 1976, *2*(2) 2–6,

The Medical Letter on Drugs and Therapeutics. September 19, 1980, *22*(19), 77–81.

The Medical Letter on Drugs and Therapeutics. February 6, 1981, *23*(3), 9–12. (a)

The Medical Letter on Drugs and Therapeutics. May 1, 1981, *23*(9), 41–44. (b)

Mednik, B.R. Breakdown in high-risk subjects: Familial and early environmental factors. *Journal of Abnormal Psychology,* 1979, *82,* 469–475.

Meissner, M. *Technology and the worker.* San Francisco: Chandler & Sharp Publishers, Inc., 1969.

Meltzer, H., & Wickert, F.R. *Humanizing organizational behavior.* Springfield, Ill.: Charles C Thomas, Publisher , 1976.

Metzger, N. Labor relations demand special attention in the multihospital systems. *Hospitals,* January 1, 1981, *55*(1), 57–59.

Milam, J.R. & Ketcham, K. *Under the influence: A guide to the myths and realities of alcoholism.* Seattle: Madrone Publishers, 1981.

Miles, R.H. A comparison of the relative impacts of role perceptions of ambiguity and conflict by role. *Academy of Management Journal,* March 1976, *19*(1), 25–35.

Miles, R.H., & Perreault, W.D., Jr. Organizational role conflict: Its antecedents and consequences. *Organizational Behavior and Human Performance,* 1976, *17,* 19–44.

Miller, G.A. Professionals—bureaucracy: Alienation among industrial scientists and engineers. *American Sociological Review,* October 1967, *32,* 755–768.

Mintzberg, H. *The structuring of organizations.* Englewood Cliffs, N.J.: Prentice-Hall, Inc., 1979.

Moch, M.K.; Bartunek, J.; & Brass, D.J. Structure, task characteristics, and experienced role stress in organizations employing complex technology. *Organizational Behavior and Human Performance,* 1979, *24,* 258–268.

Mohl, P.C. Group process interpretation in liaison psychiatry nurse groups. *General Hospital Psychiatry,* 1980, *2,* 104–111.

Molberg, L.M. Trustees take leadership role in community health policy making. *Hospitals,* August 16, 1981, *55*(16), 103–113.

Monat, A., & Lazarus, R.S. (Eds.) *Stress and coping.* New York: Columbia University Press, 1977.

Moore, T., & Wood, D. Power and the hospital executive. *Hospitals and Health Services Administration,* Spring 1979, *24*(2), 30–41.

Morano, R.A. How to manage change to reduce stress. *Management Review,* November 1977, 23.

Morris, J.H., & Snyder, R.A. A second look at need for achievement and need for autonomy as moderators of role perception-outcome relationships. *Journal of Applied Psychology,* 1979, *64,* 2, 173–178.

Morris, J.H.; Steers, R.M.; & Koch, J.L. Influence of organization structure on role conflict and ambiguity for three occupational groupings. *Academy of Management Journal,* March 1979, *22*(1), 58–71.

Myers, J.K.; Lindenthal, J.J.; & Pepper, M.P. Life events and mental status: A longitudinal study. *Journal of Health and Social Behavior,* 1972, *13,* 398–406.

National Commission on Nursing: Initial report and preliminary recommendations. Chicago: American Hospital Association, Hospital Research and Educational Trust, 1981.

National Council on Alcoholism. Personal communication. St. Louis, Missouri, May 19, 1983.

Nelson, E.G., & Henry, W.F. Psychosocial factors seen as problems by family practice residents and their spouses. *The Journal of Family Practice,* 1978, *6*(3), 581–589.

Newman, J.E. Understanding the organization structure-job attitude relationship through perceptions of the work environment. *Organizational Behavior and Human Performance,* 1975, *14,* 371–397.

Newman, J., & Beehr, T. Personnel and organizational strategies for handling job stress: A review of research and opinion. *Personnel Psychology,* Spring 1979, *32*(1), 1–44.

Nie, N.H.; Hull, C.H.; Jenkins, J.G.; Steinbrenner, K.; & Bent, D.H. *Statistical package for the social sciences* (2nd ed.). New York: McGraw-Hill Book Company, 1975.

Nix, H.L., & Bates, F.L. Occupational role stresses: A structural approach. *Rural Sociology,* 1962, *27,* 7–17.

Nuckolls, K.B. Who decides what the nurse can do? *Nursing Outlook,* October 1974, *22,* 630–631.

Numerof, R.E. Assertiveness training for nurses in a general hospital. *Health and Social Work,* February 1978, *3*(1), 80–102. (a)

Numerof, R.E. The expanded nurse role from the perspective of the new medicine. *Health Care Management Review,* Summer 1978, *3*(3), 45–52. (b)

Numerof, R.E. *Nurses, management, and interpersonal needs: A preliminary study.* Unpublished paper, Washington University, 1981.

Numerof, R.E. *The practice of management for health care professionals.* New York: AMACOM, American Management Association, 1982.

Numerof, R.E., & Abrams, M.N. Before impairment: Physician stress and the organization's responsibility. *Health Care Management Review,* Fall 1981, *6*(4), 77–82.

Numerof, R.E., & Abrams, M.N. *Sources of stress among nurses: An empirical investigation.* Washington University, 1982. Paper presented to the 43rd Annual Academy of Management Meeting, August 1983.

Numerof, R.E., & Gillespie, D.F. *Developing a measure of burnout.* Washington University, unpublished paper, 1983.

Numerof, R.E.; Shachar Hendin, S.A.; & Cramer, K.D. The impact of organizational stressors on nursing, health, and medical administrators. Paper presented to the Second Annual Symposium on Research in Nursing and Health Administration. Medical College of Virginia, Richmond, Virginia, April 1983.

Numerof, R.E.; Shachar Hendin, S.A.; & Cramer, K.D. Stress in health administrators: An analysis of stress situations, stress symptoms, and coping strategies. Paper presented at the 43rd Annual Academy of Management Meeting. Dallas, August 1983.

Oaklander, H., & Fleishman, E.A. Patterns of leadership related to organizational stress in hospital settings. *Administrative Science Quarterly,* 1964, *8*(4), 520–532.

Oates, W. *Confessions of a workaholic.* New York: World Publishing Company, 1971.

O'Connell, M.J.; Cummings, L.L.; & Huber, G.P. The effects of environmental information and decision unit structure on felt tension. *Journal of Applied Psychology,* 1976, *61,* 493–500.

Organ, D.W., & Greene, C.N. Role ambiguity, locus of control, and work satisfaction. *Journal of Applied Psychology,* 1974, *59,* 101–102.

Ornstein, R.E. *The psychology of consciousness.* New York: W.H. Freeman and Company, 1972.

Oskins, S.L. Identification of situational stressors and coping methods by intensive care nurses. *Heart and Lung,* 1979, *8,* 953–960.

Parasuraman, S., & Alutto, J.A. An examination of the organizational antecedents of stressors at work. *Academy of Management Journal,* March 1981, *24*(1), 48–67.

Parasuraman, S.; Drake, B.H.; & Zammuto, R.L. *Primary versus team care, and shift assignments in nursing: Impact on work stressors and job attitudes.* Paper presented to the 41st annual meeting of the Academy of Management, San Diego, August 1981.

Parkington, J.J., & Schneider, B. Some correlates of experienced job stress: A boundary role study. *Academy of Management Journal,* June 1979, *22*(2), 270–281.

Patten, T.H. *Organizational development through teambuilding.* New York: John Wiley & Sons, Inc., 1981.

Paykel, E.S. Life stress and psychiatric disorder: Applications of the clinical approach. In B.S. Dohrenwend & B.P. Dohrenwend (Eds.), *Stressful life events: Their nature and effects.* New York: John Wiley & Sons, Inc., 1974.

Pearlin, L.L. Alienation from work: A study of nursing personnel. *American Sociological Review,* June 1962, *27,* 314–326.

Pearson, M.M. Drug and alcohol problems in physicians. *Psychiatric Opinion,* April 1975, *12*(4), 14–18.

Pelletier, K.R. *Mind as healer, Mind as slayer.* New York: Delacorte Press, 1977.

Pendleton, B. Coping with managerial stress. *Management World,* January 1981, *10,* 25.

Peskin, D. *The doomsday job: The behavioral anatomy of turnover.* New York: AMACOM, American Management Associations, 1973.

Perrow, C. The analysis of goals in complex organizations. In A. Etzioni (Ed.), *Readings on modern organizations.* Englewood Cliffs, N.J.: Prentice-Hall, Inc., 1969.

Peterson, M.F., & Cooke, R.A. *Potential sources and outcomes of strain and intergroup tension experienced by emergency unit staff.* Paper presented at the 41st annual meeting of the Academy of Management, San Diego, August 1981.

Pettigrew, L.S., & Raney, D.C. *Job-related stress in the medical residency across two points in time.* Paper presented to the 42nd annual meeting of the Academy of Management, New York, August 1982.

Pfeffer, J. Power and resource allocation in organizations. In B. Stow & G.R. Salancik (Eds.), *New directions in organizational behavior.* Chicago: St. Clair Press, 1976.

Pines, A., & Maslach, C. Characteristics of staff burnout in mental health settings. *Hospital and Community Psychiatry,* April 1978, *29*(4), 233–237.

Pitts, F.N.; Schuller, A.B.; & Rich, C.L. Suicide among U.S. women physicians, 1967–1972. *American Journal of Psychiatry,* 1979, *136,* 694–696.

Quick, J.C. Dyadic goal setting and role stress: A field study. *Academy of Management Journal,* June 1979, *22*(2), 241–252.

Rabkin, J.G., & Struening, E.L. Life events, stress, and illness. *Science,* December 3, 1976, *194,* 1013–1020.

Rahe, R.H. Life change events and mental illness: An overview. *Journal of Human Stress,* September 1979, *5*(3), 2–10.

Rahe, R.H., & Arthur, R.J. Life change and illness studies: Past history and future directions. *Journal of Human Stress,* March 1978, *4*(1), 3–15.

Rahe, R.H.; Meyer, M.; & Smith, M. Social stress and illness onset. *Journal of Psychosomatic Research,* 1964, *8,* 35–44.

Rahe, R.H.; Ryman, D.H.; & Ward, H.W. Simplified scaling for life change events. *Journal of Human Stress,* December 1980, *6*(4), 22–27.

Randolph, W.A., & Finch, F.E. The relationship between organization technology and the direction and frequency dimensions of task communications. *Human Relations,* 1977, *30,* 1131–1145.

Reid, K. *An exploratory study of the burnout syndrome in the social work profession.* Kalamazoo, Mich.: Western Michigan University, School for Social Work, 1977.

Reiner, B.S., & Kaufman, I. *Character disorders in parents of delinquents.* New York: Family Service Association of America, 1959.

Reiser, S.J. *Medicine and the reign of technology.* Cambridge, England: Cambridge University Press, 1978.

Richards, G. Where grow tomorrow's CEO's? *Hospitals,* March 16, 1982, *56*(6), 86–92.

Ricklefs, R. Many executives complain of stress. *The Wall Street Journal,* September 29, 1982, p. 27.

Rockwell, F.P.A.; Sommer, B.; Sassenrath, E.N.; Rozee-Koker, P.; & Stinger-Moore, D. Job stress and health in working women. *Journal of Human Stress,* December 1981, *7*(4), 19–26.

Roeske, N.C.A. Stress and the physician. *Psychiatric Annals,* July 1981, *11*(7), 245–258.

Rogatz, P. The case for the medical director. *Trustee,* June 1979, *32*(6), 21–25.

Rogers, D.L., & Molnar, J. Organizational antecedents of role conflict and ambiguity in top-level administrators. *Administrative Science Quarterly,* 1976, *21,* 598–610.

Rose, D.K., & Rosow, I. Marital instability among physicians. *California Medicine,* March 1972, *116*(3), 95–99.

Rosenman, R.H.; Brand, R.J.; Jenkins, C.D.; Friedman, M.; Strauss, R.; & Worm, M. Coronary heart disease in the western collaborative group study: A follow-up experience of 4½ years. *Journal of Chronic Diseases,* 1970, *23,* 173–190.

Rousseau, D.M. Technological differences in job characteristics, employee satisfaction, and motivation: A synthesis of job design research and sociotechnical systems theory. *Organizational Behavior and Human Performance,* 1977, *19,* 18–42.

Scheffler, R.M.; Weisfeld, N.; Ruby, G.; & Estes, E.H. A manpower policy for primary health care. *The New England Journal of Medicine,* May 11, 1978, *298*(19), 1058–1062.

Schildkraut, J.J., & Kety, S.S. Biogenic amines and emotion. *Science,* April 7, 1967, *156,* 21–30.

Schneider, D.P., & Foley, W.J. A systems analysis of the impact of physician extenders on medical cost and manpower requirements. *Medical Care,* April 1977, *15*(4), 277–297.

Schuler, R.S. Role perceptions, satisfaction, and performance: A partial reconciliation. *Journal of Applied Psychology,* 1975, *60,* 683–687.

Schuler, R.S. The effects of role perceptions on employee satisfaction and performance moderated by employee ability. *Organizational Behavior and Human Performance,* 1977, *18,* 98–107. (a)

Schuler, R.S. Role conflict and ambiguity as a function of the task-structure-technology interaction. *Organizational Behavior and Human Performance,* 1977, *20,* 64–74. (b)

Schuler, R.S. Role perceptions, satisfaction, and performance moderated by organizational level and participation in decision-making. *Academy of Management Journal,* March 1977, *20*(1), 159–165. (c)

Schuler, R.S.; Aldag, R.J.; & Brief, A.P. Role conflict and ambiguity: A scale analysis. *Organizational Behavior and Human Performance,* 1977, *20,* 113–115.

Schutz, W. *The interpersonal underworld: FIRO-B.* Palo Alto, Calif.: Science and Behavior Books, Inc., 1966.

Scotch, C.B. Sex status in social work: Grist for woman's liberation. *Social Work,* July 1971, *16,* 3, 5–12.

Scully, R. Stress in the nurse. *American Journal of Nursing,* 1980, *80,* 912–913.

Sells, S.B. On the nature of stress. In J. McGrath (Ed.), *Social and psychological factors in stress.* New York: Holt, Rinehart & Winston, Inc., 1970.

Selye, H. *The stress of life.* New York: McGraw-Hill Book Company, 1956.

Selye, H. *Stress without distress.* Philadelphia: J.B. Lippincott Co., 1974.

Selye, H. *Stress in health and disease.* Reading, Mass.: Butterworth Publishers, Inc., 1976.

Selznick, P. *Leadership in administration.* New York: Harper & Row, 1957.

Sheridan, J.E., & Vredenburgh, D.J. Predicting leadership behavior in a hospital organization. *Academy of Management Journal,* December 1978, *21*(4), 679–89.

Sheridan, J.E., & Vredenburgh, D.J. Structural model of leadership influence in a hospital organization. *Academy of Management Journal,* March 1979, *22*(1), 6–21.

Shevrin, H. Brainwave correlates of subliminal stimulation, unconscious attention, primary- and secondary-process thinking, and repressiveness. *Psychological Issues,* 1973, *8*(2), 56–87.

Shulin, S. Burnout: The professional hazard you face in nursing. *Nursing,* 1978, *8,* 22–27.

Shulin, S. Rx for stress—your stress. *Nursing,* January 1979, *9,* 53–55.

Siegal, H.A., & Faryna, A.F. Strategies for early intervention with the alcoholic patient. *Urban Health,* November 1980 , 42–45.

Siegel, B., & Donnelly, J.C. Enriching personal and professional development: The experience of a support group for interns. *Journal of Medical Education,* November 1978, *53,* 908–14.

Simborg, D.W., Starfield, B.H., & Horn, S.D. Physicians and nonphysician health practitioners: The characteristics of their practices and their relationships. *American Journal of Public Health,* January 1978, *68*(1), 44–48.

Simmel, G. [*The sociology of George Simmel.*] (K.H. Wolff trans.). Glencoe, Ill.: The Free Press, 1950.

Simon, H. *Administrative behavior. A study of decision-making processes in administrative organization* (3rd ed.). New York: The Free Press, 1976.

Simonton, O.C., & Simonton, S. Belief systems and management of the emotional aspects of malignancy. *Journal of Transpersonal Psychology,* 1975, *7*(1), 29–48.

Sloss, P.F. Medical staff privileges: Time for another look. *Trustee,* February 1979, *32*(2), 8–13.

Small, G.W. House officer stress syndrome. *Psychosomatics,* October 1981, *22,* 10, 60–69.

Smith, M.J.T., & Selye, H. Stress-reducing the negative effects of stress. *American Journal of Nursing,* 1979, *79*(10), 1953–1956.

Solomon, G.F. Emotions, stress, the central nervous system, and immunity. *Annals of the New York Academy of Science,* 1969, *164*(2), 335–43.

Sperling, M. *The major neuroses and behavior disorders in children.* New York: Aronson, 1974.

Springer, E., health care attorney, Horty, Springer, and Mattern. Pittsburgh personal communication, October 1980; December 1982.

Stein, L.I. Male and female: The doctor-nurse game. *Archives of General Psychiatry*, June 1967, *16*, 202–211.

Steppacher, R.C., & Mausner, J.S. Suicide in male and female physicians. *Journal of the American Medical Association*, 1974, *228*, 323–328.

Sterman, M.B. Neurophysiological and clinical studies of sensorimotor EEG biofeedback training: Some effects on epilepsy. In L. Birk (Ed.), *Seminars in psychiatry*, Vol. 5(4). New York: Grune & Stratton, Inc., 1974, 507–525.

Stern, J.L. Public sector bargaining in 1985. *Labor Law Journal*, May 1977, *28*, 264–275.

Suinn, R.M. How to break the vicious cycle of stress. *Psychology Today*, December 1976, *10*(7) 59–60.

Sullivan, H.S. *Conception of modern psychiatry*. London: Tavistock Publications, 1955.

Sullivan, J.A.; Dachelet, C.Z., Sultz, H.A., Henry, M., & Carrol, H.D. Overcoming barriers to the employment and utilization of the nurse practitioner. *American Journal of Public Health*, November 1978, *68*(11), 1097–1103.

Suls, J., & Mullen, B. Life events, perceived control and illness: The role of uncertainty. *Journal of Human Stress*, June 1981, *7*(2), 30–34.

Szasz, T. *The myth of mental illness*. New York: Dell Publishing Company, Inc., 1961.

Szasz, T. Bad habits are not diseases. *Lancet*, July 8, 1972, *2*, 7767, 83–84.

Szilagyi, A.D. An empirical test of causal inference between role perceptions, satisfaction with work, performance and organizational level. *Personnel Psychology*, Autumn 1977, *30*(3), 375–388.

Szilagyi, A.D.; Sims, H.P.; & Keller, R.T. Role dynamics, locus of control, and employee attitudes and behavior. *Academy of Management Journal*, June 1976, *19*(2), 259–276.

Taubman, R. (cited by M.M. Manber). Being a doctor may be hazardous to your health. *Medical World News*, August 20, 1979, 68–78.

Taxay, E.P. The health care team. *Journal of the American Medical Association*, December 1978, *239*, 1137.

Tennant, C., & Andrews, G. The pathogenic quality of life event stress in neurotic impairment. *Archives of General Psychiatry*, 1978, *35*, 859–863.

Thomas, C.B., & Duszynski, K.R. Closeness to parents and the family constellation in a prospective study of five disease states: Suicide, mental illness, malignant tumor, hypertension and coronary heart disease. *The Johns Hopkins Medical Journal*, May 1974, *134*(5), 251–70.

Thompson, R.F. *Foundations of physiological psychology*. New York: Harper and Row, 1967.

Toffler, A. *Future shock*. New York: Bantam Books, Inc., 1970.

Tokarz, J.P., Brenner, W., & Peters, K. *Beyond survival*. Chicago: American Medical Association, 1979.

Tosi, H.W. Organizational stress as a moderator of the relationship between influence and role response. *Academy of Management Journal*. March 1971, *14*(1), 7–20.

Trick, K. Maintenance of nurse's mental health under stress. *Nursing Mirror*, December 10, 1965, i–ii.

Twaddle, A.C., & Hessler, R.M. *A sociology of health*. St. Louis: The C.V. Mosby Company, 1977.

Umbdenstock, R.J. Governance: Trustees are closing the gap between hospitals and consumers. *Hospitals,* April 1, 1979, *53*(7), 111–115.

Umbdenstock, R.J. Hospital governance comes of age. *Hospitals,* April 1, 1980, *54*(7), 85–88.

Vaillant, G.E. *Health of the healer.* Keynote address, Fourth Annual AMA Conference on the Impaired Physician, Baltimore, October 30, 1980.

Vaillant, G.E.; Brighton, J.R.; & McArthur, C. Physicians use of mood-altering drugs. *The New England Journal of Medicine,* Feburary 12, 1970, *282*(7), 365–370.

Vaillant, G.E.; Sobowale, N.C.; & McArthur, C. Some psychologic vulnerabilities of physicians. *The New England Journal of Medicine,* August 24, 1972, *287*(8), 372–375.

Valenzi, E., & Dessler, G. Relationships of leader behavior, subordinate role ambiguity, and subordinate job satisfaction. *Academy of Management Journal,* December 1978, *21*(4), 671–678.

Van Vorst, C.B. Quality assurance: The buck stops with the board. *Trustee,* May 1979, *32*(5), 25–28.

Vash, C.L. *The burnt-out administrator.* New York: Springer Publishing Co., Inc., 1979.

Vinokur, R., & Selzer, M.L. Desirable versus undesirable life events: Their relationship to stress and mental distress. *Journal of Personality and Social Psychology,* 1975, *32,* 329–337.

Von Brauchitch, H. The physicians' suicide revisited. *Journal of Medical Disorders,* 1976, *162,* 40.

Vreeland, R., & Ellis, G.L. Stresses on the nurse in an intensive care unit. *Journal of the American Medical Association,* 1969, *208*(2), 332–334.

Vroom, V. *Work and motivation.* New York: John Wiley & Sons, Inc., 1964.

Weiner, M.F., & Caldwell, T. Stresses and coping in ICU nursing: Nurse support groups on intensive care units. *General Hospital Psychiatry,* 1981, *3,* 129–134.

Werblun, M.N.; Deshler, J.; & Martin, L.R. Building identity in a family practice residency program. *The Journal of Family Practice,* August 1977, *5,* 278–80.

Werner, E.E., & Smith, R.S. *Vulnerable but invincible: A longitudinal study of resilient children and youth.* New York: McGraw-Hill, 1982.

Werner, E.R., & Korsch, B.M. Professionalization during pediatric internship: Attitudes, adaptation, and interpersonal skills. In E.C. Shapiro & L.M. Lowenstein (Eds.), *Becoming a physician: Development of values and attitudes in medicine.* Cambridge, Mass.: Ballinger Publishing Co., 1979, pp. 1–125.

White, R., & Lippit, R. *Autocracy and democracy.* New York: Harper & Row, 1960.

Williams, M.; Ho, L.; & Felder, L. Career patterns: More grist for women's liberation. *Social Work,* July 1974, *19,* 463–67.

Winick, C. Physician narcotics addicts. *Social Problems,* 1961, *9,* 174–186.

Wolfe, S. Strikes by health workers: A look at the concept, ethics, and impacts. *American Journal of Public Health,* 1979, *69*(5), 431–433.

Wurmser, L. *A psychotherapist's view of problems of drug abuse.* Baltimore: Johns Hopkins Drug Abuse Clinic, 1975.

Wyler, A.R.; Masuda, M.; & Holmes, T.H. Seriousness of illness rating scale. *Journal of Psychosomatic Research,* 1968, *11,* 363–374.

Yodfat, Y.; Fidel, J.; & Eliakim, M. Analysis of the work of nurse-practitioners in family practice and its effects on the physicians' activities. *The Journal of Family Practice,* February 1977, *2*(2), 345–350.

Index

A

Abrams, M.M., 166
Absenteeism, 42, 285
  alcoholism and, 217
  burnout and, 212
  discipline and, 268-269, 271
  teamwork and, 251
Accident proneness, 103
Accountability
  evaluation climate and, 256-257
  group, 250
  of medical directors, 108
  performance appraisal and, 264
Administrators. *See also* Chief
  executive officer (CEO); Managers
  associate, 94
  board of trustees and, 192-193,
    199, 200-204
  conflict negotiations and, 197-200
  evolution of position of, 192-193
  health care sector and, 191
  impaired physicians and, 145
  isolation of, 204-206
  management development and,
    61-62, 63
  nurse-physician-administrator
    relationships and, 162, 178-180
  performance appraisal and, 43-44
  physicians and, 146-150

stress research on
  background and purpose of,
    78-81
  coping strategies and, 111-115
  findings summary and, 129-131
  overview of, 75-78
  the sample for, 81-82
  sex and position and, 86-102
  stress events questionnaire and,
    102-107
  stress model and, 131-133
  stress situations and, 82-86
  symptomology and, 107-111
  symptoms and demographic
    variables and, 115-125
  vulnerability and, 125-129
  value system conflicts and, 193-196
Adrenalin, 11, 12
Adrenocortical involvement, 12-13,
  15
Adrenocorticotropic hormone
  (ACTH), 10, 11
Adults, 22, 23
Affection, nurse stress study and, 176
Age
  administrator stress study and, 81,
    117, 121, 122, 123, 130, 131
  nurse stress study and, 174
  of physician administrators, 148
Aggressive individuals, 57
Aiken, L.H., 180

Alarm (Phase I of GAS), 15
Alcoholics Anonymous, 221
Alcoholism, 141, 143, 145, 224, 228, 223
  analysis of, 217-221
  assistance program for, 285-286
  physicians and, 219, 234
Alutto, J.A., 172, 182
Ambiguity (job), 65-66
American Academy of Medical Directors, 150
American Hospital Association, 182
American Medical Association, 143
  alcoholism and, 218
  Resident Physicians Section of, 136
American Nurses' Association, 184-185
Amphetamines, 223-224
Anger, 56, 284
  nurses and, 160, 231
Animals, 9, 14
Anxiety, 280
  amphetamine abuse and, 224
  performance, 188
Assessment. See Evaluation; Performance appraisal
Assistance programs for employees, 285-287
Autogenic training, 276
Autonomic nervous system, 9
Autonomy issue
  administrators and, 195
  nurses and, 157-158, 161, 163, 165, 179, 181, 182, 183, 193
  teams and, 244
Avoidance, 21, 231-232
  of confrontation, 232-233

Barbiturates, 224-225
Bardo, burnout and, 211
Barnard, J., 159
Bates, E.M., 138

Beattie, H., 139
Beehr, T.A., 236-237, 274
Behavior
  alcoholism and, 219, 220
  burnout and, 210
  communications and, 47
  drug addiction and, 223
  emotional disturbances and, 226-227
  evaluation and defensive, 52-56
  external, 103, 105, 107, 121-122
  inappropriate, 142
  negative appraisal avoidance and, 21
  nurse training programs and, 159-160
  passive-aggressive and aggressive, 56-57, 160
  perceptions and, 23
  self-destructive, 30-32
  snapping, 142
  stress at personal level and, 41-42, 67-72
  stress reduction and, 278-285
  thinking and, 24-25
  tolerated physician, 262-263
Behavior modification, 64-65, 279
Belasco, J.A., 182
Beliefs. See Values
Bem, D.J., 159
Bem, S.L., 159
Bensen, H., 275
Biofeedback, 9, 277
Block, A., 211
Bloom, J.R., 183
Board of trustees, 192-193, 199, 200-204
Boredom, 122, 244
Brain, 6-8, 14, 18-19, 23, 24, 26
Brodsky, A., 212-213
Burnout, 248
  characteristics of, 210-211
  multiple dimensions of, 211-217

C

Caldwell, T., 170
Cancer, 152
  holistic medicine and, 153-154
  immune system and, 13
  personality and, 70-71
Cannon, Walter B., 5, 9
Career development, 244-248
Centralization, 257-258
Central nervous system, 26, 221, 224
CEO. *See* Chief executive officer
  (CEO)
Cerebral cortex, 7, 8, 26
Certainty, 56
Certainty vs. provisionalism defensive
  behavior (evaluation), 56
Change
  in administrative roles, 192
  in drug addicts, 223
  nurses and, 161, 163
  organizational, 260
    employees and, 247
  stress and health status, 37-39
  vulnerability to stress and, 32-33
Charns, M., 139
Chief executive officer (CEO). *See
  also* Administrators
  management development and, 63
  stress analysis and, 94-102, 111,
    115, 121, 122, 198
Children, 21
  cancer and trauma in, 71
  coping and, 22
  nurse stress study and, 174
  stress and experiences of, 274
  stress and number of, 117, 121,
    123, 130
Clark, W.D., 233
Clinical issues, 91
  vs. administrative issues, 146-148
  staff and, 98
Cognition, 21
  perceived stressors and, 8, 14
  perception and sensation and, 23
  perceptual problems and, 45

stress management and, 278-285
Communication
  administrators and, 205
  board and administrators and, 201
  burnout and interpersonal, 214-215
  defensive behaviors and, 54, 55, 56,
    57
  directed, 283-285
  distortion of, 101
  emotional problems and, 233
  hospital and nurses and, 181
  interdepartmental, 240
  interpersonal environment and,
    46-52
  keeping channels open and, 279
  nurses and physicians and, 179
  staff and, 98
  stress management and, 241,
    257-259
  teamwork and, 250, 253
  upward, 256
Compensation (defense mechanism),
  232
Compensation (nurses), unions and,
  180-181
Competition, 199, 258
  career development and, 247
  CEO-board, 202
  internal, 62
  nurses and, 161
  organizational stress and, 66-67
  personality and, 69
Conflict
  administrators and value, 193-196
  communications and, 284
  drug addiction and, 222-223
  individual values and, 21
  interdisciplinary work, 94-95
  managerial personality, 64-65
  negotiation (administrator), 197-200
  physician and nurse, 97, 100, 101,
    145, 150, 162, 178, 179, 182, 231,
    249
  power, 194
  resolution of, 150
  role, 66, 149

staff, 96
team, 254
value, 21, 150, 193-196
Context survey (McLean's model), 35
Control, 54, 280, 281
  evaluation climates and, 54
  holism and, 153
  nurse stress study and, 167,
    174-175
  stress management and, 263-272
  teamwork and, 252-253
  trustees and administrators and,
    192-193, 201
Control vs. problem orientation
  defensive behavior (evaluation), 54
Conversion, 231
Coombs, R.H., 137
Coping strategies, 1, 39, 73, 81, 263.
  See also Stress management
  administrator stress study and,
    111-115, 117, 125, 130-131
  board and administrator and,
    201-202
  burnout and, 214
  checklist (McLean's model), 34-35
  children and, 22
  examples of, 304-311
  general strategies for, 278-280
  model of stress and, 131-133
  nurse stress study and, 175
  residency and, 139
  teaching of (nurse managers), 188
  vulnerability and, 128
Coronary heart disease (CHD)
  IPS and, 36
  personality and, 68-69, 70, 152
Cost containment, 60, 140, 184, 185,
  196
Costs
  job enlargement and, 248
  stress and turnover, 42
Counseling, 286, 287
Cramer, Kathryn D., 36
Credentialing, 203
Culture, 27
  as stressor, 260-261
Cunningham, R.M., 204

D

Dana, B., 154
Deadlines, 101, 115
Death, 42, 153, 154, 166, 170-172,
  175, 177
Decentralization, 257-258
Decision making
  middle management and, 65
  nurses and, 157, 159, 178, 182, 184
  nursing administrators and, 183
  perception and, 45-46
  Type B personality and, 70
Defense mechanisms, 229-232
Defensive behavior, evaluation and,
  52-56. See also Behavior
Degrees (academic titles). See also
  Training
  compensation and, 180
  health care, 238
  nurse stress study and, 166, 172
  nurse training programs and, 161
  organizational hypotheses (nurse
    stress study) and, 167
  professional issues and, 181
  stress in nurses and, 119
Demographics
  administrator stress study and,
    81-82, 103, 115-125
  Global Vulnerability to Stress
    Index (GVSI) and, 125-129
  nurse stress hypotheses and, 174
  nurse stress study and, 166-167
Denial, 115, 122, 129, 144, 145
  alcoholism and, 221
  as defense mechanism, 230
  myth of infallibility and, 108
  residency and, 139
Dependency needs, 139, 144-145. See
  also Needs
Depressive disorders, 38, 103, 107,
  117, 123, 210
Description vs. evaluation defensive
  behavior (evaluation), 53-54
Developmental stages (life
  experiences), 26-27

Diagnosis, 162, 163
Diagnostic and Statistical Manual III (American Psychiatric Association), 227
Disability, 22-23
Discipline, 267-272
Discrimination stress, 86
Disease. *See also* Illness
  administrator's view of, 195
  alcoholism as, 218-219
  General Adaptation Syndrome and, 16
  immune system and, 13
  life events and, 37-39
  models (holistic vs. vitalistic) of, 151-155
  nature of, 5-6
  personality and heart, 68-69, 70
  personal level and stress-related, 70-72
  physician dissociation and, 145
  physician residency and, 137
  risk factors and, 36
The Disease Concept of Alcoholism (Jellinck), 218
Displacement, 231
Drug addiction, 141, 143, 145, 233
  analysis of, 221-226
E.I. du Pont de Nemours & Co., 285

E

Eastman Kodak Company, 285
Edelwich, J., 212-213
Education. *See* Training
Elliot, C.L., 183
Emotional disturbance, 226-232
Emotions, 14
  administrator stress study and, 103, 105, 107, 117
  bodily changes and, 5
  burnout and, 210, 211
  limbic system and, 7
  nurse stress study and, 170-172
  patient care and nurses and, 166

physician stress and, 136, 137, 143
psychological causes of stress and, 20
subcortex and, 6
Empathy vs. neutrality defensive behavior (evaluation), 55
Employees. *See also* Staff
  alcohol assistance program and, 285-286
  assistance programs for, 285-287
  discipline and, 267-272
  group retaliation and, 271
  injury and, 75
  organizational change and, 247
  organizational interdependence and, 245
  personnel analysis and, 245-246
  quality of work life and, 59
  subordinate and superior relations and, 256-257, 264-267
  support systems and, 261-263
  working space analysis and, 43-45
Endocrine system, 10-12, 13, 14
Environment, 25
  psychological causes of stress and, 18-20
  reticular activating system and, 8
  as source of stress, 42-52
  stressors and, 2
  stress prevention and, 243-244
Epictetus, 273
Epileptic seizures, 7
Equality vs. superiority defensive behavior (evaluation), 55
Etzioni, A., 157
Eustress, 2
Evaluation. *See also* Professional appraisal
  assistance program, 287
  CEO-board and, 203
  defensive and supportive climates and, 52-56
  stress reduction and climate of, 256-257
Exhaustion (Phase III of GAS), 15-16

Expectations
    administrator stress and, 86, 129
    burnout and job, 210, 214, 216
    nurse managers and, 188
    unreasonable, 99

F

Family
    alcoholism and, 221
    physician administrators and,
        149-150
    residency and, 139
    work and stress and, 91, 95
Females. See Women
Fight-flight response
    adaptive syndrome and, 14-16
    physiological mechanisms and,
        9-10
Freidson, E., 194
French, J.D., 8
Freud, Sigmund, 136, 227, 231, 232
Friedman, M., 68, 69

G

Gastrointestinal system, alcohol and,
    220
General Adaptation Syndrome, 15-16
Genetic factors, 22-23, 30, 39
Georgopoulos, B.R., 191
Gibb, J.R., 53
Gillespie, D.F., 211-212
Global Vulnerability to Stress Index
    (GVSI), 125-129, 131. See also
    Vulnerability to stress
Glucocorticoids, 13
Goals
    management development and, 240
    middle management and, 96
    staff and, 100
    teamwork and, 250-251
    unclear, 94
Goffman, E., 50

Gonadotropic hormones (GTH), 11.
    See also Hormones
Government regulations, 95, 111
Group activities. See Teamwork

H

Harrison, R., 11-12, 198
HASS (Health Administrator Stress
    Study). See Administrators, stress
    research on
Health
    administrators' views of, 195
    mental, 227-228
    nature of, 5-6
Health administrators. See
    Administrators
Health Administrators Stress Study
    (HASS). See Administrators,
    stress research on
Health care sector
    administrators and stress and, 191
    alcoholism in, 219
    growth of, 58
    interhospital arrangements and,
        62-64
    management development and,
        60-62, 237-243
    organizational stress sources in,
        58-59
    physicians and, 143-146
    quality circles and, 254
    technology lag and, 60
    unsuitable role problem and, 64
Health maintenance, 151, 154
Henry, W.F., 138
Heredity. See Genetic factors
Heroin, 222, 226. See also Drug
    addiction
Holistic approach
    health care and, 5
    physicians and, 141, 153-155
Holmes, T.H., 2, 37-38, 39
Hormones, 11-13, 15

Hospitals
administrator's power base in,
192-193
burnout victims and, 212
communication with nurses and,
181
HASS and type of, 82
impaired physicians and, 145
insensitivity to nurses and, 184
interhospital arrangements and,
62-64
management development and, 242
multihospital systems and, 204, 260
nurses' issues and, 186
organization of departments in,
195
stress and costs and, 42
Hypnosis (self), 276-277
Hypothalamus, 6-7, 8, 10-11, 14

I

Identification, 230
Illness, 42. *See also* Disease
administrator stress study and,
103, 105, 115, 120-121
burnout and, 210, 212
hereditary, 22-23
holism and, 152-153
life events and, 37-39
nature of, 5-6
stress and predisposition to, 16
stress and psychosomatic, 3
terminal, 166
Immune system, 13, 70
Independent actions, 145
Individual Profile of Stressors (IPS),
33, 36
administrator stress study and, 81,
125-129
copy of, 314-316
Infertility, 11-12
Injury, 75
Innovation
accepting, 100

clinical, 95-96
Intellectualization, 230
Interdisciplinary work conflict, 94-95
Interpersonal relationships
administrators and, 200, 205-206
administrators stress study and, 86,
103, 105-107, 122
burnout and, 210, 212, 214-215
communication problems and,
46-52
corporate executives and, 279
nurses and, 163, 167, 174
nurse stress hypotheses and,
170-172, 174-176
perception problem and stress and,
45-46
residency and, 139
stress reduction and, 248-249
Intervention strategy list, 237
Interviews
administrator stress study, 80-81
nurse stress study, 165
Introjection, 230
Isolation, 230
administrators and, 204-206

J

Jacobson relaxation technique, 275
Jellinek, E.M., 218
Job. *See* Position (job)
Job analysis, 245-246
Job challenge, 27
Job design, 243-244
Job enlargement, 248
Job overload, 29
Job switching, 65
Johns Hopkins Medical Journal, 72
Joint Commission on the
Accreditation of Hospitals (JCAH),
203
Jourard, S.M., 160
Judgment errors, 95
Judgment questioned by colleagues,
101

K

Kahn, R.L., 66, 75
Kanter, R.M., 188
Katz, D., 66, 75
Korsch, B.M., 138

L

Labor-management, 58. *See also*
    Unions
Laing, R.D., 228
Lateness, 271
Lawrence, P.R., 165, 172
Leadership
    administrators and, 199
    nurse-physician-administrator and,
        162-163
    nurses and, 158-159, 178, 188
    physicians and hospital, 193
    quality circle, 255
    teamwork and, 250, 252-253, 254
Learning experiences, 25
Levinson, Harry, 57, 147, 199
Librium, 225-226
Life experiences
    psychological causes of stress and,
        26-27
    vulnerability to stress and, 37-39
Lighting, 44
Limbic system, 7
Lorsch, J.W., 165, 172
Lynn, N.B., 159

M

McArthur, C., 72
McKenna, J.F., 42, 172
McLean, A., 33, 34-35, 274
McLean model of vulnerability, 33-35
Magical undoing, 230
Males. *See* Men
Malpractice, 108, 140, 142

Management
    board and CEO and, 201
    burnout and, 216-217
    labor and, 58, 59-60
    quality circles and, 255
    sources of stress and, 58
    stress and middle, 65, 91-102, 107
    stress problem and, 41-42, 61
Management audit, 240, 241, 242
Management development, 60-62
    stress prevention and, 237-243
Management-by-objectives (MBO),
    254-255, 265
Managers. *See also* Administrators
    competition and, 62
    emotional problems and, 232
    negative response to stress and, 41
    nurses as, 186-189
    organizational stress and, 64-65
    physicians as, 148-150, 199-200
    productivity and stress and, 28-29
    quality of work life and, 59
Marital discord, 141, 142, 143
Marketing, 150, 196, 239
Maryland Health Service Cost
    Review Commission, 184
Maslach, C., 210
Mawardi, B.H., 138
Medicaid, 185
Medical directors, 107, 149, 279
    coping and, 111-115
Medical staff, 149, 262
    board and, 202-204
Medical staff presidents, 108-111,
    115, 121
Medicare, 185
Meditation, 275, 277
Memory, 22
    keeping notes and, 266
Men, 56
    administrator stress study and, 81,
        86-102, 122, 130, 131
    heart disease and, 68
    leadership positions and, 162-163
    perceived stress level and, 117
    suicide and, 141

Mental illness, 227-228
Meprobamate, 225
Miller, G.A., 211
Minorities, 91
Mission statement, 63
Missouri Nurses Association, 185
Models
 administrator stress study and
  stress, 131-133
 communication (DESC), 284
 delivery of care and medical,
  196-197
 dynamic (stress), 76-78
 holistic vs. disease (medicine),
  151-155
 McLean's vulnerability, 33-35
 Selye's stress, 15-16
Moore, B.N., 138
Morphine, 226. *See also* Drug
 addiction
Motivation
 defensive behavior and, 54
 management development and, 241
 psychological causes of stress and,
  21-22, 27
 teamwork and, 251
Myers, J.K., 38
Myths
 of infallibility, 108, 141, 143
 professional, 67-68, 99
 role, 282

N

Narcotics. *See* Drug addiction
National Commission on Nursing,
 177-178, 180, 183, 249
National Council on Alcoholism, 217
National Institute of Occupational
 Safety and Health (NIOSH), 75
Needs. *See also* Dependency needs
 assessment, 240
 communication and, 47
 hospital's sensitivity to patient, 45
 nurses' access to power and, 163

nurse stress study and, 167,
  174-176
 physicians' denial of own, 144
 psychological causes of stress and
  internal, 21-22
 women and family, 91
Nelson, E.G., 138
Neurophysiologic aspects of stress, 3,
 70
Neutrality vs. empathy defensive
 behavior (evaluation), 55
Newman, J., 274
Nightmares, 103
Noise, 8, 48
Noradrenalin, 12
Numerof, R.E., 166, 212
Nurse clinicians, 161, 162
Nurse practitioners, 161, 162
Nurses
 autonomy issue and, 157-158, 161,
  163, 165, 179, 181, 182, 183, 193
 health maintenance and, 151
 impaired physicians and, 145
 job enlargement and, 248
 as managers, 186-189
 National Commission on Nursing
  and, 177-178
 nurse-physician-administrator
  relationships and, 178-180
 patients and, 158, 160, 162, 163,
  166, 178
 physicians and, 97, 100, 101, 150,
  157, 162, 178-180, 179, 182, 231,
  249
 professional myths and, 67-68
 professional socialization and role
  of, 158-163
 role definition and, 157-158
 shortage of, 184
 sources of stress and, 164-167
 stress incidents and, 279
 stress levels and, 119
 stress study hypotheses and, 166,
  167-177
 suing of, 163
 union bargaining and, 180-186

unsuitable role problem (clinical
and administrative) and, 64
working space and appraisal of,
43-44
Nursing directors
decision making and, 183
stress analysis and, 94-102
unionization and, 182

O

Organizational factors in residency,
138-140
Organizational structure, stress
management and, 257-259
Organizations
affiliation with, 259
burnout and, 213-214
disorganization in, 101
nurses and barriers in, 162-163
physician managers in, 149
politics and, 200
stress levels and, 27
stress management
monitoring and control and,
263-267
overview of, 235-237
prevention and, 237-248
socialization and, 259-263
stress reduction and, 248-257
stress and nature of, 236
stress sources in, 41-42
health care sector and, 58-59
identifying, 58
interhospital arrangements and,
60-62
labor-management and, 58
unions and, 59-60
management and, 58
management development and,
59-60
managers and, 64-65
middle management and, 65
quality of work life and, 59
suboptimization and, 66-67

Orientation programs, 67
management staff and, 247
for nurse managers, 187-188
Outcomes
administrator stress study and,
102-107
middle management and, 96

P

Pain, 23
Parasuraman, S., 172
Parasympathetic nervous system,
9-10
Passive-aggressive individuals, 56-57,
160
Patients
burnout and, 211
holism and, 153
hospital's sensitivity to needs of, 45
nurses and, 158, 160, 162, 163,
166, 178
perception of, 152
physician administrators and,
149-150
physician values and, 147
quality care and, 97
as real consumer of health care,
194
satisfaction of, 58-59
stress as a function of sex and, 86
Pay, 97
nurses and unions and, 180-181
Pearson, M.M., 141
Pelletier, K.R., 3, 5, 7, 68, 72
Perception
defensiveness and distortions in, 52
emotional responses and, 280-281
interpersonal relationships and,
45-46
of patient, 152
psychological causes of stress and,
23-25
of stress, 76, 117, 129-130, 131-133
of stress vulnerability, 128

Performance appraisal. *See also*
Evaluation
climate for, 256-257
stress management and, 264-267
working space and, 43-44
Perrow, Charles, 192
Personality, 39
aggressive, 57
cancer and, 13, 70-71
communication and, 49
managers and conflict and, 64-65
nurse stress study and, 176, 177
passive-aggressive, 56-57, 160
residency and, 139
self-concept and, 25
Type A, 68-69, 70, 86, 91, 152,
279-280
Type B, 69-70
Personal Stress Symptom
Assessment, 102-107, 126, 299-302
Physicians
alcoholism and, 219, 234
changing values and, 146
clinical vs. administrative
perspective and, 146-148
cynicism among, 137
dominance of, 193, 197, 198
health care system and, 143-146
holistic approach and, 153-155
impaired, 140-143
defining, 135-136
emotional problems and, 234
nonreporting of, 145-146
management and administration
and, 148-150, 199-200
management training and, 107-108
nurses and, 97, 100, 101, 145, 150,
157, 162, 178-180, 179, 182,
231, 249
power of, 194, 196
professional myths and, 67-68
residency and, 135-140
stress levels and, 119
tolerated behaviors of, 262-263
vitalistic approach and, 151-153
vulnerability and, 143

Physician's assistants, 161, 162
Physiological mechanisms
adrenocortical involvement and,
12-13
the brain and, 6-8
endocrine system and, 10-13
fight-flight response and, 9-10
adaptive syndrome and, 14-16
immune system and, 13
nature of health and illness and,
5-6
physiologic keys to, 8-9
Physiological stress management,
274-278
Pituitary gland, 10-11, 14
Planning
coping strategies and, 278
long-range, 246-247
strategic, 61
Position (job)
administrator stress study and, 81,
86-102, 103-105, 108, 129
ambiguity and rigidity and, 65-66
coping and, 115
nurse stress study and, 177
work-related vulnerability and,
34-35
Power
administrator's base of, 192-193,
194-195
allocation and function of, 198-199
distribution of, 202
managerial nurses and, 163
physicians and, 194, 196
teamwork and, 252-253
Prevention, 153
Problem orientation defensive
behavior (evaluation), 54
Productivity, 42, 65, 186, 255
alcoholism and, 217-218
organizational stress and, 58
socioemotional components of
stress and, 27-29, 31
Professionalism, 99, 194, 198
Provisionalism vs. certainty defensive
behavior (evaluation), 56

Psychological causes of stress, 13.
    See also Stress
    environmental events and, 18-20
    feelings and emotions and, 26
    genetic factors and, 22-23
    life experiences and, 26-27
    memory and, 22
    motivation and, 21-22
    perception and sensation and,
        23-25
    self-concept and, 25-26
    sensory receptors and, 18-20
    values and, 20-21
Psychological stress management,
    274-275
Psychosomatic illness, 3, 16. *See also*
    Illness

Q

Quality care, 97, 108, 194, 249, 251
Quality control circles, 254-256
Quality control mechanisms, 263-264
Quality of work life, 59
Questionnaire (stress study), 81,
    102-107, 289-297

R

Radiation, 43
Rahe, R.H., 2, 36, 37-38
Rationalization, 231
Reaction formation, 230
Reflexive reactions, 9
Regression, 231
Regulations. *See* Government
    regulations
Reid, K., 211
Relaxation techniques, 275
Repression, 231
Research
    nurses and, 158, 162, 164-177
    residency and, 138, 140

on stress in health administrators
    background and purpose of,
        78-81
    coping and, 111-115
    findings summary and, 129-131
    overview of, 75-78
    the sample for, 81-82
    sex and position and, 86-102
    stress events, outcomes and
        symptoms (questionnaire) and,
        102-107
    stress model and, 131-133
    stress situations and, 82-86
    symptomology and, 107-111
    symptoms and demographic
        variables and, 115-125
    vulnerability and, 125-129
Residency
    organizational factors and, 138-140
    self-management and, 137-138
    stressors and, 135-137
    stress vulnerability and, 144
Resistance (Phase II of GAS), 15
Resource scarcity, 94
Responsibility, 288
    communication and, 284
    job, 98
    of medical directors, 108
    patient care, 97
    performance appraisal and, 266
Reticular activating system, 8
Rewards
    structure of, 61
    unsuitable role problem and, 64
Rigidity (job), 65-66
Risk
    administration and, 63
    burnout and, 210
    disease, 36
    residency and, 137
Role
    conflict in, 66, 149
    definition of nurses', 157-158
    expansion of nurses', 161-162
    myths of, 282
    unsuitable managerial, 64

Role model
  stress and CEO, 204
  stress and women and, 86, 91
Rosenman, R.H., 68, 69, 70
Rules, 269-270

S

Sabotage, passive-aggressive behavior
  and, 57
Sample in administrator's stress
  research, 81-82
Sandler, infertility and stress and, 11
Self-alienation (nurse), 160
Self-concept, 23
  psychological causes of stress
    and, 25-26
Self-confidence, 56
Self-esteem, 53
Self-fulfilling prophecy, 23
Self-hypnosis, 276-277
Selye, Hans, 1, 2, 15, 16, 273
Selzer, M.L., 38
Seminars (management development),
  240-241
Sensation, 23-25
Sensory motor cortex, 7
Sensory receptors, 18-20
Services, sharing of, 62-63
Sex. *See* Men; Women
Simon, Herbert, 258
Skills, ambiguity and rigidity and,
  65-66
Sleep deprivation, residency and, 137
Sleep drugs, 225
Snapping behaviors, 142. *See also*
  Behavior
Sobowale, N.C., 72
Socialization, 238, 249
  nurses and, 158-163
  stress management and, 259-263
Social Security, 185
Solomon, George, 13
Specialists, 138, 244
  nurses and, 167-172, 248

Spontaneity vs. strategy defensive
  behavior (evaluation), 54-55
Staff. *See also* Employees
  attracting qualified, 102
  communicating with, 98
  complaints of, 99
  conflicts with, 96
  dealing with stress of, 97
  goals and, 100
  incompetence, 98
  information and, 100
  interdisciplinary work and, 94-95
  middle management as buffer to,
    99
  new, 97, 261
  power and clinical, 198-199
  shortages, 101-102, 115
  unions and, 184, 201, 260
Stein, L.I., 179
Sterman, M.B., 7
Strategy vs. spontaneity defensive
  behavior (evaluation), 54-55
Stress. *See also* Coping strategies;
  Stressors; Stress management;
  Vulnerability to stress
  alcohol addiction and, 141, 143,
    145, 224, 228, 234
  analysis of, 217-221
  burnout and, 210-217
  confronting problems of, 232-234
  defensive and supportive climates
    and, 52-56
  defining, 1-2
  drug addiction and, 141, 143, 145
  analysis of, 221-226
  elastic limits and, 29-32
  emotional disturbances and,
    226-232
  examples of work-related, 209
  health administrator study of
    background and purpose of,
      78-81
    coping and, 111-115
    findings of, 129-131
    overview of, 75-78
    sex and position and, 86-102

stress and, 82-86, 102-107,
  131-133
symptoms and, 107-111, 115-125
vulnerability and, 125-129
high-pressure scenario and,
  263-264
individual variants and, 17-18
as management or personal
  problem, 41-42
negative effects of, 2-3, 14, 31, 37,
  128, 129, 136, 141, 263, 274
neurophysiology and, 3, 70
nurses and, 164-177, 182-183
organizational response to
  monitoring and control and,
    263-267
  overview of, 235-237
  prevention and, 237-248
  socialization and, 259-263
  stress reduction and, 248-257
physiological mechanisms and, 5-13
positive effects of, 2
productivity and, 27-29, 31
psychological causes of, 18-27
Selye's model for, 15-16
sources of
  defensive and supportive climates
    and evaluation and, 52-56
  interpersonal environment and,
    45-52
  at organizational level, 41-67
  passive-aggressive and aggressive
    personalities and, 56-57, 160
  at personal level, 41-42, 67-72
  physical environment and, 42-45
Stress Center (St. Louis University
  School of Medicine), 33
The Stress of Life (Selye), 15
Stress management, 288. *See also*
  Coping strategies
  health care system and, 144
  interventions and, 128-129
  organizational response to
    monitoring and control and,
      263-267
    overview of, 235-237

prevention and, 237-248
socialization and, 259-263
stress reduction and, 248-257
techniques for, 278-287
Stressors
  checklist (McLean's model) for, 35
  cognitively perceived, 8
  consequences of, 3-4
  culture as, 260-261
  individual reactions to, 17-18,
    235-236
  IPS and, 33, 36, 81, 125-129,
    314-316
  major administrator, 129, 198
  moderator variables and, 76, 131
  nurses and unions and, 182-183
  research on nursing, 164
  residency and, 135-137
  social support and, 263
  stress management and, 129
  stress reaction and, 3
  as stress triggers, 2
  vulnerability and relevance of, 33
Stress tolerance, 29-32
Subcortex, 6-8
Sublimation, 232
Suboptimization. *See* Unit
  suboptimization
Substitution, 232
Suicide, 141
Superiority vs. equality defensive
  behavior (evaluation), 55
Supervisor and subordinant
  relationships, 256-257, 264-267
  discipline and, 267-272
Supervisory training, 287
Support groups (nurse stress study),
  175
Support system (internal), 261-263
Suppression, 231
Survival system, 14
Sympathetic nervous system, 9-10
Symptoms
  administrator stress study and,
    107-111, 115-125
  of alcoholism, 219-221

of burnout, 210-211, 212
disease model and, 151-152
of drug addiction, 221-226
stress study questionnaire and,
102-107
of work-related stress, 209
Szasz, Thomas, 228

T

Teamwork, 111
analysis of, 249-254
autonomous teams and, 244
interprofessional, 178
staff stress and, 97-98
stress reduction and, 249-254
Technology, 60, 140, 178, 197
Tenure, 121, 122, 130, 131
nurse stress hypotheses and,
172-173
Termination, 247
discipline system and, 268-269, 270
team, 253-254
Thinking, 24
control over others and, 281
lack of flexibility in, 96-97
Thyrotropic hormone (TTH), 11
Time demands, 82, 100, 129, 144
Toffler, Alvin, 260
Tokarz, J.P., 136, 139
Total New Coping Strategies
(TNCS), 126. *See also* Coping
strategies
Total New Stress Situations (TNSS),
125-126, 128
Total Personal Stress Symptom
Score (TPSS), 126
Traditionalism (nurse), 158-159
Training, 42. *See also* Degrees
of administrators, 194, 200
assistance programs and, 287
in management, 238-243
of nurse administrator, 187
nurse socialization and, 159-160

nurses and union bargaining and,
181
organizational hypotheses (nurse
stress study), 170
physician and management,
107-108
physicians' and administrators'
ideas concerning nursing, 178
Trait assessment, 265
Tranquilizers, 225-226
Transcendental meditation, 275, 277
Transference, 25-26
Trust, 257, 262
burnout and lack of, 215-216
teamwork and, 250
Trustees. *See* Board of trustees
Turnover, 42, 184, 238
Type A and Type B personalities.
See Personality, Type A;
Personality, Type B

U

Unions, 260
discipline system and, 267, 268
labor-management and, 58
sources of stress and, 59-60
nurses
compensation and, 180-181
the future and, 183-186
professional issues and, 181-182
stressors and, 182-183
staff protection and, 201
Unit suboptimization
career development and, 246
competition and stress and, 66-67
decentralization and, 258
socialization and, 238
University of Michigan Institute for
Social Research, 235
U.S. Department of Labor, 75

V

Vacations, 117, 121, 123, 130, 131
Vadem, A.G., 159

Vadem, R.E., 159
Vaillant, G.E., 72, 143, 144
Valium, 225
Values
    administrators and, 193-196
    burnout and, 217
    job design and, 243
    orientation of, 146-148, 161
    physicians and changing, 146
    physicians and conflicts in, 150
    psychological causes of stress and,
        20-21
Vasopressin, 11
Ventilation, 44
Vinokur, R., 38
Vitalistic approach to medicine,
    151-153
Vulnerability to stress, 81. *See also*
    Stress
    administrator stress study and,
        125-129
    change and, 32-33
    Individual Profile of Stressors
        (IPS) and, 36, 125-129
    life events and, 37-39
    McLean's model of, 33-35
    model of stress and, 131-133
    physicians and, 139, 143, 144
    stressor relevance and, 33

W

Weiner, M.F., 170
Wellness, 136
Werner, E.R., 138
Women, 27, 56
    access to leadership positions and,
        162-163
    administrator stress study and, 81,
        86-102, 103, 122, 130, 131
    heart disease and, 68
    leadership and, 158-159, 188
    minority, 91
    perceived stress level and, 117
    role conflict and, 66
    suicide and, 141
Working hours, 117
Working space
    performance appraisal and, 43-44
    waiting room example of, 44-45

Y

Yoga, 277

About the Author

RITA E. NUMEROF is an assistant professor at the George Warren Brown School of Social Work and adjunct assistant professor of Health Administration and Planning, the School of Medicine, Washington University in St. Louis.

She has authored numerous articles on management and organization development in the health care industry as well as two other books, *Accent on People* and *The Practice of Management for Health Care Professionals*. As a faculty member of the Estes Park Institute, Dr. Numerof has conducted a variety of seminars on such topics as team building, effective leadership, and managing organizational stress for administrators, trustees, and medical directors. As a consultant Dr. Numerof leads seminars and provides consulting services focusing on productivity improvement through effective human resource management.

Prior to her appointment at Washington University, Dr. Numerof designed and directed the graduate program in health administration at LaSalle College in Philadelphia, Pennsylvania. She also spent five years as a manager in a major East Coast hospital and has over ten years' experience as a practicing psychotherapist.

Rita Numerof graduated magna cum laude from the Honors College, Syracuse University in 1969, and received her M.S.S. (1971) and Ph.D. (1979) from Bryn Mawr College. She is listed in *Who's Who of American Women*.